1987

ALCOHOL AND BIOLOGICAL MEMBRANES

THE GUILFORD ALCOHOL STUDIES SERIES
HOWARD T. BLANE AND DONALD W. GOODWIN, EDITORS

ALCOHOL AND BIOLOGICAL MEMBRANES
  Walter A. Hunt

ALCOHOL PROBLEMS IN WOMEN: ANTECEDENTS, CONSEQUENCES,
  AND INTERVENTION
  Sharon C. Wilsnack and Linda J. Beckman, Editors

DRINKING AND CRIME: PERSPECTIVES ON THE RELATIONSHIPS
  BETWEEN ALCOHOL CONSUMPTION AND CRIMINAL BEHAVIOR
  James J. Collins, Jr., Editor

ALCOHOL AND BIOLOGICAL MEMBRANES

Walter A. Hunt

THE GUILFORD PRESS
New York   London

LIBRARY OF CONGRESS CATALOGING IN PUBLICATION DATA

Hunt, W. A. (Walter A.)
  Alcohol and biological membranes.

  (The Guilford alcohol studies series)
  Bibliography: p.
  Includes index.
  1. Alcohol — Physiological effect. 2. Cell membranes —
Effect of drugs on. 3. Brain damage — Etiology.
I. Title. II. Series. [DNLM: 1. Alcohol, Ethyl —
pharmacodynamics. 2. Brain — drug effects. 3. Cell
Membrane — drug effects. QV 84 H943a]
QP801.A3H86 1985   574.87′5   84-25317
ISBN 0-89862-165-8

To
D. HELEN HUNT
without whose financial support
this book could not have been written

Acknowledgments

I would like to thank the following people for their valuable comments and discussions of various parts of this book: Drs. Floyd E. Bloom, Jane H. Chin, Dora B. Goldstein, Gerhard Freund, R. Adron Harris, Paula L. Hoffman, Robbe C. Lyon, Edward Majchrowicz, Michael J. McCreery, Michael J. Mullin, Terry C. Pellmar, George R. Siggins, Charles E. Swenberg, Boris Tabakoff, and numerous other scientists who freely supplied me with preprints of their latest work.

Preface

Alcoholism is a serious health and social problem in many countries throughout the world and inflicts numerous problems on their societies. These problems include medical complications ranging from addiction and damage to various organs of the body to other significant costs, related to fatal accidents, violent crimes, and loss to the national economy.

As with any disease, the key to the successful treatment of alcoholism is through research into the mechanisms underlying the disease. A number of advances have been made over the last decade that have led to a better understanding of how alcohols interfere with cellular function. One area of alcohol research that has shown considerable promise is the study of the structure and function of membranes and how they can be altered by alcohols.

Since I last wrote a review on alcohol–membrane interactions in the mid-1970s (Hunt, 1975), the number of studies involving alcohol–membrane interactions has exploded. Keeping track of the recent developments in this field has been difficult because of fast-evolving advances made using a variety of different experimental approaches. Although a few reviews have been published, they have tended to involve studies derived from only one perspective, for example, the use of molecular probes. To date, there are no multidisciplinary reviews of the whole field of alcohol–membrane interactions. Such a review is needed now in order to put into perspective the varied results obtained from different disciplines.

The purpose of this book, therefore, is to provide an up-to-date multidisciplinary treatise of the state of the art of this important field of research. Although alcohols can alter the properties and function of many types of membranes in various organ systems, most of the studies and consistent findings across several scientific disciplines deal with the effects of alcohols on membranes of neuronal origin. Consequently, this book will be oriented toward this area. However, when relevant, related membrane effects in other organs will be discussed.

The approach taken in writing this book is to provide a conceptual analysis of the research performed, including both the underlying rationale of the studies and the basis for an experimental approach. Because of the multidisciplinary nature of the research involving alcohol–membrane interactions, information on the theory and execution of experiments will be presented to help readers with diverse backgrounds put in context the results presented. Of course, if the reader is already familiar with a particular technique, that section of a chapter can be skipped. Also, since different readers may be used to a particular nomenclature for expressing alcohol concentrations, concentrations will be expressed both in millimolar (mM) and in milligrams/deciliter (mg/dl) and alcohol doses as grams/kilogram (g/kg). In addition to summarizing the various research findings, critical analyses will be included in an attempt to determine consistencies and discrepancies in proposed mechanisms of action, as well as suggestions of possible approaches to future research. An attempt has been made to refrain from being too technical and "jargonesque." Therefore, this book should appeal not only to investigators in alcoholism research, but to pharmacologists, neuroscientists, clinicians, students, and other people interested in the drug abuse field in general.

Many scientific disciplines have been used to explore the ways in which alcohol can interact with membranes. These have included physical chemistry, biochemistry, physiology, anatomy, and pathology. Different chapters of this book will examine data accumulated by these various approaches. Discussions of direct measurements of alcohol–membrane interactions, electrophysiological properties of cells, movements of ions and other cellular constituents, activities of functional components of membranes, neurotransmitter receptors, and how the chronic ingestion of alcohol can lead to brain damage will be presented. Also, with the use of the information derived, an examination of possible therapeutic approaches to the problems of alcohol intoxication, overdose, and dependence will be made.

The study of alcohol–membrane interactions has become an exciting area of research. It is hoped that the reader will find this book both timely and stimulating.

Contents

Chapter 1. Introduction   1

General Properties of Alcohols   *1*
Experimental Design   *3*
Criteria for Mechanisms of Action   *4*
Structural Models of Biological Membranes   *4*
General Aspects of Anesthetics   *7*
Similarities between Alcohols and Anesthetics   *9*

Chapter 2. Membrane interactions   14

General Studies of Alcohol–Membrane Interactions   *14*
Principles Underlying the Use of Molecular Probes   *15*
Use of Molecular Probes in Alcohol–Membrane
    Studies   *23*
Changes in Membrane Composition with Chronic
    Ethanol Treatment   *30*
Commentary   *35*

Chapter 3. Membrane electrophysiology   41

General Considerations   *41*
Methodological Procedures   *44*
Effects of Alcohols on Invertebrate Preparations   *44*
Single-Unit and Multiple-Unit Activity In Vivo   *47*
Electrical Activity Measured In Vitro   *58*
Electrical Activity of Cells Grown in Culture   *61*
Commentary   *63*

Chapter 4. Ion movements   66

Monovalent Ions   *66*
Calcium   *70*
Commentary   *75*

Chapter 5. Membrane-bound enzymes   78

Methodological Considerations   *78*
Sodium- and Potassium-Activated Adenosine
    Triphosphatase   *81*

Adenylate Cyclase and Other Enzymes Related to
  Cyclic Nucleotides   *87*
Other Enzymes   *98*
Uptake Mechanisms   *99*
Commentary   *100*

Chapter 6. Neuroreceptors   103

Methodological Considerations   *103*
Catecholamine Receptors   *105*
Serotonin Receptors   *110*
Acetylcholine Receptors   *112*
GABA Receptors   *114*
Glutamate Receptors   *119*
Opiate Receptors   *121*
Commentary   *125*

Chapter 7. Brain damage   130

Morphological Studies   *131*
Electrophysiological Studies   *133*
Biochemical Studies   *135*
Similarities to Aging   *136*
Fetal Alcohol Syndrome   *137*
Mechanisms of Brain Damage   *139*
Commentary   *142*

Chapter 8. Therapeutic approaches   145

Hyperbaric Environments and Hypothermia   *146*
Membrane Stabilizers   *147*
Pharmacological Manipulation of Neuroreceptors   *149*
Drug Replacement Therapy   *153*
Commentary   *154*

Chapter 9. Summary   156

References   161

Author Index   199

Subject Index   212

1. Introduction

Ethanol, the active ingredient of alcoholic beverages, is a member of a class of short-chain aliphatic alcohols that is characterized by one or more hydroxyl groups attached to a hydrocarbon chain. Because of their small molecular size and simple structure, alcohols do not appear to act on receptors in the normal pharmacological sense. To appreciate this, one needs only to examine Figure 1-1 to see that, when compared to another depressant drug such as pentobarbital, ethanol is quite small. Usually, drugs have specificity for receptors because they can assume many unique conformations, only one of which will allow binding to the receptor. Ethanol has a limited number of conformations, none of which is likely to be unique.

Alcohols seem to act in many respects like general anesthetics. About 50 years ago, Meyer and Gottlieb (1926) suggested that anesthetics exert their action by disrupting normal membrane structure, thereby depressing neuronal function. Throughout the course of this book, we shall explore the many ways in which alcohols have been shown to interact with membranes. These will include physical studies utilizing very sophisticated techniques that allow one to assess the structural integrity of membranes, electrophysiological and ion flux measurements to address basic neuronal mechanisms, analyses of the properties of functional entities in membranes, such as membrane-bound enzymes and neuroreceptors, and finally, the consequences of chronic exposure of membranes to alcohols, which may result in brain damage.

In order to have an appropriate orientation for the following discussions, a number of considerations need to be presented. In this introductory chapter, we shall discuss the general properties of alcohols, develop the criteria for evaluating published data, review the structure of membranes and theories of anesthesia as they pertain to the understanding of the actions of alcohols, and examine some of the similarities between alcohols and anesthetics.

General properties of alcohols

As mentioned at the beginning of this chapter, aliphatic alcohols are simple organic molecules containing one or more hydroxyl groups on a hydrocarbon chain. The hydrocarbon chain can be straight or branched

1

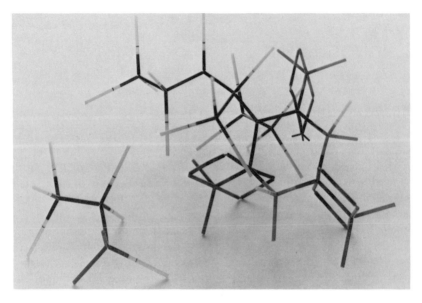

Figure 1-1. Molecular structures of ethanol (left) and pentobarbital (right).

and can contain double as well as single chemical bonds between the carbons. Since hydroxyl groups are "hydrophilic" (water soluble, lipid insoluble) and hydrocarbons are "hydrophobic" (water insoluble, lipid soluble), alcohols can assume the physical and chemical properties of both moieties and thus are also amphiphiles.

The hydroxyl groups of alcohols are undissociated under physiological conditions. The alcohols are polar and can form hydrogen bonds readily with water, properties that raise the boiling points of the alcohols relative to their corresponding hydrocarbons. The hydrocarbons, on the other hand, are nonpolar and can associate only by van der Waals forces. The degree of such associations is greater as the chain length of the hydrocarbons increases. The physical and chemical properties of alcohols are a balance between these polar and nonpolar properties and depend again on the length of the hydrocarbon chain. Short-chain alcohols, such as methanol, ethanol, and propanol, are water soluble and assume properties similar to water. As the chain length increases, the properties of the alcohols become more like those of a hydrocarbon. These properties greatly influence the partition coefficients, to which we shall refer a number of times during the course of this book. The "partition coefficient," as we shall use it here, is the ratio of the solubilities of a compound at equilibrium in lipid to that in water. The concentrations obtained are a function of the concentrations of the compound in each phase.

Experimental design

In order to put reported data into the proper perspective, close examination of the experimental design must be made. This is necessary because of a number of factors related to addictive drugs in general, and in some cases to ethanol in particular.

When dealing with the mechanism of action of a drug, it is presumed that its effect is dependent on its interaction with some biological site and that the duration of this effect depends on the time during which this interaction occurs. This general principle appears to be valid for the acute effects of alcohols. However, the analysis of the chronic effects of alcohols requires that additional considerations be applied. When successive doses of the drug are administered, the possible summation of single responses resulting from single doses must be taken into account. One possible consequence of this might include a delayed recovery from the pharmacological effects, even though the drug has been eliminated from its site of action.

Characteristic of addictive drugs is the development of "tolerance" and "physical dependence." Tolerance is the progressive loss of sensitivity of an organism to a given dose or concentration of a drug with repeated use. Physical dependence is a state exhibited by a series of withdrawal signs and symptoms following the abrupt cessation of chronic drug administration. Each of these phenomena may be mediated by its own set of mechanisms.

Finally, the direct cellular toxicity of alcohols must be considered, especially with long-term treatment. In Chapter 7, the discussion will be focused on ethanol-induced brain damage. The mechanism of such damage may be different from those that may underlie tolerance or physical dependence.

In summary, the analysis of studies dealing with the effects of alcohols on the body must attempt to differentiate among the various factors that may contribute to the observed responses. This would provide a better understanding of just what aspect of drug action is being examined.

One aspect of chronic ethanol treatment that will recur often in this book is the method used to administer ethanol. A variety of approaches has been employed in an attempt to induce tolerance and physical dependence (see review of Pohorecky, 1981). These have included mostly oral intubation, inhalation, and liquid diets. Oral administration of one to five doses of ethanol a day with a gastric feeding tube is used for relatively short treatment periods, usually for less than a week. Inhalation involves having ethanol in the inspired air in a closed chamber. Here again, lengths of treatment generally last about 3–10 days. With longer-term treatments, lasting from one week to several years, ethanol is administered in the drinking fluid. This fluid is often a liquid diet, which provides all of the nutrients needed by the experimental animals. To what extent these different treatment regimens and possible problems of malnutrition may influence the results obtained is not clear.

Criteria for mechanisms of action

When considering possible mechanisms of action of alcohols, a number of criteria need to be addressed in order to adequately evaluate their relevance. These criteria have been described by Hunt (1975) and can be reiterated here:

> (1) Biochemical and biophysical changes induced by alcohols have to occur at the sublethal concentrations found *in vivo* after ethanol ingestion [100 mM (460 mg/dl)] and in physiologically important magnitudes to be considered relevant. (2) The time course of these changes must correlate with the appearance and disappearance of CNS depression and with changes in blood (brain) alcohol levels, since the time course of depression corresponds with these changes. (3) The increasing potency of alcohols with increasing lipid solubility must be explained. And (4) the changes involved must be relevant to mechanisms responsible for neuroexcitability. (p. 195)

When evaluating a potential mechanism for any of the chronic effects of ethanol, some of the above criteria are relevant. For example, the time course of development and dissipation of such phenomena as tolerance and physical dependence should correlate with a similar time course of the reported biological change. Also, the biological change has to be relevant to an underlying mechanism that could mediate any of the specific aspects of the phenomena.

Structural models of biological membranes

The main purpose of membranes, which are generally 75–90 Ångströms (Å) thick and surround a cell, is to separate the contents of a cell from the surrounding environment. However, at the same time, selective passage of certain ions, water, and metabolites is another function of membranes. In order to do this, membranes are composed of a complex array of substances, predominantly lipids and proteins, that are organized in such a manner as to provide an effective barrier between the inside and outside of the cell. Various activities of membranes will be discussed throughout this book and will include the movement of ions, enzymatic reactions, active transport systems, and the translation of information. All of these functions depend on the unique membrane structures of a cell.

The exact structure of membranes is not entirely known, but probably depends on the general function of the cell. Many models of membrane structure have been suggested and have been reviewed elsewhere (Hendler,

MINI SPEECH
Preview of Persuasion

Name: _Cari_

Main Points:

1. _UNsafe wAste_

2. _$_

3. _Safety via Accidents_

Source: _Science, etc._

Grade: _A_

1971). For the purpose of the discussion here, emphasis will be placed on the most accepted model of membranes advanced by Singer and Nicholson (1972).

The model described by Singer and Nicholson suggests that membranes are a fluid mosaic of lipids and proteins (Figure 1-2). The basic lipid structure is a bilayer of phospholipids consisting of carboxylic polar head groups and nonpolar hydrocarbon chains. Since water bathes both the inside and outside surfaces of the membrane, the polar head groups are oriented toward the surfaces, while the hydrocarbon chains are oriented away from the aqueous medium and toward the interior of the membrane. The fatty-acid chains of the phospholipids, generally 16–24 carbons in length, are believed to be aligned perpendicular to the surface of the membrane, thus maximizing hydrophobic interactions.

The orientation of proteins imbedded in membranes is based on the same thermodynamic considerations as for lipids. The ionic groups are in contact with the aqueous environment, while the remainder of the more hydrophobic portions of the proteins are clustered in the interior of the membrane. The three-dimensional structure of these proteins depends, in part, on their length and amino acid composition. For example, if a protein is long enough, it can traverse the entire width of the membrane with the ionic groups located at the outer and inner surfaces. Otherwise, the

Figure 1-2. Singer–Nicholson model of membrane structure. From S. J. Singer & G. L. Nicholson, The fluid mosaic model of the structure of cell membranes. *Science*, 1972, *175*, 720–731. Copyright 1972 by the American Association for the Advancement of Science. Reprinted by permission.

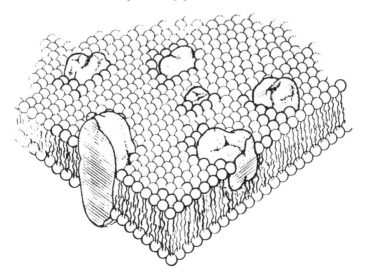

proteins fold in a manner in which the most stable configuration would be attained. In this case, the ionic groups at both ends of the protein would be in contact with the same surface of the membrane.

Membranes contain other constituents besides phospholipids and proteins. Oligosaccharides associated with proteins or lipids are found on the surface of membranes. Cholesterol, which can comprise up to 25% of the membrane lipid, can intercalate between the phospholipids with the steroid ring of cholesterol, containing a single hydroxyl group, being oriented toward the polar head groups of the phospholipids (Figure 1-3). The branched aliphatic chain would protrude into the lipid core. Cholesterol can render the surface of membranes quite rigid.

The structure of the membrane bilayer may be asymmetric in erythrocytes (Bretschner, 1973) and synaptosomal plasma membranes (Fontaine, Harris, & Schroeder, 1980). It appears that the lipid composition differs between the outer and inner surfaces of the membrane. Along the outer surface, the lipids are generally choline phospholipids and glycolipids, while along the inner surface, they are more likely to be serine or ethanolamine

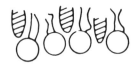

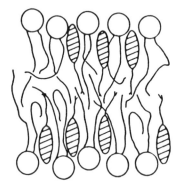

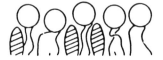

Figure 1-3. The orientation of cholesterol in biological membranes. From C. Tanford, *The hydrophobic effect: Formation of micelles and biological membranes*. New York: Wiley, 1973. Reprinted by permission.

phospholipids. Also, protein either extends completely through the membrane or is associated with the inner surface.

Because the fatty-acid chains of phospholipids have freedom of movement within the membrane, membrane constituents can have a certain degree of mobility as well (Edidin, 1974). There are three ways in which they can move, which include rotational and translational movement and "molecular tumbling." In a given axis, molecules can rotate in a fluid environment. This can be for the molecule as a whole or can occur around carbon–carbon single bonds. With translational movement, a molecule can diffuse in a zigzag fashion through the lipid bilayer, in a path parallel to the surface of the membrane. This phenomenon is also called "lateral diffusion." Finally, molecular tumbling refers to the ability of a molecule to move randomly in all directions with any angle of axis. This type of motion does not generally occur in membranes because the ionic charges on many molecules would keep them close to the surface and because of the varying physical properties of molecules structured within the membrane itself.

The movement of any molecule within a membrane depends on how ordered the membrane structure is. Based on various physical conditions and molecular interactions, the membrane can be very ordered, in which little movement of molecules can occur, or can be rather fluid, with considerable movement possible. This general concept is referred to as "fluidity." The fluidity of membranes and alterations in fluidity induced by alcohols has become an important area of research and will be discussed in depth in Chapter 2.

In light of the foregoing discussion, it should be emphasized that the true structure of biological membranes has not been conclusively demonstrated for membranes in general (Tanford, 1973) and for neural membranes in particular. Consequently, all studies that imply changes in the structure or properties of biological membranes must make certain assumptions about membrane structure that may or may not be true.

General aspects of anesthetics

Since alcohols have a number of properties in common with general anesthetics and have mechanisms of action based on these properties, a short review of the theories of anesthesia should help understand how alcohols may exert their actions, especially on membranes. Should a more comprehensive discussion of this topic be desired, the reader should consult Cohen and Dripps (1965), Seeman (1972), or Roth (1979).

A thoroughly convincing definition of anesthesia has not been validated. However, the most accepted definition has been that an anesthetic reversibly blocks the action potentials of neurons without affecting the resting membrane potential (Seeman, 1972). How anesthetics accomplish this is still unknown in spite of over 100 years of research on the subject. A number of theories have been advanced to explain how they work. Interestingly, the most popular one is based on studies with alcohols.

At the turn of the century, Meyer (1899, 1901) and Overton (1896, 1901) proposed that the potencies of anesthetics are dependent on their lipid solubility. This concept formed the basis of what is now known as the Meyer–Overton rule of anesthesia. The premise of this rule is the requirement that anesthetics must dissolve in the hydrophobic portions of membranes, and to do so they must be lipid soluble. Hence, the more lipid soluble the anesthetic is, the greater its potency as an anesthetic. Developed further, Meyer and Gottlieb (1926) and Meyer (1937) proposed that anesthesia occurs when a certain molar concentration of the anesthetic is attained in the lipid regions of the cell.

Since it is difficult to determine the amount of anesthetic in the membrane, Ferguson (1939) attempted to resolve this problem with the use of "thermodynamic activities." Thermodynamic activity of an anesthetic refers conceptually to the amount necessary to induce a biological effect and is defined as

$$a = \gamma X$$

where a is the thermodynamic activity, γ the activity coefficient, and X the concentration of the anesthetic. At equilibrium, the thermodynamic activities of the anesthetic in its various phases are equal. Therefore, the effective concentration of the anesthetic in the membranous phase can be calculated. With this approach, Ferguson (1939) and Brink and Posternak (1948) demonstrated that thermodynamic activity coefficients of anesthetics increase with increasing lipid solubility and that anesthesia will occur at a particular thermodynamic activity in the membrane.

Going one step further, Mullins (1954) suggested that the volume occupied by the anesthetic in the membrane is an important factor. Once a certain volume of the membrane is occupied by the agent, anesthesia will occur. An extension of this idea presumes that the membrane actually expands in response to the presence of the anesthetic dissolved in the membrane. This hypothesis has some support based on the ability of anesthetics to expand artificial membranes, bulk phase solvents, oils, and rubber (Seeman, 1972).

One phenomenon that has provided support for the membrane expansion hypothesis of anesthesia is the ability of hyperbaric environments to reverse anesthesia (Halsey, 1982). High pressure is believed to oppose the anesthetic-induced membrane expansion and may actually restore the order of the membrane components (Chin, Trudell, & Cohen, 1976; Lever, Miller, Patton, & Smith, 1971).

A more recent development in the understanding of the mechanism of action of anesthetics is the study of fluidity of membranes. As discussed earlier, fluidity is a physical property of membranes that can describe the intrinsic order of membranes. Anesthetics have been shown to fluidize membranes (Trudell, 1977), a concept to be developed in greater detail in Chapter 2.

So far, the various theories presented have addressed anesthetic interactions with membranes only with the lipid components. As discussed earlier, biological membranes are composed of a variety of substances. Proteins, another major constituent of membranes, are also believed to be sites of action of anesthetics (Trudell, 1977). In neural tissue, this can include such entities as ion channels, membrane-bound enzymes, and receptors. Since ethanol can modify the functional units of membranes, subsequent discussions in Chapters 4, 5, and 6 will deal with the effects of alcohols on these subjects.

Similarities between alcohols and anesthetics

Alcohols have a number of properties in common with anesthetics. The main similarity is the relationship between potency and lipid solubility. The potencies of alcohols to alter a variety of endpoints will be discussed in a number of chapters of this book. Those discussed here will focus on general biological and behavioral parameters.

The early studies examined the effects of different alcohols on microorganisms and invertebrates (Bills, 1924; Cole & Allison, 1930; Dethier & Chadwick, 1947; Rang, 1960; Tilly & Schaffer, 1926, 1928). The results of all of these experiments demonstrated that alcohols with increasing chain lengths and increasing solubilities were more potent in inducing the studied biological endpoint. In some cases, the effectiveness of longer-chained alcohols (C7–C10) was progressively diminished. This phenomenon has been designated as "cut-off." The mechanism of cut-off is unknown. Ferguson (1939) has suggested that the thermodynamic activities of the longer-chain alcohols is not great enough for sufficient amounts to enter the membrane and exert a biological effect (Pringle, Brown, & Miller, 1981). Another explanation may relate to the difficulty in solubilizing these alcohols in the aqueous compartments of the body to allow for adequate transfer of the alcohol to its active sites. This may make these studies experimentally difficult to perform, since little alcohol could interact with the membrane.

More recent reports have examined the behavior of animals after alcohol injection (LeBlanc & Kalant, 1975; McCreery & Hunt, 1978; Wallgren, 1960). When measuring the ability of alcohols to induce various levels of intoxication, the potencies of the alcohols increased as the hydrocarbon chain was lengthened. Figure 1-4 shows the results of a study in which 68 different alcohols and related compounds were tested for their ability to induce ataxia (McCreery & Hunt, 1978). A linear relationship was obtained over a wide range of membrane/buffer partition coefficients. The three-dimensional structure of the alcohol did not seem to influence potency other than how it contributed to the lipid solubility of the alcohol. The concentrations of the alcohol in the membrane, volumes of the membrane occupied by the alcohols, and thermodynamic activities were equal at the intoxication endpoint used and indicated that the potency of an alcohol over a wide range of partition coefficients could be predicted from its lipid solubility. Cut-off was also observed with alcohols with high partition coefficients. Their actions resembled that of hydrocarbons. Finally, intoxication similar to that obtained with alcohols was observed with other amphiphilic compounds. This suggests that the balance of the hydrophilic and hydrophobic properties of alcohols provides a very important contribution to their pharmacological properties.

Figure 1-4. Relationship of intoxicating potencies of various hydroxyl-containing compounds to their membrane/buffer partition coefficients. From M. J. McCreery & W. A. Hunt, Physico-chemical correlates of alcohol intoxication. *Neuropharmacology*, 1978, *17*, 451–461. Copyright 1978 by Pergamon Press, Ltd. Reprinted by permission.

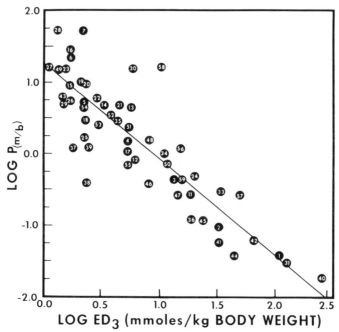

The importance of the lipid solubility of alcohols has also been applied to the development of alcohol tolerance and physical dependence. It has been known for a long time that cross-tolerance and cross-dependence can develop between ethanol and other alcohols. This means that if tolerance develops to ethanol, tolerance also develops to other alcohols, even though an animal may have never been treated with them. With cross-dependence, other alcohols will suppress an ethanol withdrawal syndrome and maintain dependence.

The potencies of short-chain aliphatic alcohols were tested in ethanol-tolerant and -nontolerant rats (LeBlanc & Kalant, 1975). When doses of the alcohols were corrected for their thermodynamic activities, the dose–response curves obtained for motor decrement on the moving-belt test were identical in nontolerant animals, consistent with other studies discussed above. When animals were rendered tolerant to ethanol, the dose–response curves for all of the alcohols shifted to the right to the same degree. These data suggest that the change in the membrane that reduces the efficacy of the alcohols with chronic ethanol treatment, does so equally for all of them.

If alcohols have a common mechanism of action, then they all should — and not only ethanol — be able to induce physical dependence. Several studies have rendered animals physically dependent on *t*-butanol (Grant & Samson, 1981; McComb & Goldstein, 1979a, 1979b; Thurman & Pathman, 1975; Wallgren, Kosunen, & Ahtee, 1973). The withdrawal syndrome that is observed after the alcohol is eliminated from the body is indistinguishable from one obtained after ethanol withdrawal. In fact, when ethanol and *t*-butanol are administered in two 3-day sequential periods, dependence is maintained with no withdrawal syndrome observed, unless both alcohols are withdrawn (McComb & Goldstein, 1979a). The order in which the drugs are administered does not change the results.

The ability of an alcohol to induce physical dependence can be related to its lipid solubility. In experiments with *t*-butanol, less drug was required as compared to ethanol to induce dependence (McComb & Goldstein, 1979b). The difference in potencies of *t*-butanol and ethanol was of the same order as the difference between their respective partition coefficients. In another study, the efficacy of aliphatic diols (alcohols with two hydroxyl groups) to suppress an ethanol withdrawal syndrome was tested (Hunt & Majchrowicz, 1980; Majchrowicz, Hunt, & Piantadosi, 1976). Of the diols examined, all of them could suppress the withdrawal syndrome and, at the right doses, do so without inducing any apparent intoxication. Furthermore, the potencies of the diols were proportional to their partition coefficients. Nonalcoholic amphiphiles, but not hydrocarbons, were also effective in suppressing the ethanol withdrawal syndrome, analogous to their ability to induce intoxication.

As discussed earlier in this chapter, anesthesia can be reversed using high pressure. The ability of high pressure to antagonize ethanol intoxication has been studied in laboratory animals, with initial experiments requiring a rather toxic 68 atmospheres (atm) of air to be effective (Halsey & Wardley-Smith, 1975). Using pure oxygen, antagonism could be observed at pressures of 30–60 atm in a pressure-dependent manner (Alkana & Syapin, 1979). Even at these pressures, oxygen toxicity was found. In a subsequent study, hyperbaric environments containing as little as 6 atm of helium–oxygen (20% oxygen) could antagonize ethanol narcosis (Alkana & Malcolm, 1980). Helium is a useful substitute for nitrogen in the experimental atmosphere, because it does not have depressant effects in the pressure ranges used (Membery & Link, 1964).

The above experiments did not control for possible hypothermic effects of helium (Membery & Link, 1964) or possible hypoxia resulting from compression at subnormal oxygen partial pressures (Mustala & Azarnoff, 1969). When the body temperature of the animals and oxygen tensions were maintained, antagonism of narcosis could be observed with 1–12 atm helium–oxygen (Alkana & Malcolm, 1981, 1982a; Malcolm & Alkana, 1982). In these experiments, narcosis was measured by "sleep-times," which is the difference between the time at which an animal first loses its righting reflex and the time when the righting reflex is regained. The blood ethanol concentrations at which the righting reflex was regained after ethanol administration were not reduced by high pressure but were, in fact, slightly elevated. This suggests that an enhanced ethanol elimination from the body was not responsible for the observed effect of high pressure on ethanol-induced depression.

Upon closer examination, the effectiveness of hyperbaric environments to antagonize ethanol intoxication depended on the level of intoxication present when the treatment was administered. As the dose of ethanol was increased, the mean percentage reduction in sleeping time provided by high pressure was progressively reduced (Alkana & Malcolm, 1981). This finding might be expected if hyperbaric environments compressed membranes previously expanded by an anesthetic. Greater membrane expansion associated with high concentrations of ethanol in the membrane would require higher pressures for antagonism. On the other hand, high pressure might be squeezing the ethanol out of the membrane (Franks & Lieb, 1982). Again, greater amounts of ethanol in the membrane would require higher pressures to remove it. Antagonism of anesthesia was also effective when hyperbaric helium–oxygen environments were administered at various times after anesthesia was produced (Alkana & Malcolm, 1982b).

In a recent set of experiments, the ability of hyperbaric environments to induce a withdrawal syndrome in ethanol-dependent mice was attempted (Alkana, Finn, & Malcolm, 1983). This is analogous to the well-known ability of naloxone, a morphine antagonist, to precipitate withdrawal in morphine-dependent animals. The logic used in the study assumed that dependence results from compensatory changes in an organism during chronic treatment with ethanol and that high pressure should not only reverse intoxication in such animals, but induce a withdrawal syndrome. Ten days after treatment with ethanol in a liquid diet, 12 atm of helium-oxygen precipitated withdrawal and intensified it as well. These data suggest that the reactions that occur with chronic ethanol administration and that lead to the development of physical dependence may take place in the cell membrane.

2. Membrane interactions

Because of the similarities between alcohols and anesthetics, alcohols may exert a primary action on the membranes of cells. This is based, in part, on the general and physical properties of alcohols. By dissolving in membranes by virtue of their lipid solubility, alcohols could disrupt normal membrane function. In this chapter, we shall examine the evidence supporting the hypothesis that alcohols alter the structure of membranes. Both indirect and direct measures of membrane properties will be reviewed with special emphasis on the use of molecular probes. The theory and the practical application of these probes will be developed and the various reported studies assessed.

General studies of alcohol–membrane interactions

A number of approaches have been used to study the ability of alcohols to interact with membranes. One indirect approach was based on the ability of lipid-soluble drugs to protect cells from lysis. Traube (1908) was first to describe the antihemolytic effect of pentanol on erythrocytes in hypotonic solutions. This protection of erythrocytes may be analogous to the stabilizing effects of many drugs, whereby neurons become resistant to depolarization (Guttman, 1940). This concept was extended to include the inhibition of a change in the resting membrane potential (Shanes, 1958).

The ability of aliphatic alcohols to protect human erythrocytes from osmotic lysis has been systematically investigated (Roth & Seeman, 1971; Seeman, 1966). Using a homologous series of alcohols from methanol to nonanol, lysis was inhibited in a concentration-dependent manner. As the chain length of the alcohols increased, the potencies of the alcohols increased accordingly. The concentration of ethanol that induced an antihemolytic effected exceeded 100 mM (460 mg/dl).

One of the theories of anesthesia states that anesthetics occupy a volume of the membrane and actually expand it (see Chapter 1). The ability of alcohols to expand membranes has been examined in both artificial and biological membranes. The surface area of monolayers of stearic acid (Booij & Dijkshoorn, 1950), phospholipids and cholesterol (Gatenbeck & Ehrenberg, 1953), and nerve–lipid films (Skou, 1958) are all expanded by alcohols. Anesthetics, including alcohols, will also expand erythrocyte ghost membranes (Roth & Seeman, 1972; Seeman, Kwant, Sauks, & Argent, 1969; Seeman & Roth, 1972) and brain synaptosomes (Seeman, 1974). In erythrocytes, however, membranes were reported to expand roughly 20 times the volume of the membranes occupied by the anesthetic. Seeman (1972) suggested that this may reflect extensive conformational changes in proteins.

The notion that these biological membranes expand more than lipid bilayers has recently been challenged (Franks & Lieb, 1981). The two anesthetics ethanol and halothane were found to occupy equal volumes in biological membranes, lipid bilayers, and water. Also, the membranes were found to expand considerably less than previously reported (Seeman, 1972, 1974). The conclusion drawn was that any expansion of membranes by anesthetics was due to the presence of the drug molecules themselves, with no additional changes in volume from protein conformational changes. This suggested that the anesthetics may have more specific targets in membranes than generally believed.

If alcohols expand membranes, this might account for their antihemolytic effects. With an increase in the membrane surface area, the pressure on the membrane exerted by hypotonic environments would be reduced, thereby reducing the chance of lysis.

In another approach, the ability of ethanol to interact with phosphatidylcholine vesicles was explored (Rowe, 1983). The temperature at which vesicles underwent transition from the gel to the liquid phase was determined in the presence and absence of ethanol. This was accomplished by monitoring changes in the optical density of scattered light with increasing incubating temperatures. In concentrations of ethanol of up to 435 mM (2000 mg/dl), the transition temperature declined in a concentration-dependent manner. At higher concentrations of ethanol, this effect was reversed to the point where the transition temperature was elevated as compared to controls. The fatty-acid composition of the phospholipid vesicles influenced some of these properties. The concentration of ethanol at which the reversal in the transition temperature occurred progressively increased. Based on thermodynamic considerations, these data suggested that ethanol was preferentially dissolving in the fluid phase of the lipid, that is, the part of the vesicle that is most fluid.

Principles underlying the use of molecular probes

Most of the studies over the last decade dealing with alcohol–membrane interactions have explored their ability to alter the fluidity of biological membranes. Fluidity refers to the mobility of molecules in membranes. As discussed in Chapter 1, biological membranes are probably fluid mosaics, which allow motion of the molecules that constitute their structure. This motion includes rotational as well as translational mobility.

Fluidity of membranes can be assessed with the use of molecular probes. Often having structures similar to the constituents of the membrane, these probes can report on the properties of the microenvironment in which they reside. In order to measure these properties, the probes must possess properties that allow them to be studied by physical techniques, such as electron paramagnetic resonance (EPR) or fluorescence spectroscopy.

Both EPR and fluorescent probes have one major distinction in common. They contain on their molecular structure a moiety whose properties can be studied by EPR or fluorescence techniques. In the case of an EPR probe, the attached moiety contains a free radical characterized by the presence of an unpaired electron. By virtue of its charge, mass, and spin, the unpaired electron possesses a magnetic moment and angular momentum. If a static magnetic field is applied, the electron will precess like a spinning top around its axis and align either parallel or antiparallel to the magnetic field. Each orientation is associated with a slightly different energy level. The rate at which the electron precesses is determined by its environment and by the strength of the magnetic field. The higher the strength of the magnetic field, the faster the electron precesses.

If an oscillating magnetic field is added at a frequency equal to the rate of precession of the electron, resonance is attained and a spin transition of the electron from one energy level to the other occurs as the electron realigns. This is associated with an absorption of energy that can be measured. In practice, the strength of the static magnetic field is varied until the precession rate of the electron equals the frequency of the oscillating magnetic field.

An often used radical is the nitroxide free radical (Figure 2-1). The unpaired electron is located in the π-orbital of the nitrogen atom (Figure 2-2) and is stabilized by surrounding methyl or alkyl groups. The EPR spectrum obtained from this type of free radical reflects the interaction of the magnetic fields generated from the spins of the free electron and the nitrogen nucleus (hyperfine coupling).

The EPR spectrum depends in part on the orientation of the free radical in the applied static magnetic field with respect to the three main axes of the nitroxide group (Figure 2-2). If the magnetic field is oriented so that it is parallel to each of these axes, the respective spectra in Figure 2-3 are obtained. (The spectrum obtained from an EPR spectrometer is the first derivative of the absorption spectrum.) The vertical deflections in each spectrum are the changes in absorption and the horizontal axis represents the change in the intensity of the applied static magnetic field.

Information concerning the mobility of a probe can be acquired using the order parameter (S). The order parameter represents the time-averaged

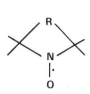

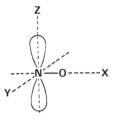

Figure 2-1. A nitroxide, spin-labeled moiety.

Figure 2-2. The molecular axes of a nitroxide moiety.

angular orientation of the probe about its axis and does not measure lateral diffusion of the probe. Quantitatively, the order parameter varies from 0 to 1, with 0 representing the most random or fluid state and 1 the most ordered or rigid state. Figure 2-4 illustrates how the EPR spectrum changes as the order parameter increases from 0 to 1.

When the nitroxide free radical undergoes isotropic motion, that is, randomly tumbles in a nonviscous solvent, such as water, the EPR spec-

Figure 2-3. EPR spectra when the applied static magnetic field is applied to each of the axes in Figure 2-2.

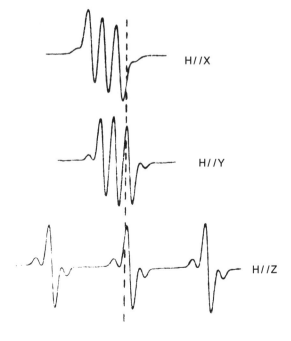

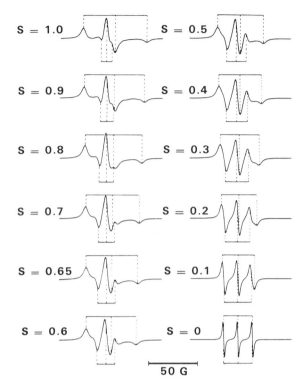

Figure 2-4. EPR spectra representing various values of the order parameter (*S*). From D. Marsh, Election spin resonance: Spin labels. In E. Grell (Ed.), *Membrane spectroscopy*. Berlin: Springer-Verlag, 1981. Reprinted by permission.

trum obtained is the average of spectra in all possible planes and consists of three lines equally spaced ($S=0$ in Figure 2-4). If the motion of the nitroxide free radical becomes anisotropic, that is, becomes progressively more restricted until it becomes immobile, the EPR spectrum broadens and the peaks become smaller and less distinct ($S>0$ in Figure 2-4) and represents the spectra of the specific orientations of the free radical molecules partially averaged and partially superimposed onto one another.

Figure 2-5 shows how the order parameter is calculated. $T'_{\parallel}$ and $T'_{\perp}$ are determined from the hyperfine splittings of the EPR spectrum as indicated. The other values are reference values for the particular probe being used in crystalline form, which represents the most rigid state that the probe can experience. Because of the difference in the polarity of the environment of the probe in the experimental preparation from that in the crystal, a correction factor (a/a') is indicated. This difference in polarity modifies the EPR spectrum, independent of changes in fluidity. The reference values for the probe in the crystal can be obtained from the literature.

The more the movement of the probe is restricted, the greater will be the difference between $T'_{\parallel}$ and $T'_{\perp}$. This index of fluidity is the one used in most of the EPR studies of alcohol–membrane interactions to be discussed later.

A number of spin-labeled compounds can be used to study membrane properties. The probes used most in alcohol studies have been the doxyl derivatives of stearic acid (Figure 2-6). Because of molecular interactions within the membrane, the axis along the acyl chain will orient parallel to the acyl chains of the phospholipids. With the free radical attached at different positions on the acyl chain, different depths of the membrane can be studied. Using these probes, a progressive reduction in the order parameter is obtained as the spin label is inserted deeper within the membrane because of the increasing fluidity gradient (McConnell & McFarland, 1972). The reference values for 5-doxylpalmitate in a crystal are used to calculate order parameters using doxylstearic acid probes.

Figure 2-5. EPR spectrum of 5-doxylstearic acid in mouse synaptosomal plasma membranes and the manner in which the order parameter (S) is calculated. T_{xx}, T_{yy}, T_{zz}, and a are reference data for the probe in a crystal. From D. B. Goldstein & J. H. Chin, Interaction of ethanol with biological membranes. *Federation Proceedings*, 1981, *40*, 2073–2076. Copyright 1981 by FASEB. Reprinted by permission.

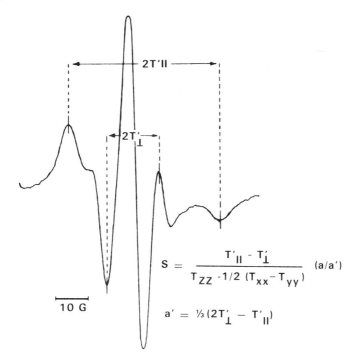

$$S = \frac{T'_{\parallel} - T'_{\perp}}{T_{zz} - 1/2\,(T_{xx} - T_{yy})} \ (a/a')$$

$$a' = \tfrac{1}{3}\,(2T'_{\perp} - T'_{\parallel})$$

2T'll

2T'⊥

10 G

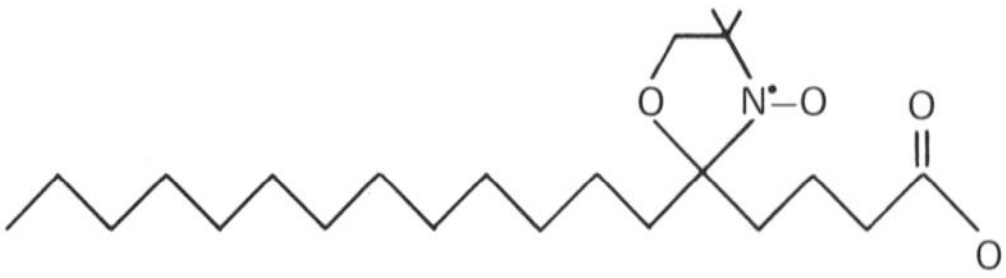

Figure 2-6. Doxyl derivatives of stearic acid. The 12- and 16-doxyl derivatives have been used in alcohol studies.

Fluorescence spectrometry can also be used to determine the fluidity of membranes. Similar to the EPR probes, fluorescent probes contain a moiety whose properties are sensitive to the microenvironment in which they reside. This moiety, like the spin labeled moieties, can be attached to different locations on a structure that will place it in a number of areas of the membrane from the surface to the inner core, depending on the properties of the molecule.

In order for fluorescence to occur, the molecule must first be excited by absorbing an appropriate amount of energy. This will elevate an electron from its normal orbital, called the ground state, to a higher, less stable orbital, called the excited state. The electron remains in this excited state for a very short time (nanoseconds) before it returns to its more stable ground state. When this occurs, light (fluorescence) is emitted. This light has a longer wavelength than that used to excite the molecule because, in addition to fluorescence, energy can be dissipated by other means, such as by molecular vibration.

The fluorescent properties of a probe are measured in a number of ways. How much light a given concentration of a probe can produce after excitation is referred to as the "quantum yield." The quantum yield is sensitive to several factors. One of these is the polarity of the environment of the probe. There is often a substantial difference in the quantum yield over a range of polarities. In some cases, the quantum yield is quite small in aqueous solutions, but very high in nonpolar solvents. These types of probes are called hydrophobic probes and can provide useful information when absorbed to proteins and membranes.

An electron can exist in an excited state for a finite period of time. Measurement of the lifetime of this excited state can provide information on the motion of the molecule rather than its orientation. Such measurements are not often done, in part because of the high cost of the equipment and the difficulty in interpreting changes in lifetimes.

The technique used most often in studies of alcohol–membrane interactions has been fluorescence polarization. With this technique the molecules are excited with polarized light. Those molecules whose electronic orientation is parallel to the plane of the polarized light will have the highest probability of being excited. The fluorescence emitted may also be polarized. Any change in the angle of the plane of the fluorescence emission depends on the degree to which the molecule rotates in the excited state. The degree of rotation is a reflection of the rotational mobility of the probe in its microenvironment. An analogous situation would be to measure, using a camera with a very fast shutter speed, how much an object moves, while the shutter is open.

Experimentally, the probe is excited with polarized monochromatic light and the extent to which the emission is polarized is determined by measuring the difference in intensity of the fluorescence at angles parallel and perpendicular to the plane of the excitation light. If the probe is in a completely rigid state, it will not rotate and little emission will be found in the plane perpendicular to the plane of the excitation light. The fluorescence would be almost completely polarized. If molecules of the probe can rotate 90° while in the excited state, fluorescence in the plane perpendicular to the excitation light will be increased. If the probe is completely mobile, no difference will be found between the fluorescence intensity in the planes parallel and perpendicular to the excitation light. Fluorescence polarization is calculated as follows:

$$P = (I_{||} - I_{\perp})/(I_{||} + I_{\perp})$$

where P is the fluorescence polarization, $I_{||}$ the emission intensity parallel to the plane of the excitation light, and $I_{\perp}$ the emission intensity perpendicular to the plane of the excitation light. It should be emphasized that when comparing the degree of fluorescence polarization between two samples, the lifetimes of the excited state must be equal.

The degree of fluorescence polarization provides information on the fluidity of the microenvironment surrounding the probe, similar to that obtained from the order parameter calculated from an EPR spectrum. If the probe moves freely in solution, no polarization is observed because the emission is equally probable in all planes. In a more structured environment, movement of the probe is restricted, thereby favoring more discrete molecular orientations. Thus, polarization will be greatest in a rigid environment. The difference in emission intensity between the parallel and perpendicular planes, reflecting polarization, is analogous to the difference in the hyperfine splitting obtained from the EPR spectrum to calculate the order parameter.

A variety of fluorescence probes have proved useful in the study of membrane fluidity (Figure 2-7). The one used most often, especially in alcohol–membrane studies, is 1,6-diphenyl-1,3,5-hexatriene (DPH). This probe will partition into hydrophobic regions of the membrane. Other probes that are used include 8-anilino-1-naphthalene-sulfonic acid (ANS), which probes the membrane surface, and 9-anthroic acid derivatives of stearic acid (Waggoner & Stryer, 1970). These latter probes are analogous to the spin-labeled stearic acid probes discussed earlier and will probe dif-

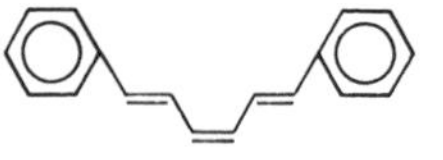

Figure 2-7. Some fluorescence probes used to measure polarization. DPH, 1,6-diphenyl-1,3,5-hexatriene; ANS, 8-anilino-1-naphthalene-sulfonic acid; 12-AS, 12-(9-anthroyl)stearic acid.

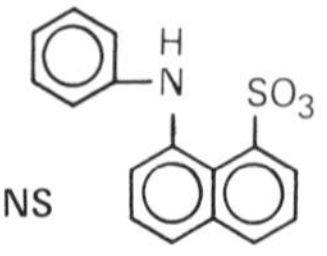

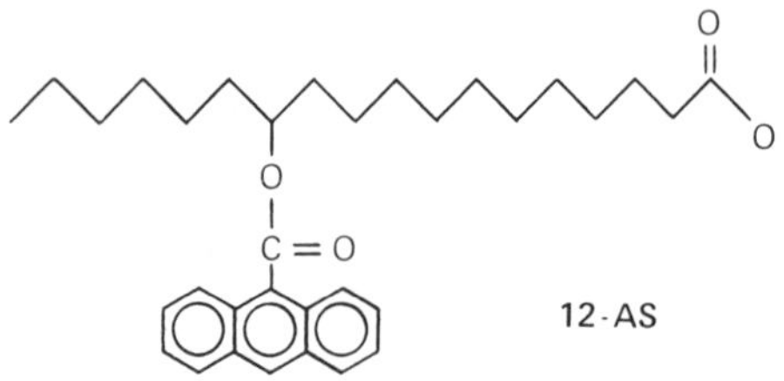

ferent depths of the membrane (Thulborn & Sawyer, 1978; Thulborn, Tilley, Sawyer, & Treloar, 1979).

Finally, the last index of fluidity that is used in both EPR and fluorescence studies as well as a variety of other biological endpoints is the "phase transition temperature." The phase transition temperature is one at which, with increasing temperatures, the membrane is transformed from a gel to a liquid state. A higher phase transition temperature is indicative of a more structured environment. The phase transition temperature is determined from a plot of the value of an endpoint measured against the reciprocal of the absolute temperature at which the measurement was made (Figure 2-8). This is known as an "Arrhenius analysis." The temperature at which the slope of the regression line changes is the transition temperature. Although Arrhenius plots are generally applied to chemical reactions, they have been used for other purposes, including the properties of molecular probes.

The preceding discussion of molecular probes was not designed to be exhaustive, but to give the reader a brief orientation of the theory underlying their use. For additional information the reader should consult the following references: Bolton (1972); Brand and Gohlke (1972); Chignell (1973); Marsh (1981); Pesce, Rosén, and Pasby (1971); Schreier, Polnaszek, and Smith (1978); Shinitzky and Barenholz (1978).

Use of molecular probes in alcohol–membrane studies

Acute effects of ethanol on membrane order

The use of molecular probes to study the effect of alcohols on membranes began in the early 1970s. Some rather crude experiments with both fluorescent and EPR probes suggested that alcohols can alter the properties of the probes when placed in membranes derived from erythrocytes and brain. Using the fluorescent probe ANS, the ability of alcohols to alter the quantum yield of ANS in erythrocyte membranes was studied. The fluorescence of ANS is very sensitive to the polarity of the environment in which it resides. In nonpolar environments, the quantum yield is high, while in polar environments, the quantum yield is high, while in polar environments, it is low (Brand & Gohlke, 1972). Since a high quantum yield is obtained after ANS is inserted in membranes, the binding sites are probably in a nonpolar environment. Thus, a change in the quantum yield could suggest a change in the polarity of this environment.

Short-chain aliphatic alcohols all reduced the quantum yield of ANS in erythrocyte membranes, especially at the lower concentrations used (Roth & Spero, 1976). Alcohols with longer chain lengths than methanol and ethanol could increase fluorescence at higher concentrations. Ethanol concentrations of at least 500 mM (2300 mg/dl) were required to be effective. No effect of alcohols was observed on the fluorescence of ANS-labeled liposomes. Because the affinity of the dye for its binding site was

Figure 2-8. Representative Arrhenius plot. V, velocity of reaction; T, temperature (°K); E, energy of activation (that which is needed to initiate a reaction); R, gas constant.

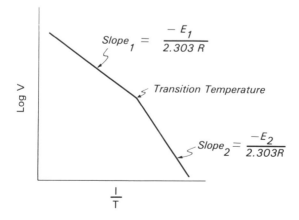

not altered, it was concluded that the reduced fluorescence reflected a lower apparent number of binding sites and probably a change in the conformation of proteins.

In another early experiment, the EPR probe 3-*spiro*-(2'-(*N*-oxyl-4', 4'-dimethyloxazolidine))cholestane, was used to study the effects of alcohols in membrane bilayers prepared from both erythrocyte ghosts and brain (Paterson, Butler, Huang, LaBalle, Smith, & Schneider, 1972). This probe was used to study the orientation of lipids and was presumed to orient itself perpendicular to the longitudinal axis of the bilayer. When high concentrations of alcohols were incubated with the membranes, the spectrum changed in a manner suggesting that the probe had tilted away from its normal perpendicular position, that is, the membrane became more disordered. This effect was greater as the chain length of the alcohol increased. Although ethanol was not used, extrapolation of the data suggested that a concentration of at least 100 mM (460 mg/dl) would be needed to observe any effect at all.

More recently, a more systematic approach has been taken using EPR probes. Using 5-doxylstearic acid, Chin and Goldstein (1977a) examined the effect of ethanol on the order parameter in synaptosomal membranes from the mouse brain. 5-Doxylstearic acid is a spin-labeled compound with a nitroxide free radical containing moiety attached to a fatty acid chain at the 5-position and is believed to orient in the membrane parallel to the phospholipid acyl chains. With this probe, ethanol reduced the order parameter in a concentration-dependent manner with concentrations as low as 10 mM (46 mg/dl). These data were interpreted to mean that ethanol disordered or fluidized the membranes. Similar results were observed with brain myelin and mitochondrial fractions and erythrocyte membranes.

To ascertain whether the potencies of different alcohols to fluidize membranes could be correlated with their lipid solubilities, the ability of different concentrations of the alcohols to decrease the order parameter was determined in synaptosomal membranes, and the slopes of these changes were calculated (Lyon, McComb, Schreurs, & Goldstein, 1981). These slopes, as well as the intoxicating potencies of the alcohols, were found to be directly related to their lipid solubilities (Figure 2-9).

To demonstrate a relationship between membrane disordering and intoxicating potencies further, order parameters were determined in membranes derived from strains of mice with different sensitivities to ethanol (Goldstein, Chin, & Lyon, 1982). Using genetic breeding techniques, strains of mice have been developed that are either highly sensitive to the intoxicating effects of ethanol (long-sleep mice) or relatively insensitive (short-sleep mice) when compared to a heterogenous strain (McClearn & Kakihana, 1973). Ethanol more easily disordered synaptosomal and erythrocyte membranes derived from the long-sleep mice than those from short-sleep mice. Furthermore, in the heterogenous strain, the strain not bred for al-

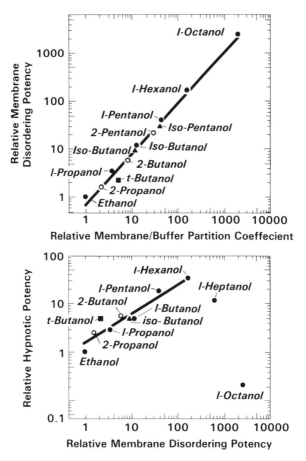

Figure 2-9. (Top) Plot of the potencies of alcohols to change the order parameter versus the lipid/water partition coefficient. (Bottom) Plot of the potencies of alcohols to induce intoxication versus the lipid/water partition coefficients. From R. C. Lyon, J. A. McComb, J. Schreurs, & D. B. Goldstein, A relationship between alcohol intoxication and the disordering of brain membranes by a series of short-chain alcohols. *Journal of Pharmacology and Experimental Therapeutics*, 1981, *218*, 669–675. Copyright 1981 by the American Society for Pharmacology and Experimental Therapeutics. Reprinted by permission.

cohol sensitivity, ethanol disordered membranes to the greatest extent in animals that were most sensitive to ethanol.

Since the experiments described above used the same probe and examined the effects of alcohols on the same area of the membrane, it is relevant to ask whether other areas of the membrane are altered by the presence of alcohols and whether different sensitivities could be observed. To test this possibility, probes with nitroxide moieties attached at the 5-, 12-, or 16-positions on the acyl chain of stearic acid were used (Chin & Goldstein, 1981; Goldstein & Chin, 1981). As expected, as the spin label extended deeper into the lipid bilayer of the membrane, the order parameter decreased, consistent with an increasingly more fluid environment. Ethanol in concentrations of 350 mM (1610 mg/dl) had a greater effect on the mobility of the spin-labeled moiety located at deeper levels of the membrane. Ethanol was also more effective for all these probes, with increases in the incubation temperature and decreases in the cholesterol content. Similar results have been reported with other anesthetics with respect to their effectiveness in deeper regions of the membrane (Lenaz, Curatola, Mazzanti, Bertoli, & Pastuszko, 1979). These data suggest that the extent to which ethanol disorders the membrane depends on the degree of order of the lipid bilayer before the ethanol is added.

To test this possibility further, Chin and Goldstein (1981) varied the fluidity of egg phosphatidylcholine vesicles by altering the cholesterol concentration, then determined the order parameter of the vesicles, spin labeled with 5- or 12-doxylstearic acid. The addition of cholesterol would be expected to increase the order parameter, that is, make the membrane more rigid (see Chapter 1). The presence of the cholesterol had a considerable influence on the fluidizing effect of ethanol. Ethanol disordered the vesicles to a lesser extent as the cholesterol concentration was increased.

The probes used in these studies primarily address alcohol–lipid interactions. Few reports systematically examined alcohol–protein interactions. One set of experiments explored the ability of ethanol to alter protein conformation using a maleimide nitroxide probe, which binds to sulfhydryl groups of proteins (Logan, Laverty, & Peake, 1983). When measured in synaptosomal or erythrocyte membranes, the protein conformations indicated by this probe were not significantly altered by physiologically compatible concentrations of ethanol.

Using fluorescence techniques, similar conclusions as those drawn using EPR techniques have been made about the ability of alcohols to disorder membranes. With the probes DPH and 1-aminopyrene, the effect of ethanol to alter the quantum yield, fluorescence polarization, fluorescence lifetime, and phase transitions of these compounds in synaptosomal and erythrocyte membranes was explored (Harris & Schroeder, 1981, 1982; Vanderkooi, 1979). The probes used report on the microenvironment in different depths of the membrane: DPH of the membrane core (Klausner, Kleinfeld, Hoover, & Karnovsky, 1980; Shinitzky & Barenholz, 1978) and 1-aminopyrene of the membrane surface (Vanderkooi, 1979).

Ethanol was differentially effective in reducing the quantum yield and fluorescence polarization of DPH in membranes at concentrations as low as 10–25 mM (46–115 mg/dl), depending on the tissue preparation (Harris & Schroeder, 1981, 1982). No effect on fluorescence lifetimes was observed at any concentration of ethanol used. Also, the excitation and emission spectra of DPH were unchanged, suggesting that the polarity of the environment on the DPH molecules was unaltered. The properties of 1-aminopyrene were unchanged, unless concentrations of at least 333 mM (1532 mg/dl) ethanol were used. These data suggest that the microenvironment surrounding the DPH molecules resides became more fluid in the presence of ethanol. In further support is the observation that the phase transition temperatures for fluorescence polarization of DPH as determined from Arrhenius plots were reduced in the presence of ethanol (Harris & Schroeder, 1981; Vanderkooi, 1979). Since intrinsic fluorescence of tryptophan residues was unaffected by ethanol, the conclusion was drawn that ethanol preferentially disorders the lipids of the membrane.

Similar disordering effects of different alcohols have been reported using microsomes obtained from the heart of chick embryos (Zavoico & Kutchai, 1980). This response was dependent on the lipid solubility of the alcohol.

Finally, since hyperbaric environments can antagonize ethanol intoxication (see Chapter 1), high pressure also might be expected to antagonize the disordering effect of ethanol. This has been tested using spin-labeled membranes derived from the claw nerves of the crayfish (Mastrangelo, Kenig, Trudell, & Cohen, 1979). Concentrations of ethanol of 1087–2174 mM (5000–10000 mg/dl) disordered these membranes, while 100 atm of helium increased their intrinsic order. In combination, high pressure reversed the effect of ethanol.

Although there is a general correlation between the disordering effects of alcohols and intoxication, it is not clear whether nonspecifically disordering membranes will induce intoxication or whether the degree of this disordering correlates with the degree of intoxication. As discussed earlier, changes in temperature can alter the structural order of membranes.

Manipulating the body temperature of animals can alter the sensitivity to ethanol. Increasing the body temperatures increases ethanol toxicity, and lowering it reduces toxicity (Dinh & Gailis, 1979; Malcolm & Alkana, 1981; Pohorecky & Rizek, 1981). When a cold-blooded animal, the fish *Gambusia affinis*, was exposed to an increased environmental temperature, ethanol-induced loss of righting reflex was enhanced (Ingram, Carey, & Dombek, 1982). Conversely, reducing the temperature antagonized this effect of ethanol, as well as its membrane disordering effect, as measured by changes in fluorescence polarization of DPH in neural membranes. However, narcotic concentrations of ethanol disordered membranes less than a 2°C increase in temperature. An increase in temperature of 8°C did not induce narcosis. These data suggested that disordering lipids in general is not a causative factor in ethanol intoxication.

Some recent data raise further questions about the relationship of membrane order and ethanol intoxication, based on the lipid-disordering effect of ethanol in mice at different ages (Armbrecht, Wood, Wise, Walsh, Thomas, & Strong, 1983). Synaptic plasma membranes, brain microsomal membranes, and erythrocyte membranes were incubated with 250–500 mM (1150–2300 mg/dl). The animals ranged in age from 3 to 24 months. Using 5-doxylstearic acid as the EPR probe of lipid order, the older mice were resistant to the lipid-disordering effect of ethanol with very little effect observed with 500 mM (2300 mg/dl), when compared to the younger mice. No alteration in the intrinsic order of the membrane was observed. However, the older animals were considerably more sensitive to the depressant effects of ethanol (Ritzmann & Springer, 1980; Wood, Armbrecht, & Wise, 1982).

Chronic effects of ethanol on membrane order

Since chronic treatment with ethanol can lead to the development of tolerance and physical dependence, the altered sensitivity of the nervous system may result from adaptive processes that occur in membranes as a response to a chronic disruption in their normal milieu. This possibility has been addressed with both EPR and fluorescence techniques. Chin and Goldstein (1977b) were first to demonstrate that the disordering effect of ethanol on synaptosomal membranes using 5-doxylstearic acid as the probe was diminished after mice had been given short-term chronic treatment with ethanol. The order parameter of the membrane without added ethanol was unaffected. However, when using 12-doxylstearic acid, which reports on the microenvironment deeper in the membrane, the order parameter had, in fact, increased, suggesting that the portion of membrane surrounding the probe had become more ordered or rigid (Lyon & Goldstein, 1983). No change in the order parameter was observed when using 5- and 16-doxylstearic acid as probes. It was reasoned that if the disordering effect of ethanol was reduced by chronic ethanol treatment, then the membrane must somehow become more rigid to compensate for the presence of ethanol. Not only could a specific portion of the membrane become rigid, this effect could influence the properties of other parts of the membrane as well.

Tolerance to the fluidizing effects of ethanol has also been observed using fluorescence techniques. The reduction in fluorescence polarization of DPH by ethanol was attenuated after short-term chronic ethanol treatment for 3 days (Johnson, Lee, Cooke, & Loh, 1979). The effect could be seen in both mice and rats (Johnson, Friedman, Cooke, & Lee, 1980), an effect that was reversible within 12 days after ethanol withdrawal (Johnson, Lee, Cooke, & Loh, 1980). In another study, no tolerance was observed in miniature swine consuming ethanol for 3 years (Harris, Fenner, Feller, Sieckman, Lloyd, Mitchell, Dexter, Tumbelson, & Bylund, 1983).

Ethanol has been found to disorder membranes from other organs of the body. For example, in the liver, concentrations of ethanol as low as 100 mM (460 mg/dl) reduced the order parameter of 5-doxylstearic acid in mitochondrial membranes, which was progressively greater at higher concentrations (Waring, Rottenberg, Ohnishi, & Rubin, 1981).

After chronic treatment with ethanol for 4–6 weeks in a liquid diet, both hepatic mitochondrial and microsomal membranes were resistant to the disordering effect of ethanol (Ponnappa, Waring, Hoek, Rottenberg, & Rubin, 1982; Waring *et al.* 1981; Waring, Rottenberg, Ohnishi, & Rubin, 1982). An increased order parameter of 5-doxylstearic acid in membranes without the addition of ethanol was also observed. In further support is the observation that the phase transition temperatures were increased with chronic ethanol treatment (Ponnappa *et al.*, 1982; Waring *et al.*, 1982). These effects correlated with parallel changes in mitochondrial respiration, ATPase activity, and enhanced microsomal calcium uptake (Ponnappa *et al.*, 1982; Rottenberg, Robertson, & Rubin, 1980) and might represent the initial events leading to liver injury (Rubin & Rottenberg, 1982). Similar mechanisms have been postulated to occur in the heart after chronic ethanol treatment (Rubin, 1982). No differences in fluorescence polarization were observed in skeletal muscle from ethanol-tolerant mice as compared to controls (Mrak, 1983).

If membranes become more rigid with chronic ethanol administration, one consequence may be the reduced ability of ethanol to partition into the membrane, thereby decreasing its action. This possibility was first suggested with the use of a spin-labeled probe that is studied by measuring how much of it is bound to a membrane as compared to its concentration in the aqueous medium. With nitroxide-labeled decane 4-butyl-2,2-dimethyl-1,4-pentyloxazolidine-N-oxyloxazolidine (5N10), a partition coefficient can be calculated based on the relative contribution of the membrane and aqueous phases to the EPR spectrum.

In rats that have received ethanol for 35 days, the partitioning of 5N10 into both brain synaptosomal membranes and liver mitochondrial membranes was significantly reduced (Rottenberg, Waring, & Rubin, 1981), while the phase transition temperatures were elevated (Waring *et al.*, 1982).

Partition coefficients for ethanol in these membranes were determined (Rottenberg *et al.*, 1982) by incubating the membranes with [^{14}C]ethanol and [^{3}H]water, and then centrifuging the mixture. The amount of [^{14}C] ethanol in the pellet in excess of that found for [^{3}H]water was considered dissolved in the membrane. The ratio of the concentration of [^{14}C]ethanol in the membrane to that in the medium was considered the partition coefficient. After ethanol treatment for 35 days, the partition coefficient for ethanol was only 33% of that found in untreated controls in both synaptosomal and liver mitochondrial membranes. The partition coefficients for both halothane and phenobarbital were also reduced, suggesting the development of cross-tolerance.

Changes in membrane composition with chronic ethanol treatment

The alterations in membrane fluidity associated with chronic ethanol treatment are in two general forms, one direct and the other indirect. The direct one relates to a change in fluidity of the membrane itself in the absence of ethanol, while the other relates to whatever change occurs in the membrane that reduces the ability of ethanol to disorder it. In this section, we shall examine the mechanisms by which such changes could occur and whether the alterations in membrane fluidity would be expected to be related to these changes.

As discussed in Chapter 1, the composition of membranes, especially lipids, is very important in determining the degree of intrinsic fluidity of a membrane. High cholesterol and long-chain saturated fatty-acid content tend to render membranes rigid, while low cholesterol and short-chain unsaturated fatty-acid content tend to render membranes more fluid. To determine how changes in the lipid content might contribute to the changes in membrane order observed, a number of studies have measured lipid content after chronic ethanol treatment.

If the development of tolerance is related to the presence of more rigid membranes, then one cause of this could be due to an increase in cholesterol content. A number of studies examined the effect of chronic ethanol treatment on cholesterol concentrations in membranes with varying results.

When mice were treated for 8 or 9 days with ethanol administered in a liquid diet, cholesterol content in both synaptosomal plasma and erythrocyte membranes was elevated (Chin, Parsons, & Goldstein, 1978; Smith & Gerhart, 1982). Similar results were observed from synaptosomal membranes obtained from rats given ethanol for 4 days by intragastric intubation and coexisted with a decrease in the membrane-disordering effect of increased incubation temperatures (Crews, Majchrowicz, & Meeks, 1983). Rapidly developing functional tolerance, induced by successive intraperitoneal injections of ethanol over 7 hr, was also accompanied by elevated cholesterol content in erythrocyte membranes from four strains of mice (Parsons, Gallaher, & Goldstein, 1982).

With a different approach, with mice treated twice daily with ethanol for 7 days, the degree of ethanol-induced increases in membrane fluidity were measured in synaptosomal membranes with or without the removal of cholesterol (Johnson et al., 1979). When the cholesterol was extracted from the membranes, the tolerance that developed to the ethanol-induced changes in fluidity was eliminated. Furthermore, when the cholesterol was added back, the tolerance could again be observed. If mice were pretreated with the cholesterol synthesis inhibitor, diazacholesterol, behavioral tolerance could not be induced (Grieve, Littleton, Jones, & John, 1979; Littleton, John, Jones, & Grieve, 1980).

In other experiments in which ethanol was administered by daily intraperitoneal injections for 7 days, by inhalation for 3 days, or orally in the drinking water for 9 months, no change in cholesterol content was seen (Alling, Liljequist, & Engel, 1982; Lyon & Goldstein, 1983; Wing, Harvey, Hughes, Dunbar, McPherson, & Paton, 1982), even though synaptosomal membranes were more rigid after chronic ethanol treatment and were resistant to the membrane-disordering effects of ethanol (Lyon & Goldstein, 1983).

If an elevated cholesterol content accounts, at least in part, for the development of tolerance, then by what mechanism could this take place? One approach to finding out has involved measuring the transfer of [^{3}H] cholesterol from plasma into erythrocytes (Daniels & Goldstein, 1982). Ethanol accelerated this transfer in a concentration-dependent manner, although the final cholesterol content was unaltered. Increasing cholesterol concentrations in the incubation medium enhanced this reaction. Ethanol also increased cholesterol transfer when prelabeled erythrocytes, low- and high-density lipoproteins, and egg lecithin vesicles were used as cholesterol donors. It has been suggested that chronic ethanol treatment might facilitate the net transfer of cholesterol from one compartment to another.

In experiments in which the fatty-acid content and composition of synaptosomal membranes were determined, studies in which mice were treated with ethanol for 10 days by inhalation demonstrated that an increase in the saturated fatty acids and a decrease in unsaturated fatty acids occurred, consistent with increased membrane rigidity (Littleton & John, & Grieve, 1979). These changes were reflected in an elevation in the content of stearic acid (18 : 0) and a reduction in the content of arachidonic (20 : 4) and docosahexaenoic (22 : 6) acids. (The numbers in parentheses refer to the number of carbon atoms and double bonds, respectively.)

However, this shift in the content from unsaturated to saturated fatty acids was not as clear in other reports. In one case, the reverse finding was observed in guinea pigs treated with ethanol in a liquid diet for 3 weeks, and depended upon whether choline or ethanolamine phospholipids were measured (Sun & Sun, 1979). In synaptosomal fractions obtained from rats given ethanol for 5 months in the drinking water, oleic acid (18 : 1) phosphatidylcholine was slightly increased and arachidonic acid (20 : 4) phosphatidylethanolamine was slightly reduced (Alling et al. 1982). These effects correlated with equivalent changes of these substances in plasma. In other studies in which ethanol was administered for 4–8 days by intragastric intubation or liquid diet, no alteration in fatty-acid composition or phospholipid content was observed (Crews et al., 1983; Smith & Gerhardt, 1982).

In tissue preparations from other organs from animals chronically treated with ethanol, varying results were reported. In mouse erythrocyte membranes and rat platelets, only small increases in stearic (18 : 0) and oleic

(18 : 1) acids were detected (Dunbar, Harvey, McPherson, & Wing, 1981; Hwang, LeBlanc, & Chanmugan, 1981; Wing *et al.*, 1982). Similar results on oleic acid content were obtained in mitochondrial membranes from rat liver (Waring *et al.*, 1981). However, much larger increases in saturated cardiolipin phospholipids containing palmitic (16 : 0) and stearic (18 : 0) acids, and decreases in the unsaturated cardiolipin phospholipid containing linoleic (18 : 2) acid were observed. Palmitic acid was moderately reduced in liver microsomal membranes (Miceli & Farrell, 1973).

Chronic exposure of HeLa cells *in vitro* to ethanol in concentrations of 86 m*M* (396 mg/dl) for 9 days significantly altered lipid composition (Keegan, Wilce, Ruczkal-Pietrzak, & Shanley, 1983). Both cholesterol and phospholipid concentrations increased. Of the phospholipid classes, the methylated phospholipids were elevated at the expense of phosphatidic acid. Of the fatty acids, the saturated and monoenoic acids (14 : 0, 16 : 0) were increased, while the major polyenoic acid (20 : 4) was reduced.

Using a different approach to the question of the role of phospholipid composition in the sensitivity to ethanol, mice were maintained for life on a diet high in saturated fats in an attempt to increase the saturated fatty acid composition in membranes (John, Littleton, & Jones, 1980; Littleton *et al.*, 1980). This treatment had no effect on fatty acid composition in the brain. However, if the mice were exposed to ethanol in an inhalation chamber for 5 hr, their sensitivity to ethanol was reduced, accompanied by an increase in the ratio of saturated to unsaturated fatty acids. No effect on the development of tolerance was observed. On the other hand, mice fed a diet high in polyunsaturated fats for 9 months were more sensitive to ethanol (Koblin & Deady, 1981). However, parallel changes in the content of unsaturated fatty acids were not found.

The relationship between sensitivity to ethanol and saturated fatty-acid content in neural membranes has been studied in *G. affinis*, obtained from the wild and living at different times of the year (Ingram *et al.*, 1982). Fish living in the summer had higher amounts of saturated fatty acids in their membranes and were less sensitive to ethanol intoxication than their counterparts living in the winter.

Finally, the role of lipids in the development of tolerance has been studied in microorganisms. An increase in cholesterol content in *Acholeplasma laidlawii* was observed after exposure for 24 hr to halothane or cyclopropane, but only with concentrations of the drugs that would be incompatible with life in humans (Koblin & Wang, 1981). In *Escherichia coli* and *Tetrahymena pyriformis* cells exposed to 54.3–870 m*M* (250–4000 mg/dl) ethanol for 48 hr, the content of phosphatidyl ethanolamine and saturated fatty acids decreased and phosphatidyl glycerol and unsaturated fatty acids increased, similar to that observed when cells were incubated at lower temperatures (Ingram, 1976, 1977; Ingram, Dickens, & Buttke, 1980; Ingram, Ley, & Hoffman, 1978; Nandini-Kishore, Mattox,

Martin, & Thompson, 1979). This is opposite from what would be expected if membranes were to become more rigid. In fact, a reduction in the incubating temperature from 39° to 15°C would have to be maintained to induce such changes in lipid composition (Dickens & Thompson, 1981). Mutants that were selected to tolerate high concentrations of ethanol, while the parent strain would not, also had higher levels of unsaturated fatty acids. Further study suggested that ethanol inhibited saturated fatty-acid synthesis in *E. coli* cells (Buttke & Ingram, 1980). However, this effect did not seem to be membrane mediated and might result from a direct inhibition of ethanol of the enzymes involved in fatty acid synthesis. In another study using *T. pyriforma* cells, changes in lipid composition after chronic ethanol exposure did not correspond with any change in the lipid-disordering effect of added ethanol (Goto, Banno, Umeki, Kameyama, & Nozawa, 1983).

In *Clostridium thermocellum*, an ethanol-producing bacterium, the growth rate could be altered by both the addition of ethanol to the growth medium and by changes in the incubation temperature (Herrero & Gomez, 1980). When cells of the ATCC 27405 strain were incubated with ethanol, the optimal growth temperature decreased. This would be expected if the optimal growth rate of the cells depended on an optimal intrinsic order of their cell membranes. If ethanol fluidized the membranes, then lowering the temperature would counteract this effect. When the C9 strain, an ethanol-resistant mutant, was used the addition of ethanol to the growth medium had no effect on the optimal growth temperature.

The lipid composition of *Zymomonas mobilis*, a microorganism that can withstand high concentrations of ethanol, was determined in order to ascertain whether the lipid composition of the cells could explain their natural ethanol tolerance (Carey & Ingram, 1983). Vaccenic acid (18 : 1) was the most abundant fatty acid in these cells. Incubation of the cells with ethanol did not alter the fatty composition, although phosphatidylethanolamine and phosphatidylglycerol concentrations were reduced and cardiolipin and phosphatidylcholine concentrations were elevated. The lipid to protein ratio was also decreased.

It would appear that microorganisms adapt to the presence of ethanol by increasing the concentrations of longer-chain unsaturated fatty acids at the expense of saturated fatty acids. This is contrary to the idea that saturated fatty-acid concentrations should increase in order to counteract the fluidizing effect of ethanol, but consistent with a number of the studies discussed earlier that used mammalian cells. The apparent paradox has been examined further using *E. coli* cells.

Using a series of fluorescent probes that report on the microenvironment at different depths of the membranes of the *E. coli* cells, ethanol was found to disorder the membrane to a greater extent near the cell surface rather than deep in the membrane, as has been shown in mammalian cells

(Dombek & Ingram, 1984). However, hexanol, a more lipid-soluble aliphatic alcohol, disordered the membrane in the lipid core. A depletion of the membrane protein or an elevation of the incubating temperature, disordered the membranes. When the cells were grown in the presence of ethanol, the membrane became more rigid at all depths. Using cells that were either deficient in lipids or protein grown in the presence of ethanol, bulk proteins contributed significantly to the subsequent rigidity of the membranes. The results suggested that the lipid to protein ratio may be important in the fluidity of membranes after exposure to ethanol in *E. coli* and possibly other cells.

Since proteins are also a major constituent of membranes, the possibility that chronic ethanol administration leads to alterations in the conformation of proteins imbedded in membranes in the brain has been investigated (Dinovo, Gruber, & Noble, 1976; Gruber, Dinovo, Noble, & Tewari, 1977). Since many proteins contain sulfhydryl groups that may be either exposed on the membrane surface or within the complex structure of the protein, its availability to react with agents such as 5,5'-dithio-(bis)-2-nitrobenzoic acid (DTNB) and N-ethyl maleimide (NEM) can be considered an index of conformational changes in the proteins. This assumes that there is either an increase or a decrease in the availability of the sulfhydryl groups for reaction. Rats that drank 10% ethanol solutions for 6–8 weeks had 16% more sulfhydryl groups reacting with DTNB or NEM in microsomal membranes than in the control membranes. No change in the total concentration of sulfhydryl groups was found. Ethanol added *in vitro* to microsomes from untreated rats exhibited the opposite response, with reductions of 2–20% obtained in the concentration of reactable sulfhydryl groups with ethanol concentrations of 5.4–217 mM (24.8–998 mg/dl). These data were interpreted to reflect conformational changes in proteins resulting from chronic ethanol administration.

Additional evidence to suggest that proteins alter their conformation in response to ethanol exposure has been derived from experiments using cultured astroblasts (Noble, Syapin, Vigran, & Rosenberg, 1976). The general approach taken was similar to that used for sulfhydryl groups. Glycoproteins and glycolipids on the surface of membranes contain sialic acid. If sialic acid molecules are oriented along the membrane surface, they can be released by reaction with neuraminidase. Therefore, alterations in neuraminidase-releasable sialic acid on the membrane surface is an index of steric modifications of the macromolecules to which the sialic acid is attached. When the astroblasts were incubated with 100 mM (460 mg/dl) ethanol for 19–110 days, the amount of sialic acid released by neuraminidase was elevated by 10–52%. The length of the incubation did not influence the magnitude of the change. Addition of ethanol to cells not previously incubated with ethanol did not alter sialic acid release.

Other glucoconjugates were studied in mice by measuring the availability of galactose for oxidation. Chronic ethanol treatment for 3 days led to an elevation in reactable galactose (Goldstein, Hungund, & Lyon, 1983).

Commentary

Through the course of this chapter, evidence was presented that demonstrates that alcohols can interact with membranes. The most consistent evidence has been related to the ability of alcohols to disorder membranes. The data were derived with the use of molecular probes that were inserted into the membrane and the properties of these probes were examined using EPR or fluorescence techniques. The validity of these studies depends on the assumptions made concerning the localization and molecular orientation of the probes.

The basic localization of a probe depends on the structure of the membrane and the physical and chemical properties of the probe. The exact structure of a membrane depends largely on its function. Whether all membranes, especially neuronal membranes, have a fluid mosaic structure is not known, although a relatively basic membrane structure would be expected. Since membranes do not dissolve in water, the assumed decreasing polarity gradient from the membrane-aqueous interface to the membrane core is reasonable. Thus, the localization of DPH in hydrophobic regions and that of ANS near the membrane surface are likely to be true based on their physical properties. The location of spin-labeled or fluorescent stearic acid derivatives assumes the membrane to have a basic bimolecular leaflet structure. If true, the probe would tend to intercalate parallel to the phospholipids in the membrane. Additionally, the spin-labeled or fluorescent moiety on the probe should not seriously distort the membrane structure.

The data presented in this chapter conclusively show that aliphatic alcohols can alter the fluidity of membranes. However, whether these alterations in membrane properties can explain their diverse actions in living animals needs to be examined. Of the four criteria needed to be satisfied for a mechanism of action of alcohols (see Chapter 1), only the direct relationship of the potencies of the alcohols to fluidize membranes to their lipid solubility has been clearly demonstrated. A correlation in time course between the fluidity changes and the appearance and disappearance of neuronal depression may not ever be testable directly. However, a demonstration of reversibility, that is, a return to control values of the fluidity after the alcohol is washed out of the tissue preparation, has not been reported.

Finding alterations in membrane fluidity at concentrations of alcohols that would be physiologically compatible with life have not been definitive or consistent. This is due in part to the extremely small changes, at least in biological terms, that are detected. The changes reported are generally less than 5% from control values. Such small changes are particularly tricky with EPR techniques. The spectra of spin-labeled membranes in the presence of physiologically relevant concentrations of ethanol are visually indistinguishable from controls. Resolution must be accomplished with computer enhancement techniques and utilizing mathematical equations for best fit of parts of the EPR spectrum needed for the determination of $T'_{\parallel}$ and $T'_{\perp}$, used to calculate the order parameter. It would not take much of a change in an important variable to drastically alter the results of an experiment. For example, a variation of sample temperature of $\pm 0.1°C$, the precision of most EPR spectrometers, could completely mask any change by the alcohol or enhance a minimal effect (Pryer, 1980). The influence of temperature fluctuations appears also to be relevant to fluorescence techniques.

Normally in pharmacology, a drug is expected to have a relatively large effect on an endpoint for that effect to have relevance to the mechanism of action of the drug. It may be difficult to accept that such a small change in membrane order as induced by ethanol could have biological significance. One study has attempted to gain insight into this problem using several anesthetics (Pang, Chang, & Miller, 1979). The ability of these drugs to disorder artificial phospholipid membranes was correlated with their ability to promote ^{86}Rb efflux from preloaded vesicles. At general anesthetic concentrations in the vesicles, both parameters correlated quite well, except a given percentage change in measured fluidity was associated with a ten-fold higher change in ^{86}Rb efflux. This suggests that a small perturbation of the membrane might be amplified into a much larger, physiologically disruptive response.

Assuming that small changes in fluidity occur at physiologically compatible concentrations of alcohols, these changes, in order to be biologically relevant, must in some way be related to cellular function. The fact that one biological change generally occurs at a time when another biological change occurs does not prove that they are causally related. Whether altered fluidity and the degree to which it occurs can account for altered cellular function has not been conclusively demonstrated. For example, on one hand, decreased fluorescence is associated with ethanol exposure and presumably neuronal depression. On the other hand, decreased fluorescence has been closely correlated with nerve excitation of squid axons (Tasaki, Carbone, Sisco, & Singer, 1973; Tasaki, Watanabe, & Hallett, 1971). The lack of a lipid-disordering effect of ethanol in aged animals at physiologically compatible concentrations, even though the animals are more sensitive to the depressant effects of ethanol, makes this question of relevance even more perplexing. The exact role of lipid disordering in the actions of ethanol needs to be studied further.

The data suggest that the greatest change in fluidity induced by alco-

hols is in the lipid core of the membrane. This, however, does not necessarily indicate that that is where ethanol is located within the membrane.
In fact, based on its physical properties, ethanol would not be expected
to be located in a highly lipid area, but would likely be located more toward the more polar membrane surface. Furthermore, hydrocarbons that
would be expected to localize in the lipid core are not very potent as depressants (McCreery & Hunt, 1978).

The answer to this dilemma could lie in an amplification of a small
change in motion of molecules near the membrane surface along the acyl
chains to the lipid core. An analogy would be the initiation of wave motion in a flexible metal rod, stationary at one end. If the rod is moved a
small amount near the stationary point, the resultant wave would be much
larger at the free end of the rod than near the stationary end. The movement of acyl chains in membranes induced by alcohols could result from
their intercalation between the fatty acids, thereby distorting the normal
alignment of the acyl chains. This could allow more opportunity for movement at the distal end of the fatty acids and could be expressed as increased
fluidity in these areas. In fact, this amplification could be a mechanism
by which small changes in membrane order in specific areas of the membrane could result in much greater effect on functional processes of the cell.

Since membranes are composed of proteins as well as lipids, more
attention needs to be directed toward interactions of alcohols with proteins. Interactions of alcohols with functional units of membranes, such
as ion channels and transport systems, will be discussed in later chapters.
Few studies have addressed the possibility that alcohols can alter protein
conformation. One report, discussed earlier in this chapter, that involved
reactable sulfhydryl groups found a small reduction in the amount of sulfhydryl groups exposed on the membrane surface with physiologically compatible concentrations of ethanol.

The availability of sulfhydryl groups has been associated with changes
in excitation. Electrical stimulation increases the binding of thiol reagents
to membranes of squid axons and walking leg nerve bundles of the spider
crab (Marquis & Mautner, 1974a, 1974b). Whether ethanol-induced changes
in protein conformation are a cause of altered neuroexcitability or a consequence of it has not been determined. However, it is possible that alcohols partition into hydrophobic regions of functionally important proteins,
thereby altering their ability for normal molecular reorientations.

Changes in fluidity are also associated with chronic administration
of ethanol. Membranes become more rigid and are resistant to the disordering effects of ethanol. These two properties appear to be localized in different parts of the membrane, since they are generally observed with different molecular probes. Whether these changes are related to one another
or reflect independent changes in the membrane is not clear.

One postulated mechanism to account for this reduced fluidity is an ethanol-induced change in the lipid composition of the membrane. It might be predicted that cholesterol content and/or the ratio of saturated to unsaturated fatty acids would increase with chronic ethanol treatment. An increased cholesterol content is an attractive possibility because the cholesterol would be located in an area of the membrane where the increased membrane order was observed (Lyon & Goldstein, 1983; Vincent, de Foresta, Galley, & Alfsen, 1982; Waring *et al.*, 1981). However, there is no consistent evidence to support an increased cholesterol content or saturated to unsaturated fatty acid ratio after chronic ethanol administration. Furthermore, changes opposite from these predictions have been reported. In fact, increased membrane order has been observed both after consumption of ethanol in a liquid diet, where changes in lipid composition were found, and after chronic ethanol inhalation, where such changes were not seen.

Since the genetic strains of mice, long sleep and short sleep, differ only in their sensitivity to ethanol, measurements of membrane lipid composition might prove useful. Such measurements have not been made in chronically treated animals, but cholesterol and phospholipid content has been determined in liver mitochondrial membranes of untreated mice (Zysset, Sutherland, & Simon, 1983). Both cholesterol and phospholipid content was higher in short-sleep mice than in long-sleep mice with no difference in the cholesterol/phospholipid ratio.

Another factor that could influence results obtained after chronic ethanol treatment is "hypothermia." Hypothermia is a well-known concomitant of ethanol intoxication (Freund, 1973b) and involves the inability of the animals to regulate their body temperature (Freund, 1973b; Lomax, Bajorek, Chesahek, & Chaffee, 1980). As discussed earlier, changing the ambient temperature of the environment in which the experimental animals are placed alters the degree of intoxication. With increases in ambient temperature, which increases fluidity, intoxication is enhanced, while decreasing ambient temperature, which decreases fluidity, reduces intoxication unless hypothermia-induced toxicity occurs.

Depending upon how long hypothermia occurs during chronic ethanol treatment, this effect may influence how a membrane would adapt. On the one hand, the disordering effect of ethanol might induce an adaptive change in membrane composition that would make it more rigid. On the other hand, hypothermia might stimulate the membrane to become more fluid. In none of the studies in which fluidity or the concentration of membrane lipids was determined after chronic ethanol treatment was body temperature controlled. Although hypothermia itself does not appear to influence the development of tolerance (Grieve & Littleton, 1979), hypothermia may account for some of the increases in unsaturated fatty acids observed in some studies. In fact, the rigidifying effect of chronic ethanol treatment may be underestimated by opposing reactions in the membrane.

Since changes in gross lipid composition do not appear to be a prerequisite for the ethanol-induced changes in fluidity, some other, more subtle change in the membrane must be considered. The alterations in the partitioning of 5N10 and [^{14}C]ethanol into membranes from chronic ethanol-treated animals might provide some clues. Both the spin-labeled 5N10 and [^{14}C]ethanol partition into membranes to a lesser extent in the chronic ethanol-treated animals. This observation argues against the membrane becoming more nonpolar as might be expected from elevated concentrations of cholesterol and saturated fatty acids. If that were true, the partitioning of nonpolar 5N10 would increase, while that of polar ethanol would decrease. Instead, the structure of the membrane might reorient in a manner such that the 5N10 and ethanol molecules physically could not penetrate the membrane.

Partition coefficients can be altered by a number of means. For example, the partition coefficient of [^{14}C]pentabarbitone can be affected by the lipid composition of the membrane (Miller & Yu, 1977), with increases in the cholesterol or phosphatidic acid content, the partition coefficient is reduced. High pressure, which would decrease fluidity, has no effect. With aliphatic alcohols, shortening the acyl chain length would reduce partitioning (Kamaya, Kaneshina, & Ueda, 1981). However, an increase in shorter-chain fatty acids after chronic ethanol treatment has not been observed.

Another way to reduce partitioning of ethanol into membranes would be for the alkyl side chain of cholesterol to become unsaturated. Using the yeast *Saccharomyces cerevisiae*, cells were more viable in ethanol solutions when the membranes were enriched with ergosterol or stigmasterol with a double bond in the 22-position in the alkyl chain, rather than cholesterol with no unsaturation (Thomas, Hossak, & Rose, 1978). Since cholesterol constrains the movement of the first 8 or 9 carbons of an acyl chain in the membrane (Phillips, 1972; Phillips & Finer, 1974), it has been suggested that a double bond in the alkyl chain of cholesterol would further restrict the movement of the distal end of the acyl chain and thereby restrict entry of ethanol into the membrane (Hossak & Rose, 1976). The possibility of such unsaturations in mammalian cholesterol molecules in membranes after chronic ethanol administration has not been reported.

If chronic ethanol administration were not to modify the gross lipid composition of membranes, then a more subtle change would have to explain it. A possible explanation is an alteration in the membrane composition or configuration in a localized area of the membrane. This may be difficult to detect with present methods. The change may be small enough that the effect is masked by the much larger amounts of lipids that are not changed. If the membrane were to become bulkier at a specific depth, especially near the membrane-aqueous interphase, there may be less room for alcohols to intercalate into the membrane, thereby reducing their ability to partition into it. The increased rigidity observed with 5- and 12-, but not 16-doxylstearic acid, supports this possibility. It might also be expected that the EPR probes themselves partition less into membranes. This possibility has not been examined.

In summary, aliphatic alcohols dissolve in hydrophobic areas of membranes, which probably leads to an increase in fluidity, but doing so in selected depths of membranes. Changes in fluidity resulting from chronic ethanol treatment seem also to be localized. Whether these changes have any biological consequences is yet to be determined. Although the action of alcohols does not appear to be through classical receptors, they may exert their relevant effects in specific areas of the membrane, rather than through a totally nonspecific action. This may include lipid regions surrounding functional proteins.

3. Membrane electrophysiology

So far in this book, we have discussed various ways in which ethanol can interact with the structural components of membranes. In order to have any meaning for the normal activity of a cell, such interactions must have functional consequences. In this chapter and those to follow, we shall examine the evidence that suggests that ethanol can disrupt a number of mechanisms in membranes that are related to normal cellular function, especially in the brain.

The nervous system and other excitable tissues require the generation and propagation of electrical impulses to perform their biological functions. To this end, the various components of cell membranes must operate in an integrated manner to maintain efficient operation. Ethanol appears to alter the electrical properties of cells, thereby presumably having adverse consequences on the function of the preparation under study.

In the brain, electrical activity can be detected and studied at a number of levels. One of the more common approaches is the use of the electro-encephalogram (EEG). An EEG measures the change in voltage generated by the brain or a part of it over a period of time. It may represent the integrated activity of millions of cells. Consequently, the activity of single cells or small groups of cells cannot be inferred from an EEG. Since this book addresses the actions of ethanol on membranes, it is important to be able to gain information at the cellular level, rather than the more macroscopic level of the whole brain or a part of the brain. Therefore, in this chapter, we shall explore the effects of ethanol in model systems in which the activity of single cells or small groups of cells can be studied. This will include the use of single- and multiple-unit recordings from tissues *in vitro* and *in vivo*, from vertebrates and invertebrates, and from cells grown in culture. For a more global treatment of the effect of ethanol on neurophysiological parameters, the reader is referred to the reviews of Begleiter and Platz (1972), Berry and Pentreath (1980), Himwich and Callison (1972), and Klemm (1979). The next section will discuss some general considerations and methodological procedures used for the studies to be presented.

General considerations

The membrane around a neuron provides the structural entity that allows for electrical properties of the neuron to exist (Koester, 1981a,

1981b). As discussed in Chapter 1, one of the functions of a membrane is to separate the aqueous constituents on one side of the membrane from those on the other side. Many of these constituents are ionized and, therefore, electrically charged. Net electrical charges exist on each side of the membrane. Since the net electrical charge of the intracellular constituents is negative and that of the extracellular constituents is positive, this separation of charge gives rise to an electrical potential across the membrane. In order to prevent the dissipation of ion gradients and, therefore, electrical gradients, ion pumps requiring the use of cellularly produced energy are required to maintain the proper concentrations of intracellular and extracellular ions.

The unequal distribution of ions on each side of the membrane is the source of an electrical gradient that comprises the membrane potential. Each ion has an equilibrium potential at which the concentration gradient of the ion across the membrane is equal and opposite to the electrical gradient generated by that ion. The weighted average of equilibrium potentials, primarily for sodium, potassium, and chloride, constitutes the resting membrane potential.

Membranes have other electrical properties. Ions move through channels that are specific for each ion and are either open all the time to allow passive movements or gated where the channel can open and close depending on physiological conditions. As an ion moves through its channel, it meets resistance because of collisions with the walls of the channel. The reciprocal of resistance is "conductance," a term that refers to the ease by which the ion moves through its channel and can be experimentally calculated from measured membrane currents and voltages. Conductance is related to but is not the same as "permeability" of the ion. Permeability is a constant property of the membrane for a particular ion, while conductance can vary with such factors as concentration and distribution of ions and channel conditions.

Finally, since the membrane acts as an insulator that separates the positive and negative charges on its outer and inner surfaces, respectively, such charges can accumulate and be stored on these surfaces. This makes the membrane a capacitor.

The properties just discussed are important in understanding how signaling can take place within neurons and between neurons. The basis of this signaling is the change in the resting membrane potential resulting from alterations in the conductance of ions (Koester, 1981c). The "action potential" represents the most prominent change and is associated with the propagation of electrical impulses throughout a neuron. This process is illustrated in Figure 3-1. Usually, some stimulus opens the gate on the sodium channel, allowing increased sodium movement into the neuron. This results in depolarization, that is, a decreased potential difference across the membrane. If sufficient depolarization occurs so that the spike threshold is reached, other types of sodium channels open (and often calcium chan-

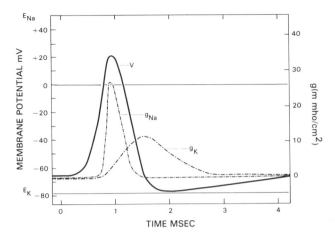

Figure 3-1. Relationship between membrane potential and changes in sodium and potassium conductances. From A. L. Hodgkin & A. F. Huxley, A quantitative description of membrane current and its application to conduction and excitation in nerve. *Journal of Physiology (London)*, 1952, *117*, 500–544. Copyright 1952 by Cambridge University Press. Reprinted by permission.

nels) leading to a further depolarization, until a reversal of membrane potential or overshoot is obtained. This depolarization spreads to adjacent areas of the membrane, allowing the action potential to be propagated throughout the neuron.

The action potential, being a transient event, is terminated by both a closing of the gate on the sodium channel and an opening of the gates of certain potassium channels, allowing potassium to flow out of the neuron. The membrane potential increases, usually exceeding the original resting membrane potential for a short time, creating the so-called afterhyperpolarization. Then, many of the potassium channels are closed, allowing the membrane potential to return to the resting state. The passive properties of the membrane discussed earlier are important in determining properties of the action potential, such as the rate at which sodium current increases and the rate at which impulses are conducted.

Once the electrical impulse reaches the end of its axon, the synapse, the signal is transferred to a postsynaptic neuron through the release of a neurotransmitter. The transmitter interacts with an appropriate receptor where the information is translated back into an electrical signal.

The interaction of a transmitter with its receptor results in changes in the resting membrane potential of the postsynaptic neuron (Kandel, 1981; Shepherd, 1979). These changes are either excitatory postsynaptic potentials (EPSPs) or inhibitory postsynaptic potentials (IPSPs). EPSPs that depolarize the neuron result from a simultaneous increase in sodium and potassium conductances, or from an increase in sodium conductance alone. Different ion channels are involved than the voltage-sensitive ones associated with the action potential. The IPSPs that are hyperpolarizing, that is, increase the membrane potential, probably result mostly from increases in potassium and/or chloride conductances. The membrane potential of a postsynaptic neuron is shifted depending on the summation of all the EPSPs and IPSPs induced by all presynaptic inputs to the neuron.

Methodological procedures

Electrophysiological methodology tends to fall into two general categories, stimulation and recording. The electrical activity of neurons can be altered by either electrical stimulation or chemical manipulation. With electrical stimulation, a neuron can be stimulated either orthodromically, where an anatomical pathway presynaptic to the neuron is stimulated, or antidromically, where the axon of the neuron itself is stimulated. With orthodromic stimulation, the forward movement of an action potential synaptically stimulates the recorded neuron. This allows for the analysis of synaptic transmission. With antidromic stimulation, the backward movement of the action potential is terminated when it reaches the cell body and attached dendrites. This allows for the study of the electrical properties of the cell body and dendrites of that neuron.

Chemical manipulation involves the exogenous application of drugs or transmitters, which can have excitatory or inhibitory influences on the activity of the neurons. This is often accomplished by "iontophoresis" or superfusion *in vitro*. Iontophoresis uses multibarreled micropipettes that can be placed in or near a cell and can contain a number of different substances. One or more barrels of the pipette can be used for applying the substances and/or for recording. The drugs, which generally have an electrical charge, are held in the pipette by an electrical current with an opposite charge. By changing the polarity of the current, an amount of drug can be released depending on the amount of current involved.

Recording techniques can vary depending on the information desired. Cellular activity can be monitored both intracellularly and extracellularly. A very important aspect of recording cellular activity is cell identification, which can be difficult. However, without it, interpretation of data obtained can be severely hampered. More detail on some of these techniques will be presented in later sections of this chapter.

Effects of alcohols on invertebrate preparations

Some of the earliest studies of neuronal activity in cellular preparations have been with invertebrates. By means of extracellular recordings of the squid giant axon, the resting membrane potential and characteristics of the action potential were measured in the presence of varying concentrations of ethanol in the bathing medium (Moore, Ulbricht, & Takata, 1964). Ethanol at concentrations of 810–2700 mM (3700–12,000 mg/dl) had no effect on the resting membrane potential, but slightly reduced the height and duration of the action potential. Using the same concentrations of ethanol, maximum sodium and potassium conductances were decreased 20–40%. In another study using the squid giant axon, 510 mM (2300 mg/dl) ethanol reduced the height of the action potential by 45% (Armstrong & Binstock, 1964).

In recent experiments, 7.5 mM benzyl alcohol reduced the height of the action potential and the rate of depolarization in the squid giant axon (Harper, MacDonald, & Wann, 1983). However, unlike the general observations with alcohols discussed in this and other chapters, the effectiveness of benzyl alcohol in inducing these physiological responses was greater as the temperature of the medium was decreased. This action was attributed to a higher number of sodium channels in the inactivated state at lower temperatures, thereby reducing sodium currents available for depolarization.

Neurons from *Aplysia*, a seal mollusk, have been used for several approaches to the study of the effects of ethanol on neurons. *Aplysia* neurons are very useful models for the study of drug effects because of their well-defined anatomical structures within ganglia and their physiological responses. Using intracellular recordings, ethanol had no significant effect on the resting membrane potential of these neurons, but did alter the action potential (Bergmann, Klee, & Faber, 1974). In concentrations of 110–1100 mM (500–5000 mg/dl), ethanol reduced the height of the action potential and inward sodium currents in a dose-dependent manner. Calcium currents were also reduced.

In other experiments, the "pacemaker" activity of *Aplysia* neurons was examined (Silver & Treistman, 1982). Pacemaker activity is spontaneous discharge of a neuron at a steady rate. When ethanol was applied to cells that were inactive, pacemaker activity could be induced, but only in concentrations of 400–600 mM (1840–2760 mg/dl). On the other hand, cells that normally exhibit pacemaker activity were depressed by ethanol in concentrations of 600 mM.

In another approach using *Aplysia* neurons, the phenomenon of posttetanic potentiation (PTP) was examined in the presence of ethanol (Traynor, Schlapfer, Woodson, & Barondes, 1979). PTP is observed after repetitive neuronal stimulation at a rate greater than once every 2 sec. The size of EPSPs becomes larger as the train of stimuli continues. After the cessation of the stimuli, single stimulations induce EPSPs with larger amplitudes than normal. These EPSPs eventually return to their usual size, generally over a period of 30 min. The rate at which PTP decays can be used as a measure of physiological responsiveness.

When recording from cell R15 in the isolated abdominal ganglion from *Aplysia*, the rate of decay of PTP was enhanced by ethanol in concentrations of 800 mM (3680 mg/dl) with no effect on the amplitude of an isolated EPSP, on an EPSP during repetitive stimulation of presynaptic neurons, or on the initial magnitude of PTP itself (Woodson, Traynor, Schlapfer, & Barondes, 1976). Other alcohols increased the rate of decay of PTP with potencies proportional to their lipid solubilities. The effect was fully reversible when the ethanol was removed.

Upon repeated applications of ethanol, the rate of decay of the PTP was less responsive, suggesting that tolerance had developed to the effect of ethanol (Traynor, Woodson, Schlapfer, & Barondes, 1976). In order for tolerance to develop, presynaptic neurons had to be stimulated in the presence of ethanol (Traynor, Schlapfer, & Barondes, 1980). Merely exposing the cells to ethanol for up to 16 hr was ineffective. The effectiveness of this stimulation in the development of tolerance depended on the concentration of calcium in the perfusion medium. Calcium is required for synaptic transmission. When calcium concentrations were increased in the perfusion medium, the amount of stimulation needed to develop tolerance was reduced. On the other hand, high concentrations of magnesium, which antagonize synaptic transmission, prevented the development of tolerance.

Because of the reports suggesting that ethanol can fluidize membranes (see Chapter 2), it was postulated that the ability of ethanol to accelerate the rate of decay of PTP might be a reflection of membranes whose constituents are less ordered, thereby allowing the mechanism for recovery from PTP to proceed more rapidly (Traynor *et al.*, 1979). One approach to test this possibility was to examine the rate of decay of PTP at lower temperatures. Lowering the temperature would increase the intrinsic order of the membrane, making biological processes run more slowly. As the perfusion temperature was reduced, the rate of decay of PTP was progressively lower, showing a sharp phase transition when the temperature decreased from 12 to 10°C. (Schlapfer, Woodson, Smith, Tremblay, & Barondes, 1975). This might reflect the membrane transforming from a liquid to a gel state (see Chapter 2). If the preparation was maintained at a lower temperature for at least 4 hr, this transition temperature was reduced. Furthermore, exposure to ethanol eliminated the transition altogether.

There are major problems using invertebrate preparations to study the mechanism of action of alcohols. One is the lack of sensitivity of these preparations to the actions of ethanol. In the studies presented, although not lethal to the invertebrate used, the concentrations of ethanol needed to exert much of any biological effect are greater than the concentrations that would be lethal in higher organisms, especially mammals.

Another problem is the question of extrapolation of data obtained from invertebrate preparations to mammals. Invertebrate preparations have contributed greatly to the basic understanding of how neurons maintain and generate their electrical properties. Mammalian brains, however, are much more complicated because of extensive intercommunications among their various regions. Invertebrate studies cannot address how ethanol affects these complex interactions of neurons in higher organisms.

Single-unit and multiple-unit activity *in vivo*

Extracellular unit recordings of electrical activity monitor the firing of action potentials from one or more neurons. Such recordings reflect the electrical activities of neurons. Single-unit recordings measure the electrical activity of single cells and can be recorded with an electrode placed near the plasma membrane. Cell identification is particularly important with this technique. Multiple-unit recordings measure the activity of small populations of cells. This activity represents the summed response of all the cells in the population. Another approach to the recording of the activity of a population of cells is the measurement of "field potentials." Field potentials represent the nearly synchronous firing of a population of cells.

Multiple-unit recordings have been used to estimate which areas of the brain are most sensitive to ethanol (Hyvarinen, Laakso, Poine, Leinone, & Sippel, 1978; Klemm, Dreyfus, Forney, & Mayfield, 1976; Klemm, Mallari, Dreyfus, Fiske, Forney, & Mikeska, 1976; Klemm & Stevens, 1974). Using unanesthetized rats or rabbits with electrodes chronically implanted in 9–14 areas of the brain, spontaneous multiple-unit activity was measured after intraperitoneal doses of ethanol (0.3–1.2 g/kg). Considerable variability in the responses was obtained between animals and within the same animals given more than one dose of ethanol. However, when the data were analyzed as a whole, clear regional sensitivities emerged. The areas of the brain most affected by ethanol with reduced multiple-unit activities were the cerebral cortex, cerebellar cortex, thalamus, midbrain reticular formation, and hippocampus. Single-unit activity recorded from neurons in the primary somatosensory cortex was not significantly altered by ethanol administration (Collins & Roppolo, 1980).

Effects of ethanol on the hippocampus

The use of the hippocampus for studying the effects of ethanol on cellular electrical activity has accelerated in the last few years, in part because of the well-described structural architecture and physiology of the hippocampus and the advent of the slice preparation (to be discussed later). Since descriptions of the hippocampus can be rather lengthy, only the general anatomical features relevant to the discussion of the effect of ethanol on the hippocampus will be presented. For a more detailed treatment, the reader should consult the reviews of Shepherd (1979) and Andersen (1975).

The hippocampus is a C-shaped body found bilaterally in the brain (Figure 3-2). The main areas of the hippocampus are called the CA1–4 regions, with the CA1 and CA3 being the largest and most studied areas. The main output cells of the hippocampus are the pyramidal cells. The pyramidal shape of their cell bodies is imparted by the attached dendritic trunks. The apical and basal dendrites give the pyramidal cells their characteristic shape. The pyramidal cells are the ones from which electrophysiologists generally record unit activity. This is due, in part, to their large size. The output of these cells, which is through the fornix, projects to areas of the hypothalamus, basal ganglia, thalamus, and septum. The hippocampus is intimately involved with many behaviors and is part of the limbic system.

Neuronal input to the hippocampus comes from three main sources. One is from the entorhinal cortex in the temporal lobe, with its projections entering the hippocampus through the perforant pathway and terminating in the dentate fascia and CA1 region. Other sources of input come from the septum and through commissural fibers from the hippocampus

Figure 3-2. Synaptic organization of the hippocampus. SO, stratum oriens; SP, stratum pyramidale; SR, stratum radiatum; SL-M, stratum lacunosum-moleculare; DF, dentate fascia; alv., alvear pathway; perf., perforant pathway; mf, mossy fiber; P, pyramidal cell; B, basket cell; Gr, granule cell. From G. M. Shepherd, *The synaptic organization of the brain: An introduction* (2nd ed.). New York: Oxford University Press, 1979. Reprinted by permission.

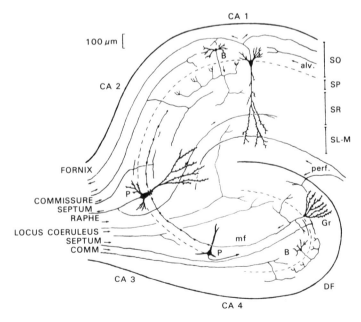

in the opposite side of the brain. Both of these pathways enter through the fornix and terminate on apical and basal dendrites in the stratum radiatum and stratum oriens, respectively. Finally, input from mossy fibers, arising from the granule cells in the dentate fascia, go to the pyramidal cells primarily in the CA3 area of the hippocampus.

The hippocampus also contains intrinsic pathways that originate and terminate within it. These include the recurrent collaterals, which are branches of the principal axon from a pyramidal cell and which synapse onto an inhibitory interneuron, which, in turn, feeds back onto other pyramidal cells and the original pyramidal cell. Other axon collaterals from the CA3 pyramidal cells that terminate in the CA1 region are called Schaffer collaterals and are excitatory.

In the hippocampus, ethanol administration resulted in a biphasic effect on multiple-unit activity (Klemm et al., 1976). Activity was initially increased, and then later decreased. Also, differences in the sensitivity to ethanol within this structure were evident. The greatest effects were observed on recordings from the CA1 neurons and hippocampal commissural fibers, and from structures sending afferent fibers to the hippocampus, such as the entorhinal cortex. Much smaller effects were apparent in the CA3 and dentate fascia.

Further analysis of hippocampal activity after ethanol administration has been accomplished using single-unit recordings (Grupp, 1980; Grupp & Perlanski, 1979). Spontaneous single-unit activity in the dorsal hippocampus was altered in a biphasic manner after intravenous doses of ethanol of 0.1–0.8 g/kg. These doses resulted in blood ethanol concentrations of 0.87–8.7 mM (4–40 mg/dl). At the lowest doses of ethanol, an increase in activity was predominant within the first 10 min after ethanol administration. At progressively higher doses, the excitatory response was followed by an inhibitory one, with only inhibitory effects on activity obtained at the highest doses of ethanol studied.

Since measurements of spontaneous single-unit activity may not take into account the importance of various neuronal inputs to an area of the brain from which recordings are made, activity resulting from stimulation of well-identified pathways would provide further information on the actions of ethanol. In the hippocampus, stimulation of two afferent pathways, the commissural pathway and the mossy fibers from the dentate fascia, was used to study the effect of ethanol on CA3 pyramidal cells (Newlin, Mancillas-Trevino, & Bloom, 1981). Both single-unit activity and field potentials were recorded.

Ethanol administration to rats under halothane anesthesia with an intraperitoneal dose of 3 g/kg increased the number of stimulus-evoked single-unit spikes (action potentials) and the size of the population spike, the excitatory component of the field potential. The duration of the inhibitory component of the field potential following the initial evoked spikes was prolonged. The effects were the same no matter which of the two afferent pathways was stimulated. Dose–response relationships were complex, with the enhancement of poststimulus inhibition showing increases with blood ethanol concentrations up to about 38.0 mM (175 mg/dl), followed by decreases above these levels. No dose–response relationship was observed for the excitatory responses induced by ethanol. Since these dose-response curves did not correlate with each other, these responses appeared to involve different mechanisms. Because the stimulus-evoked inhibitory component of the field potential may reflect recurrent collateral inhibition (Anderson, Eccles, & Loyning, 1964), these results were suggested to reflect stimulation by ethanol of this type of inhibitory response to the pyramidal cells.

Recurrent collateral inhibition has also been studied in the goldfish with interesting, but different results from those above (Faber & Klee, 1976). In the goldfish, the startle reflex is mediated by a network of cells that include the Mauthner cell. The activity of the Mauthner cell is regulated, in part, by collateral inhibition. Extracellular and intracellular recordings were obtained from Mauthner cells of unanesthetized, paralyzed goldfish. The cells were activated by stimulation of the VIIIth nerve. To study the effects of ethanol, the gills were perfused with 217–435 mM (1000–2000 mg/dl) ethanol solutions. Ethanol inhibited collateral inhibitions of the Mauthner cells. However, brain ethanol concentrations at this point correlated in other goldfish with hyperexcitability, characterized by hyperreflexia, including an enhanced startle reflex. Higher brain ethanol concentrations were associated with gross behavioral depression. Collateral inhibition was still depressed. The effect of ethanol on collateral inhibition may depend on the neural circuitry involved and its function.

Possible direct effects of ethanol on pyramidal cells of the hippocampus were examined in two strains of mice selectively bred for their sensitivity to ethanol. Those that sleep longer when given a dose of ethanol are called the long-sleep mice, and the others are called the short-sleep mice. Ethanol was applied directly onto the cells by micropressure ejection (Sorensen, Dunwiddie, McClearn, Freedman, & Hoffer, 1981). The concentration of the ethanol in the micropipette was 750 mM (3450 mg/dl). The concentration of ethanol in contact with the cell could not be determined. Ethanol depressed spontaneous activity *in situ* equally in both the long-sleep and short-sleep mice in a dose-dependent manner.

In other studies using halothane-anesthetized rats, locally applied ethanol from pipettes containing concentrations of 1000–3000 mM (4600–13,800 mg/dl) had a predominantly excitatory effect on 55% of the hippocampal pyramidal cells tested (Berger, French, Siggins, Shier, & Bloom, 1982). Inhibitory and biphasic effects (excitation followed by inhibition) were also observed in 42% of the cells.

Chronic treatment with ethanol may also alter stimulus-induced inhibitory responses in the hippocampus. Stimulation of the stratum radiatum of the CA1 region activates commissural fibers and Schaffer collaterals originating in the CA3 region, both of which terminate on apical dendrites of pyramidal cells of the CA1 region (see Figure 3-2). When ethanol was administered in a liquid diet for 20 weeks and recordings made 8 weeks after withdrawal, population spikes were significantly increased over those observed in controls, pair-fed the liquid diet without added ethanol (Abraham, Hunter, Zornetzer, & Walker, 1981). Furthermore, the population spike after stimulus-induced tetani (analogous to PTP discussed previously) was also enhanced. These results were interpreted as being consistent with a reduction in recurrent collateral inhibition. In another laboratory in which rats were treated for 18 weeks with ethanol in a liquid diet, these effects were not observed (Lee, Dunwiddie, Deitrich, Lynch, & Hoffer, 1981). Although the experimental designs were similar, the aspect of chronic ethanol administration reflected by the results above, whether it be tolerance, dependence, or brain damage, is unclear. The results may be related to some of the physiological consequences of brain damage (see Chapter 7).

Effects of ethanol on the cerebellum and vestibular system

The cerebellum has also been a useful model for studying the effect of ethanol on the electrical properties of membranes. This is, in part, because of the role of the cerebellum in motor coordination and control of posture and of its well-defined neuronal circuitry. The cerebellum receives its primary afferent input from the spinal cord, brain stem, and cerebral cortex. It is composed of three general parts: the cerebellar cortex, white matter, and deep nuclei. The deep nuclei provide the main output relays from the cerebellum.

The cerebellar cortex, which is of most interest to electrophysiologists, contains three layers: the molecular layer, Purkinje layer, and granular layer (Figure 3-3). All excitatory input to the cortex is provided from the climbing and mossy fibers, which ultimately synapse through granule and parallel fibers onto the Purkinje cells. The Purkinje cells, the main output cells of the cerebellar cortex, are inhibitory and project to the deep cerebellar nuclei and vestibular nuclei. There are also interneurons that provide inhibitory input to Purkinje cells and to the granule cells. For a more comprehensive treatment of cerebellar anatomy and physiology, the reader should consult the reviews of Eccles, Ito, and Szentágothai (1967) and Ghez and Fahn (1981).

The Purkinje cell is the one from which electrical recordings are most often obtained. It is characterized by its spontaneous and relatively high rate of discharge. It receives its major excitatory input from parallel fibers arising from granule cells activated by the mossy fibers and from climbing fibers originating in the inferior olivary nucleus in the brain stem. Stim-

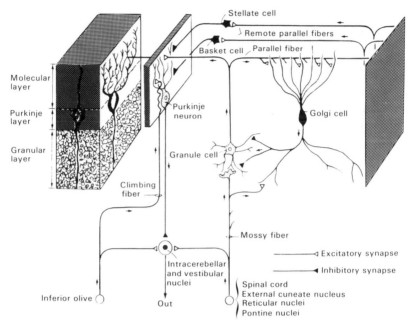

Figure 3-3. Synaptic organization of the cerebellar cortex. From C. Ghez & S. Fahn, The cerebellum. In E. R. Kandel & J. H. Schwartz (Eds.), *Principles of neural science*. New York: Elsevier/North Holland, 1981. Reprinted by permission.

ulation of climbing fibers results in bursts of discharge in Purkinje cells, whereas parallel fibers evoke single spikes.

The earliest report to address the effect of ethanol on cerebellar Purkinje cells used decerebrate, unanesthetized cats (Eidelberg, Bond, & Kelter, 1971). When ethanol was injected intravenously at a dose of 0.6 g/kg, spontaneous firing of Purkinje cells, as determined by means of single-unit recordings, was transiently elevated and then reduced, a short-lived effect. The interspike interval, the time between spikes, was increased. De-afferented cerebella, accomplished with electrolytic lesions of the cerebellar peduncles, were still sensitive to ethanol, suggesting a direct effect of ethanol on the cerebellum (Forney & Klemm, 1976). In addition, the blockade of the metabolism of ethanol to acetaldehyde with *d*-penicillamine did not alter the response of Purkinje cells to ethanol administration, further indicating a direct effect of ethanol (Mikeska & Klemm, 1979).

Direct effects of ethanol onto cerebellar Purkinje cells were studied in mice genetically bred for their sensitivity to ethanol in a manner similar to that done with hippocampal pyramidal cells, as discussed earlier (Sorensen, Palmer, Dunwiddie, & Hoffer, 1980). Ethanol applied locally by pressure from pipettes induced a dose-dependent depression of spontaneous

Purkinje cell activity in both strains of mice. However, unlike the hippo-campal pyramidal cells, cerebellar Purkinje cells in the long-sleep mice were twice as sensitive to ethanol as those in short-sleep mice. This is not sur-prising considering that the mice are bred based on their ability to right themselves, a cerebellar-mediated process. In addition, when comparing the depressant effect of ethanol on behavior and Purkinje cell activity among a number of other genetic strains, there was a direct relationship between behavioral and physiological depression (Spuhler, Hoffer, Weiner, & Palmer, 1982).

Some more recent reports suggest that the actions of ethanol may not be so simple as discussed above. Systemic ethanol administration to in-tact, halothane-anesthetized rats produced different results. When rats were injected with single intraperitoneal doses of ethanol (1–4 g/kg), the num-ber of simple spikes recorded from Purkinje cells, representing spontaneous activity, was little changed or slightly increased (Rogers, Siggins, Schul-man, & Bloom, 1980). The mean interspike interval for simple spikes was significantly reduced. However, the number of climbing-fiber bursts was significantly elevated in a dose-dependent manner. When ethanol was ad-ministered for 11–14 days either by gastric intubation or inhalation, the frequency of climbing-fiber bursts was unchanged from controls, suggest-ing that tolerance had developed. However, as the ethanol was eliminated from the body, the frequency of these bursts decreased below control levels.

In another laboratory, spontaneous discharge rates were transiently elevated, and then reduced in urethane-anesthetized rats after 1- to 4-g/kg intraperitoneal doses of ethanol (Sorensen, Carter, Marwaha, Baker, & Freedman, 1981). Peak blood ethanol concentrations reached a maximum of 43.5 mM (200 mg/dl). From frequency distribution histograms, it ap-peared that the activity of cells firing at slower rates was increased and that of cells firing at faster rates was reduced. The transient elevated activity was observed only while the blood ethanol concentrations were rising. Since at this time the concentration of ethanol in the locus ceruleus was higher than in the cerebellum, it was suggested that ethanol interferes with the normal tonic inhibitory noradrenergic influence from the locus ceruleus on Purkinje cells. This hypothesis was based on observations that ethanol can reduce the firing rates of neurons in the locus ceruleus (to be discussed later). To test this possibility, animals were pretreated with 6-hydroxydopa-mine or propranolol in order to reduced noradrenergic–receptor interac-tions. As expected, the mean discharge rates were elevated. However, no further elevation of activity was observed after ethanol administration.

In another study in which urethane-anesthetized rats were treated with 1.5-g/kg intravenous doses of ethanol, spontaneous simple spike activity was elevated and became more regular, accompanied by almost complete suppression of climbing-fiber bursts (Sinclair, Lo, & Tien, 1980). Inhibi-tion of the activity of Purkinje cells by local surface electrical stimulation of the cerebellum, which is believed to stimulate inhibitory interneurons synapsing onto Purkinje cells, was also reduced by ethanol administration (Sinclair & Lo, 1981). When repeated in unanesthetized rats, climbing-fiber bursts were depressed, but the inhibition of activity by local stimulation could not be observed. These results suggested that ethanol induced alterations in synaptic transmission. Sixteen hours after withdrawal from chronic treatment with ethanol in a liquid diet for 14 days, no alteration in the rate of Purkinje cell discharge was observed. It was suggested that this finding reflected the development of tolerance (Sinclair et al., 1980).

The apparently opposite results between some of these studies may depend on the manner in which the experiments were designed. The study of Rogers et al. (1980) injected bolus (10–20 sec) intraperitoneal doses of ethanol (1–4 g/kg), while Sinclair et al. (1980) infused 1.5-g/kg doses of ethanol intravenously over 10 min. Both experiments were repeated in which the blood ethanol concentrations were monitored over time after ethanol administration (Sinclair & Lo, 1982). The rate of increase in and highest concentrations of ethanol in the blood were quite different between the modes of ethanol administration. Fast intraperitoneal injections resulted in peak blood ethanol concentrations more than three times greater than those obtained after slow intravenous infusions [109 mM (500 mg/dl) administered over 9 min after intraperitoneal injection as compared to 32.6 mM (150 mg/dl) over 30 min after intravenous infusion]. The blood ethanol concentrations also increased more rapidly after intraperitoneal injections. A bursting discharge pattern was observed after the intraperitoneal dose of ethanol, similar to the study of Rogers et al. (1980). Respiratory depression and hypotension were also observed. Most of the animals died within 15 min after the injection. Such adverse effects were not observed by Rogers et al. (1980) after ethanol administration. On the other hand, the intravenous infusions of ethanol produced the same results described previously in the study of Sinclair et al. (1980).

The involvement of the olivocerebellar climbing fibers that synapse on Purkinje cells in the effect of ethanol has been studied further. Initially, experiments were performed in order to determine whether the responsiveness of Purkinje cells is in some way altered after ethanol treatment (Sinclair, Lo, & Harris, 1982). Climbing-fiber bursts in Purkinje cells can be induced by electrical stimulation near the fastigial nucleus, one of the deep cerebellar nuclei. The Purkinje cells are also probably being stimulated antidromically, but may also be stimulated through excitatory afferents to Purkinje cells, including climbing fibers. Ethanol administration at an intravenous dose of 1.5 g/kg over 10–22 min had no effect on the threshold of juxafastigial stimulation to induce climbing-fiber bursts. The data were interpreted to indicate that ethanol does not directly inhibit Purkinje cells and that they can respond normally when stimulated. However, since the mechanism of how the Purkinje cells were activated is not entirely clear, this conclusion is not fully justifiable. On the other hand, in other experiments, direct application of ethanol to Purkinje cells reduced spontaneous activity, but only at unphysiologically high concentrations (Siggins & French, 1979). It was suggested that ethanol exerted a nonspecific local anesthetic effect on the neurons of these studies.

In other experiments, the possibility that the climbing fibers themselves are less active after ethanol treatment was examined indirectly by determining whether ethanol could reverse the actions of harmaline, a drug that stimulates climbing-fiber activity and induces tremors (Llinas & Volkind, 1973). Ethanol administration completely antagonized the harmaline-induced tremor, but could only partially block the complex discharges (Sinclair et al., 1982), providing inconclusive results. In the study of Rogers et al. (1980), the increased Purkinje cell bursts were similar to those obtained after harmaline administration.

In further experiments, complex discharges in Purkinje cells were recorded after stimulation of the cerebral cortex or the firing frequency of cells in the inferior olivary nucleus was determined after ethanol administration (Sinclair, Lo, & Harris, 1983). Ethanol reduced the discharges in both areas. On the other hand, after 2-g/kg intraperitoneal doses of ethanol, firing rates of neurons in the inferior olivary nucleus were elevated (Rogers, Siggins, Aston-Jones, Koda, & Bloom, 1982).

The data that have been presented on the effect of ethanol on the cerebellum appear inconclusive. Different groups of investigators report opposite results on both simple and complex electrical discharges in Purkinje cells after ethanol treatment. These differences seem largely due to various experimental designs, where the anesthetic used and ultimate blood ethanol concentration and the rate at which they rise may be major factors. Sinclair and Lo (1982) claim to be able to duplicate the results of Rogers et al. (1980) in addition to their own previous experiments and suggest that the results in the Rogers et al. study may be a consequence of extreme toxicity of ethanol at such high doses. However, Sinclair and Lo (1982) used only the highest 4-g/kg intraperitoneal dose of ethanol in the Rogers et al. study, a dose that usually is not lethal. Rogers et al. (1980) used doses of 1–4 g/kg, which had a dose-dependent effect on Purkinje cell bursts. Although they did not report blood ethanol concentrations, the lower doses of ethanol should produce concentrations in the range of those found by Sinclair and Lo (1982). Therefore, the comparisons of the studies may not be quite so straightforward.

Functionally, the integrity of the afferent input to Purkinje cells could be more important than their spontaneous intrinsic activity. The role of the cerebellum in coordinating movement depends on input from the cerebral cortex, brain stem, and spinal cord. With one climbing fiber synapsing onto one Purkinje cell and the ability of a single impulse from a climbing fiber to induce a burst of activity in the Purkinje cell, small influences from the cerebral cortex through the inferior olive and the climbing fibers would have profound effects on cerebellar function. With this in mind, it therefore seems reasonable to suggest that an effect of ethanol on neurons that modify the inhibitory output of Purkinje cells would play an important role in the mechanism of action of ethanol. Synaptic input to Purkinje cells from other neuronal origins would also be important to study. In fact, there is a report indicating that ethanol might excite inhibitory interneurons in the cerebellum, thereby inhibiting Purkinje cell activity (Eidelberg et al., 1971), although it is not clear how these cells were identified.

Taken together, the data obtained from single-unit and multiple-unit recordings in vivo suggest that ethanol can exert both excitatory and inhibitory actions on the Purkinje cells of the cerebellum depending on the experimental conditions. It remains to be determined which of these actions contributes to the behavioral effects obtained after ethanol administration.

Another area of the brain related to motor coordination that might be depressed by ethanol is the vestibular system. The vestibular system detects the position of the body and its movement through space by receiving and integrating information from receptors in the inner ear and from cerebellar nuclei and Purkinje cells. Single-unit recordings in the vestibular nuclei have been obtained after ethanol administration. Ethanol was found to reduce both the spontaneous activity of the cells and the responses elicited by stimulation of the lateral vestibular nerve (Eidelberg et al., 1971; Ikeda, Sasa, & Takaori, 1980).

Effects of ethanol on the locus ceruleus

Another area of the brain that appears to be sensitive to the actions of ethanol is the locus ceruleus. The locus ceruleus is a small nucleus in the brain stem, which sends numerous noradrenergic projections throughout the brain and may function to modulate sensory input to higher centers, especially during stressful conditions (Amaral & Sinnamon, 1977) or during the presentation of novel stimuli (Foote, Bloom, & Aston-Jones, 1983). An initial study with ethanol in which single-unit recordings from unanesthestized, paralyzed rats were obtained indicated that intraperitoneal doses of 2 g/kg reduced the firing rate by as much at 80% (Pohorecky & Brick, 1977).

In more recent experiments, ethanol was studied in rats anesthetized with chloral hydrate or halothane (Aston-Jones, Foote, & Bloom, 1982). Intraperitoneal doses of ethanol of 0.5–3 g/kg had no effect on the rate of single-unit discharges or on spikes obtained from 1-Hz antidromic stimulation of the medial or lateral neocortex or of the dorsal noradrenergic bundle. However, ethanol modified the response of the locus ceruleus to sensory stimulation. The evoked responses elicited by applying electrical shocks to the foot were significantly reduced in a dose-dependent manner. In addition, the latencies of the successive responses, which are normally quite consistent, were considerably more variable, thereby rendering cell firing more asynchronous. In addition, with 10-Hz antidromic stimulation, the resultant activity was reduced by ethanol administration. Since this type of stimulation is suggested also to activate recurrent collateral inhibition of norepinephrine-containing neurons (Aghajanian, Cedarbaum, & Wang, 1977), ethanol may inhibit stimulus-induced spikes through an activation of this mechanism. These results, it is suggested, relate to a possible reduction in the ability of an animal after ethanol administration properly to focus on and respond to novel stimuli.

A major difference between the study of Pohorecky and Brick (1977) and that of Aston-Jones *et al.* (1982) may depend on the awareness of and responsiveness to the environment of the experimental animals and the spontaneous activity on neurons in the locus ceruleus. The unanesthetized, paralyzed, and artificially respired animals in the study of Pohorecky and Brick (1977) exhibited higher spontaneous activity of the recorded neurons than those in the study of Aston-Jones *et al.* (1982). Aston-Jones *et al.* (1982) suggested that this might reflect greater tonic orthodromic input to noradrenergic neurons of the locus ceruleus possibly due to stress. This, they further suggest, would make the results of the two studies compatible.

Effects of ethanol on neurotransmitter responses

Neuronal firing is modulated by the summation of all excitatory and inhibitory inputs. The ability of neurotransmitters to induce appropriate electrical events in postsynaptic neurons is critical to this process. Few studies have addressed the interaction of ethanol with transmitters or their receptors as related to neuronal firing rates.

In an early report, an isolated spinal cord preparation from the frog was perfused with ethanol in concentrations of 32.6–97.8 mM (150–450 mg/dl) and the ability of γ-aminobutyric acid (GABA) to alter primary afferent depolarization was determined (Davidoff, 1973). Ethanol enhanced primary afferent depolarization, as indicated by increased dorsal root potentials and the responsiveness of dorsal root terminals to dorsal or ventral root stimulation. This effect was also observed when GABA was applied to the preparation. Ethanol in concentrations of 97.8 mM (450 mg/dl) consistently augmented the response of GABA.

In another study, ethanol was applied to somatosensory cortical neurons by electroosmosis in methoxyflurane–N_2O-anesthetized rats (Lake, Yarbrough, & Phillips, 1973). Ethanol had little effect on the firing rate of single units. However, inhibitory responses induced by iontophoretic application of norepinephrine, serotonin, or acetylcholine were blocked by ethanol. Ethanol did not block GABA inhibition.

In more recent experiments, ethanol was locally ejected into neurons of the pericruciate cortex of methoxyflurane-anesthetized cats and single-unit activity was recorded (Nestoros, 1980a, 1980b). Different results from those of Lake *et al.* (1973) were reported. No alteration in the inhibitory action of glycine, serotonin, or dopamine on these neurons was found. On the other hand, ethanol potentiated GABA inhibition, as expressed by prolongation of the time course of GABA-induced inhibition. Potentiation of the actions of GABA was also reported after sequential, intravenous injections of 0.002 and 0.008 g/kg of ethanol (Nestoros, 1980a). Such an effect is difficult to evaluate because no measurable blood ethanol concentrations should be detected. (None were reported.) Also, intoxication should not be expected.

Finally, when ethanol was locally applied to cerebellar Purkinje cells, the effectiveness of norepinephrine and GABA to inhibit the activity of these cells was unaltered, unless sufficiently high amounts of ethanol to inhibit cellular activity nonspecifically was applied (Siggins & French, 1979).

The major differences between the studies of Lake *et al.* (1973) and Nestoros (1980a, 1980b) are the amounts of ethanol and transmitters applied to the cells. The study of Lake *et al.* (1973) applied higher amounts of ethanol and apparently lower amounts of transmitters than did Nestoros (1980a, 1980b). However, in both cases the inhibitory effect of GABA was maximal, and so a direct measurement of any potentiation of the GABA response by ethanol could not be observed. Also, the significance of the reported results is difficult to determine because of a major drawback with the iontophoretic approach. Since the amount of the drug applied depends on a number of factors, including the amount of current applied to release the drug and the length of application, one cannot determine the concentration of the substances in contact with the cells at a given time. Therefore, interpretations can be misleading. In spite of these limitations, the possible interaction of ethanol with various neurotransmitters is an important one and deserves thorough and systematic investigation.

Electrical activity measured *in vitro*

One of the newer approaches to the study of electrical properties of cells is the use of brain slices. An area of the brain, such as the hippocampus, is sliced into 300- to 500-μm sections and placed in a perfusion chamber containing an appropriate medium. Intracellular or extracellular recordings from cells are taken from the slice placed on a mesh net or filter paper. The top surface of the slice is either exposed to moist 95% CO_2/ 5% O_2 ("dry top") or the whole slice is completely submerged in the continuously flowing perfusion medium. This allows the usual electrophysiological parameters to be measured as well as the application of drugs either in the bathing fluid in known concentrations or by iontophoresis.

This approach has some major advantages over *in vivo* preparations. One advantage is the ability to study cells from mammalian brains in relative isolation, but in a somewhat "normal" environment. In addition, synaptic input to the cells can be controlled within the slice by electrical stimulation of defined neural pathways. Synaptic transmission can be blocked by using a perfusion medium containing tetrodotoxin (a drug that blocks sodium channels; see Chapter 4) or high concentrations of magnesium in order to study possible direct effects of drugs on the cells from which electrical recordings are obtained. On the other hand, slicing tissue may result in the presence of toxins from dead cells, which may alter electrical activity. Also, it is not clear whether the composition of the medium adequately reflects the conditions of the brain *in vivo*. On the whole, however, this technique allows for studies of cellular function less complicated by neural input from other areas of the brain.

A few reports have appeared that have examined the effect of ethanol on electrophysiological responses *in vitro*. Using the dry top method, field potentials were recorded from pyramidal cells in the CA1 region of hippocampal slices after stimulation of the stratum radiatum (Durand, Corrigall, Kujtan, & Carlen, 1981). When ethanol was added to the bath in concentrations of 10–100 mM (46–460 mg/dl), the orthodromic population spike, but not the antidromic population spike, was reduced in a dose-dependent manner. There was also an increase in orthodromic spike thresholds, although considerable variability of the response was observed. Ethanol did not have a consistent effect on the size of the population EPSP. The variability in the magnitude of the population spike seemed to depend on the amount of intrinsic inhibition present in the slice before the ethanol was added. When intrinsic inhibition in the slice was greater, the effectiveness of ethanol was also greater.

The degree of intrinsic recurrent collateral inhibition can be estimated by measuring the reduction in amplitude of the second of a pair of responses evoked by paired stimuli separated by varying lengths of time. The second population spike is smaller than the first due to this type of inhibitory influence. Ethanol at concentrations of 20 mM (96 mg/dl) significantly increased the amount of this paired pulse inhibition (Durand *et al.*, 1981).

Hippocampal field potentials have been measured in slices taken from rats chronically treated for 16–20 weeks with ethanol in a liquid diet (Carlen & Corrigall, 1980). Ethanol added *in vitro* could reduce the population spike in slices from control animals, as in the above studies, except ethanol was not as effective. When slices from chronically ethanol-treated rats were subjected to the same procedure, ethanol added *in vitro* was even less effective, suggesting the development of tolerance.

Using intracellular recordings from hippocampal slices, more detailed study of the possible role of changes in the conductance of different ions was undertaken (Carlen, Gurevich, & Durand, 1982). In this preparation, with the top surface of the slices exposed, ethanol was applied focally by pipette to appropriate areas of the hippocampus or in the perfusion medium. In concentrations of 5–20 mM (23–92 mg/dl), ethanol increased both EPSPs and IPSPs recorded from CA1 cells. A direct effect of ethanol on the cells was suggested, since a moderate hyperpolarization was observed even when synaptic transmission was blocked. However, in other studies, 175–350 mM (1000–2000 mg/dl) of ethanol was required in order to observe either depolarization or hyperpolarization of hippocampal pyramidal cells (Siggins & Bloom, 1980).

The ethanol-induced hyperpolarizations were examined further to determine whether the conductance of a given ion might play a role in this response (Carlen et al., 1982). Since potassium and chloride movements are most often associated with hyperpolarization, these ions were chosen for study. Injection of chloride ions into the cells did not modify the effect of ethanol. The hyperpolarizing effect of GABA, which acts through chloride channels in CA1 cells (Eccles, 1977; Eccles, Nicoll, Oshima, & Rubia, 1977), was also not altered by ethanol, in contrast to the reports of Nestoros (1980a, 1980b).

The important ion mediating this action of ethanol appeared to be calcium, especially as it affects potassium efflux. Calcium has been shown to induce a long-lasting afterhyperpolarization by increasing potassium efflux from invertebrate neurons (Meech, 1978). Such a mechanism has been suggested to account for the afterhyperpolarization seen in hippocampal CA1 cells after repetitive firing (Alger & Nicoll, 1980; Gustafsson & Wigstrom, 1981; Hotson & Prince, 1980). This afterhyperpolarization was enhanced by ethanol (Carlen et al., 1982). Calcium-induced spikes, which are observed after blocking sodium spikes with tetrodotoxin, were not affected by ethanol, but the afterhyperpolarization was still enhanced (Carlen et al., 1982). However, when calcium was completely removed from the medium to examine calcium-independent processes, the reduced and shorter-lived, stimulus-induced afterhyperpolarization was no longer affected by the application of ethanol. These data suggested that ethanol-induced hyperpolarizations were caused by potassium efflux, which is stimulated by intracellular calcium. However, more direct analyses of ionic currents, such as the voltage clamp technique, will be required for verification of this suggestion. The voltage clamp technique measures ionic conductances without changes in the membrane potential normally accompanying ion movements.

Using intracellular recordings, the bioelectric properties of hippocampal CA1 and granule cells in vitro were studied in rats treated with ethanol for 20 weeks, then withdrawn for 3 weeks (Durand & Carlen, 1984). The only effects observed were on the sizes and durations of orthodromically stimulated IPSPs and afterhyperpolarizations in granule cells were smaller, while the durations were reduced in both cell types. No changes were observed in the excitatory properties of the cells.

The study of the effect of ethanol on electrical activity from slices of the cerebellum has recently begun (Basile, Hoffer, & Dunwiddie, 1983). The slices were obtained from the mice with different sensitivities to ethanol-induced depression. The mean spontaneous firing rates of Purkinje cells in the long-sleep, short-sleep, and heterogeneous strains were not significantly different from one another, nor from those recorded from slices in media with high magnesium concentrations found to block synaptic transmission. However, the firing rates were slower than those obtained from Purkinje cells *in vivo*.

In concentrations of 10–1000 mM (46–4600 mg/dl), ethanol had a predominant depressant effect in a concentration-dependent manner on the majority of Purkinje cells in the presence of high magnesium concentrations in all three strains. Excitatory, followed by inhibitory responses were observed in some cells. Occasionally, pure excitations were observed. The sensitivity of the Purkinje cells to ethanol varied across the mouse strains. The cells from long-sleep mice were most sensitive [$ED_{50} = 75.9$ mM (349 mg/dl)], while the short-sleep mice were least sensitive [$ED_{50} = 325$ mM (1500 mg/dl)]. The differences in sensitivities were much less than those observed *in vivo*. In addition to discharge rates, action potentials had smaller amplitudes and longer durations when depressed activity was studied. No change in either parameter was found during periods of excitation. The variable sensitivities of Purkinje cells across the strains appears to be intrinsic and not dependent on synaptic transmission.

Electrical activity of cells grown in culture

Within the last few years, investigators have begun using neuronal cell cultures to study the effects of ethanol on the intrinsic electrical properties of cells in isolation. The cell lines can be derived from fetal brains (primary cultures), from tumor cells, or from normal cells hybridized to dividing cells of neuronal origin.

The first studies reported were performed using cultures of the cerebellum and cerebral cortex taken from newborn mice (Seil, Leiman, Herman, & Fisk, 1977). In cerebellar cultures, incremental additions of ethanol in concentrations of 121–337 mM (560–1550 mg/dl) had a complex effect on the spontaneous electrical activity of these cells. Initially, the discharge rate increased and became more regular, accompanied by a reduction in the amplitude of the units. After 2 min, the discharge rate decreased, until eventually the cells did not fire at all. After removal of the ethanol, normal discharge patterns resumed. In cortical cultures, ethanol had only an inhibitory effect. Although the effects observed were not unlike some of those described earlier for *in vivo* studies, the concentrations of ethanol required to obtain a reduction in electrical activity were generally well in excess of physiologically compatible concentrations.

In a more recent report, intracellular recordings were obtained from cultured cells derived from fetal mouse spinal cord neurons (Gruol, 1982), in which synaptic contact exists between cells. The concentrations of ethanol used in the medium were 10–100 mM (46–460 mg/dl). Various electrical properties were measured including membrane potential, input resistance, amplitude of the action potential, and the sensitivity of the cells to a number of neurotransmitters. The predominant effect of ethanol in concentrations as low as 20–30 mM (92–138 mg/dl) was to reduce spontaneous activity, including the frequency of EPSPs, IPSPs, and action potentials, and to reduce synaptic activity obtained after the application of glutamate onto presynaptic cells. No significant effect was observed on the membrane potential, input resistance, or the amplitude of the action potential. Responses to direct application of the transmitters, glutamate, GABA, and glycine to the recorded cells were unaffected by ethanol at low concentrations. The data suggest that ethanol exerts its action in these cells predominantly on synaptic transmission, presumably through a presynaptic mechanism.

Another series of experiments was undertaken to examine the effect of ethanol on cultures of dorsal root ganglia derived from rat embryos. This preparation was used to study the direct actions of ethanol on cells, since it appears that these cells do not synapse onto one another (Scott, Englebert, & Fischer, 1969). Intracellular recordings from cells exposed to 10.7–65.2 mM (50–300 mg/dl) ethanol indicated no alteration in the resting potential, spike amplitude, or rate of depolarization (Oakes & Pozos, 1982a). However, the duration of the action potential was prolonged and the rate of depolarization and the duration of the afterhyperpolarization were reduced. Based on similarities to the effects of channel blockers and alterations in the composition of the culture medium on the parameters measured, it was suggested that ethanol might reduce calcium conductance with a secondary decrease in potassium conductance (Oakes & Pozos, 1982a, 1982b). All the changes induced by ethanol were reversible. Voltage clamp analysis will be needed to verify this possibility.

Finally, one study has been reported in which cultured cells derived from adult mouse dorsal root ganglia were incubated with 37.0–148 mM (170–680 mg/dl) of ethanol for 12 days and the electrophysiological effects recorded (Scott & Edwards, 1981). A number of effects were observed including decreased membrane resistance, increased membrane capacitance, and reduced overshoot, afterhyperpolarization, and rate of rise of the action potential. These effects seem to correlate with cell survival and suggested that the results indicated cell damage. The effect of ethanol added acutely to cultured cells not previously exposed to ethanol was not reported.

Commentary

The data obtained from electrophysiological techniques used to study the effects of ethanol on the functional properties of membranes are inconclusive. A variety of *in vitro* and *in vivo* approaches have been utilized to examine cellular function, but the results reported do not yet provide a clear picture of what action ethanol has on the electrical properties of cells at the membrane level.

The bulk of the data to date suggests that ethanol can have either an excitatory or inhibitory action on most cell types studied, depending on the way the experiments are designed. However, ethanol in physiologically compatible concentrations often appears to act on synaptic transmission rather than directly on postsynaptic elements. The possible alteration by ethanol of the ability of neurotransmitters to induce their appropriate electrical responses has not been resolved. Although ethanol may act on the presynaptic terminals, electrophysiological analyses are not yet available in vertebrate preparations to elucidate the mechanisms involved.

The most conspicuous problem with the studies in this area is the lack of uniform experimental designs. Since there are not yet many reports at the membrane level to examine, comparisons of results between laboratories have been difficult. Some results appear contradictory, possibly due to different experimental designs. More precise statements of designs and better verifications of the tissue ethanol concentrations would likely make comparisons much easier.

What might be the experimental approach that could provide the most relevant information on the action of ethanol at the membrane level? Let us look at this question by reexamining the various techniques that have been used, starting those which produce the most general, but least precise information. This technique would be the multiple-unit recording *in vivo*. Multiple-unit recordings, as discussed earlier, measure the activity of small groups of cells. In effect, the recorded activity is the sum of the various excitatory and inhibitory influences that contribute to cellular excitability. This is particularly true because of the lack of identification of the cells that contribute to the electrical recordings. Therefore, it is difficult to distinguish, for example, excitation of excitatory neurons from inhibition of inhibitory neurons. Both phenomena could lead to increases in discharge rates. Also, the contributions of areas of the brain remote to the area where the recordings are made has to be taken into account. The use of appropriate brain lesions might be helpful. These types of recordings might provide information on the general status of activity of a cell population, which might be useful to know but would provide little information on the mechanisms involved.

Single-unit recordings *in vivo* are a bit more precise because activity is being studied in a single cell, especially if the cell can be identified. However, its activity still reflects all of the presynaptic excitatory and inhibi-

tory inputs to that cell. Still, the contributions of excitatory and inhibitory influences are more easily separated than in multiple-unit recordings,
although these influences may be from other areas of the brain. Also, there
is the problem of statistical sampling. Critical cell identification would reduce the variability of responses recorded from a number of cells. Enough
differences between cells in a given animal, though, exist that the sampling
of many cells in the same animal is needed, adding to the labor intensive-
ness of the approach.

Another advantage of single-cell studies is the ability to record intracellularly. This allows for better cell identification and more fundamen-
tal evaluations of membrane properties, such as resistance, resting potentials, and action potentials. Also, by means of micropressure application,
iontophoresis, and perfusion, the response of the cell to transmitters can
be examined in more detail, in spite of possible difficulties in interpretation, as discussed earlier. In addition, voltage clamping allows for the study
of the role that ionic currents play in the action of a drug.

A major variable in both multiple-unit and single-unit recordings *in
vivo* is the use of anesthetized preparations. In anesthetized preparations,
it is not clear whether the anesthetic itself may act synergistically with ethanol or alter its response. Different anesthetics may interact differently with
ethanol. Unanesthetized preparations avoid these difficulties, but have
problems of their own. With immobilization, where paralysis and local
anesthesia are used, it is not clear to what extent the mental status of the
animals is affected. For example, stress may confound the results observed.
In freely moving animals, movement artifacts can be encountered. In these
cases, does ethanol alter behavior, and then the activity of the recorded
neurons, or vice versa?

Electrical recordings from cells *in vitro* are particularly interesting
techniques. These have involved use of cell cultures and tissue slices from
various areas of the brain. They allow for the study of cells in relative isolation so that environments can be more easily manipulated, and drugs can
be applied in known concentrations. Cell cultures can allow for the study
of direct effects of a drug on a population of relatively homogeneous cells
with predefined properties. No other technique can provide this advantage. However, cultures from neuronal origin are either derived from tumor cells, hybrids of such cells, or prenatal tissue. This raises the issue of
relevance similar to that raised for the invertebrate preparations. On the
other hand, cells grown from fetal tissue may be particularly useful in studying such phenomena as the fetal alcohol syndrome (see Chapter 7).

Electrical recordings from brain slices appear to be a particularly ad-
vantageous technique to examine the properties of neuronal membranes.
The stimulation of well-defined neuronal pathways and alterations in the
composition of the medium can lead to better information about actions
of a drug at the membrane level and can differentiate between direct ac-

tions and indirect ones involving synaptic transmission. Resolving the best methodological approach to recording from cells (e.g., slices with top surfaces exposed vs. slices totally submerged in perfusion medium) is an important step in validating the technique. However, this technique seems most likely to eventually provide the best evidence on the action of ethanol at the membrane level on central neurons.

4. Ion movements

In Chapter 3, evidence was presented demonstrating that ethanol can exert profound effects on the electrical properties or neurons. The basis of such properties involves the movement of ions through membranes in a very precise manner. The movement of ions is also important in the normal functioning of other organs. This movement can be either passive, in which ions move along a concentration gradient, or active, in which a system in the membrane binds the ion and transports it through the membrane. This latter process requires energy. In this chapter, we shall examine the effects of alcohols on the ability of ions, especially sodium, potassium, and calcium to move through membranes.

Monovalent ions

The monovalent ions that are used most by cells are sodium, potassium, and chloride. In neurons, the movement of these ions contributes to the excitability of the cell when it is stimulated. Also, the propagation of action potentials and subsequent recovery back to a resting state involves the movement of ions.

The generation and propagation of action potentials in neurons depend primarily on the movements of sodium and potassium across the neuronal membrane (Hodgkin & Huxley, 1952). As discussed in Chapter 3, changes in membrane potential in neurons are associated with the generation of action potentials and result from a transient increase in the permeability of the membrane to sodium. This allows for sodium to flow along its concentration gradient from the outside to the inside of the neuron (Figure 3-1). This activation phase controls the rate of depolarization. Subsequently, the permeability of the membrane to sodium reverts back to the resting state and outward potassium permeability increases. At this point, the neuron repolarizes, a process called inactivation or recovery. Finally, the permeability of the membrane to both cations returns to the resting state.

Sodium and potassium move through pores in the membrane that open as a result of depolarization. These holes are called channels. Sodium channels are particularly important in the normal functioning of the neuron. For example, if they do not open sufficiently wide or if an insufficient number open at all, the neuron may not depolarize enough to "fire,"

66

that is, to generate an action potential. On the other hand, if the sodium channels do not close or do so at a slower rate, excitability may be enhanced.

Sodium channels and the mechanisms by which they function have been studied extensively. The factor that has aided greatly in characterizing sodium channels has been the availability of neurotoxins that specifically modify the ability of the channels to be activated or inactivated (Catterall, 1980). Using these neurotoxins, three active sites associated with the sodium channel have been identified. Toxins such as tetrodotoxin and saxitoxin have been widely used in the study of voltage-dependent sodium currents (Kao, 1966; Narahashi, 1974). These toxins block the transient increase in inward sodium conductance resulting from neural stimulation and bind to Site I. Sodium channels can be activated by toxins such as veratridine and batrachotoxin, which bind to Site II (Albuquerque & Daly, 1976; Straub, 1954; Ulbricht, 1969). Still other toxins such as scorpion toxin and sea anemone toxin, without having any effect on sodium permeability themselves, enhance the effects of veratridine and batrachotoxin by preventing inactivation (Koppenhofer & Schmidt, 1968; Narahashi, Moore, & Shapiro, 1969). These toxins bind to Site III.

Sodium influx can be stimulated by other methods, generally of a less specific nature. Two commonly used means are electrical and potassium stimulation, which nonspecifically depolarize membranes. Another agent that can be used is the excitatory amino acid, L-glutamate. Glutamate promotes sodium influx through a non-voltage-dependent process (Chang & Michaelis, 1980; Ozeki, Freeman, & Grundfest, 1966).

In order to maintain proper concentration gradients of sodium and potassium for normal neuronal function, the accumulated intracellular sodium and extracellular potassium must be transported back through the neuronal membrane. This is accomplished by means of an active transport system (Escueta & Appel, 1969; Ling & Abdel-Latif, 1968). The system that integrates and supplies energy for this process is a sodium- and potassium-activated adenosine triphosphatase (ATPase). This enzyme complex will be discussed in greater detail in Chapter 5.

Few direct studies have been reported on the effect of alcohols on the movement of monovalent ions. Electrophysiological data, especially from invertebrates, would suggest that alcohols should inhibit stimulated sodium influx. In squid giant axon and *Aplysia* neurons, alcohols reduce the size of an action potential and sodium conductance (Armstrong & Binstock, 1964; Bergmann *et al.*, 1974; Moore *et al.*, 1964).

In the early 1970s, the effect of ethanol and *t*-butanol on the movement of sodium and potassium into and out of electrically stimulated brain slices was investigated (Nikander & Wallgren, 1970; Wallgren, Nikander, von Boguslawsky, & Linkola, 1974). Net movement of ions between the intracellular and extracellular spaces *in vitro* was calculated from the total tissue content by first determining the volume of the extracellular space with inulin, which does not penetrate cellular membranes. Assuming that the concentrations of ions in the extracellular space were equal to those in the incubation medium, the intracellular concentrations were determined by subtracting the ion content attributable to the extracellular space from the total ion content in the tissue. Both ethanol [109 mM (501 mg/dl)] and t-butanol [34 mM (156 mg/dl)] reduced electrically stimulated sodium uptake into intracellular spaces without altering unstimulated uptake. Outward potassium movements were unaffected. Injections of ethanol *in vivo* did not significantly change sodium and potassium distribution (Kalant, Mons, & Mahon, 1966).

In recent experiments, the effect of alcohols on sodium channels has been studied more directly by measuring neurotoxin-stimulated sodium uptake into synaptosomes. When synaptosomes are incubated with veratridine, which specifically opens sodium channels, analogous to increases in inward sodium conductance induced by electrical stimulation of neurons, they will rapidly take up ^{22}NaCl (Tamkun & Catterall, 1981). This effect is blocked by tetrodotoxin, which also blocks electrically stimulated inward sodium currents.

Ethanol was quite effective in reversibly reducing both veratridine- and batrachotoxin-stimulated sodium uptake into rat brain synaptosomes (Mullin & Hunt, 1984, 1985). Nonstimulated uptake was unaffected. Inhibition of uptake was observed at concentrations of ethanol as low as 25 mM (115 mg/dl), the concentration in the blood at which behavioral depression was first observed when animals were injected with different doses of ethanol. With increasing concentrations of ethanol, sodium uptake was decreased in a concentration-dependent manner. A concentration of 345 mM (1587 mg/dl) was required for 50% inhibition of veratridine-stimulated sodium uptake and 583 mM (2681 mg/dl) for batrachotoxin-stimulated uptake. This effect could be observed only with incubation times of 3–7 sec. No changes were observed with longer incubations.

The inhibitory action of ethanol on neurotoxin-stimulated sodium uptake was due to a reduction in the maximal effect of the neurotoxins (Mullin & Hunt, 1985). The potencies of a homologous series of aliphatic alcohols were proportional to their lipid solubilities. Ethanol appeared not to interact with Sites I and III of the sodium channel. Consequently, the alcohols probably interact with Site II.

Similar results were obtained in another laboratory, which demonstated that in concentrations of 400 mM (1840 mg/dl) ethanol inhibited veratridine-stimulated sodium uptake by 43% (Harris, 1984). Furthermore, ethanol had a greater inhibitory effect in the cerebral cortex than in the cerebellum (Harris & Bruno, 1985).

In addition to normal inactivation after neuronal stimulation, further potassium efflux can be activated by a calcium-dependent process. This leads to a long-lasting afterhyperolarization and tends to reduce neural excitability (Meech, 1978). Ethanol increases this calcium-dependent potassium conductance in hippocampal slices (Carlen *et al.*, 1982) (see Chapter 3).

To determine whether ethanol-induced alterations in calcium-dependent potassium movements could be detected, the efflux of ^{86}Rb, a tracer for potassium, was examined in the presence and in the absence of ethanol from erythrocytes and synaptosomes (Yamamoto & Harris, 1983a). The isolated cells were lysed and resealed with different concentrations of calcium and EGTA to regulate the intracellular calcium concentration. They were then labeled with ^{86}Rb and the rate of efflux determined. Calcium-dependent ^{86}Rb efflux was the difference between that in the presence and in the absence of calcium.

When ethanol was incubated with erythrocytes or synaptosomes, calcium-dependent ^{86}Rb efflux was enhanced by ethanol [50–200 mM (230–920 mg/dl)] in a concentration-dependent manner (Yamamoto & Harris, 1983a). This effect was most pronounced at low intracellular concentrations of calcium. Calcium-independent efflux was unchanged. Also, other alcohols increased ^{86}Rb efflux with potencies directly related to their lipid solubilities. Using apamin, an inhibitor of calcium-dependent potassium conductance (Banks, Brown, Burgess, Burnstock, Claret, Cocks, & Jenkinson, 1979), the effect of ethanol was abolished. Furthermore, intraventricular injections of apamin into ethanol-intoxicated animals reduced sleeping times in a dose-dependent manner, but could not block the loss of the righting reflex completely.

As mentioned earlier in the chapter, neurons maintain low intracellular sodium and low extracellular potassium concentrations by means of an active transport system. The effect of ethanol [110 mM (506 mg/dl)] on potassium uptake into cortical slices has been examined. When the slices were incubated with the ethanol for 10 min, uptake was inhibited as much as 72% (Israel, Kalant, & LeBlanc, 1966). Other alcohols were also effective with their potencies proportional to their lipid solubilities. Longer incubations and increases in the potassium concentrations diminished this effect. When slices were incubated with ethanol and electrically stimulated, the uptake of potassium was reduced after the cessation of stimulation with no effect observed on sodium efflux (Wallgren *et al.*, 1974). The relationship of these findings to the transport system that is responsible for these ion movements and their significance will be discussed in Chapter 5.

Studies of the movements of the monovalent cations have not been reported in animals chronically treated with ethanol. Also, chloride movements have not been investigated after acute or chronic ethanol treatment because of the lack of a satisfactory experimental system.

Calcium

Calcium serves two major purposes in neurons: (1) to maintain a permeability barrier to passive sodium influx and thus maintain neuroexcitability (Rothstein, 1968), and (2) to act as a stimulus for neurotransmitter release (Rubin, 1970). Calcium has a fairly large hydrated radius and, therefore, membranes are not very permeable to it. In fact, most calcium is in a bound state, generally to the exterior surface of the neuronal membrane. Calcium probably binds to phospholipids and possibly proteins and may do so in combination with ATP (Hemminki, 1974; Kimizuka & Koketsu, 1962).

When the neuron is active, calcium will pass through the membrane in response to stimulation or depolarizing agents (Blaustein, 1975; Cooke & Robinson, 1971; Stahl & Swanson; 1971). In order to maintain a low intracellular concentration of calcium, transport systems, which are all ATP-dependent, move calcium into organelles, such as mitochondria and endoplasmic reticula (Diamond & Goldberg, 1971; Lust & Robinson, 1970; Tjeol, Bianchi, & Haugaard, 1970). Also, calcium can be removed by means of a mechanism that exchanges calcium for sodium in the extracellular fluid (Blaustein & Ector, 1976; Blaustein & Oborn, 1975; Blaustein & Weismann, 1970). In addition, intracellular calcium binding proteins may help keep intracellular levels of free calcium low.

Studies concerning the effect of alcohols on calcium in the brain have centered around measurements of tissue content, uptake into synaptosomes, and binding to membranes. The calcium content in various areas of the brain has been measured by several investigators after acute and chronic ethanol treatment. Initial studies suggested that ethanol was very effective in reducing calcium levels throughout the brain (Ross, Medina, & Cardenas, 1974). Reported doses as low as 1.5 mg/kg, administered intraperitoneally, were reported to decrease calcium content by more than 40%. In addition, this effect was blocked by prior treatment with naloxone, suggesting that the action of ethanol on calcium content might be mediated through opiate receptors. Other alcohols were capable of depleting calcium, but their effects did not appear to be related to their lipid solubilities (Ross, 1976).

More recently, these findings have been challenged by investigators who found little or no effect of ethanol on calcium content in the brain. Although the experimental designs of all of the studies were relatively equal, acute ethanol treatment did not alter synaptosomal calcium content (Hood & Harris, 1979) nor that in brain regions, except at high doses of ethanol (Boggan, Meyer, Middaugh, & Sparks, 1979; Ferko & Bobyock, 1980). In these latter cases, both small increases and decreases in calcium content were observed. No effect on calcium content was found after 10 days of ethanol inhalation (Ferko & Bobyock, 1980).

Of more apparent relevance to physiological function, the effects of alcohols on calcium uptake have been investigated in serveral reports. In one study, ethanol [80 mM (368 mg/dl)] *in vitro* was found to stimulate K$^+$-stimulated calcium uptake into synaptosomes derived from mouse brains (Friedman, Erickson, & Leslie, 1980). A small increase in unstimulated uptake was also observed. The effect was seen only if the tissue was preincubated with the ethanol for just 2 min before the ^{45}Ca uptake step was begun. Twelve-minute preincubations abolished the effect.

In other reports, ethanol in concentrations as low as 45 mM (207 mg/dl) *in vitro* inhibited mouse synaptosomal K$^+$-stimulated calcium uptake in a concentration-dependent manner (Harris & Hood, 1980; Stokes & Harris, 1982). The effect was independent of how long the synaptosomes were preincubated with ethanol (0.5–12 min) and the time of calcium uptake (1–6 min). If ethanol was administered to animals 5 min, but not 60 min, before preparing the synaptosomes, K$^+$-stimulated calcium uptake was also reduced. An Arrhenius analysis (see Chapter 2) indicated that in the presence of ethanol, calcium uptake was similar to that observed at higher temperatures, consistent with a more disordered environment within the membrane. An increase in the calcium but not the potassium concentration could overcome the inhibitory effect of ethanol on uptake. Calcium efflux was unaffected by ethanol in concentrations up to 400 mM (1840 mg/dl).

Other aliphatic alcohols could block K$^+$-stimulated calcium uptake with their potencies proportional to their lipid solubilities (Stokes & Harris, 1982). The concentration of ethanol that produced 50% inhibition of uptake was 1330 mM (6118 mg/dl). Of several brain regions studied, K$^+$-stimulated calcium uptake in the cerebellum and corpus striatum was most affected by ethanol.

K$^+$-stimulated calcium uptake results from depolarization across the synaptosomal membrane. Other means by different mechanisms can promote calcium uptake. For example, glutamate can induce calcium uptake by increasing calcium conductance without an accompanying depolarization (Nicoll & Alger, 1981), veratridine by inducing sodium influx and membrane depolarization (Catterall, 1980), and phosphatidic acid by acting as a calcium ionophore (Harris, Schmidt, Hitzemann, & Hitzemann, 1981). Ethanol was effective in reducing calcium uptake induced by glutamate and veratridine, but not by phosphatidic acid (Stokes & Harris, 1982). Ethanol was especially potent in reducing veratridine-stimulated calcium uptake in the cerebral cortex. Using the uptake of [^{3}H]tetraphenylphosphonium as an index of the membrane potential (Lichtschtein, Kaback, & Blume, 1979), ethanol did not alter the membrane potential in either K$^+$-stimulated or nonstimulated synaptosomes (Harris & Stokes, 1982).

Some recent evidence suggests that the uptake of calcium into nerve endings may have two components, a fast phase and a slow phase (Gripenberg, Heinonen, & Jansson, 1980; Nachshen & Blaustein, 1980). It is suggested that the fast phase of stimulated calcium uptake better reflects normal physiological processes during which ion movements occur quickly and transiently. The slow phase may be related more to circumstances where there is prolonged depolarization, such as during tetanic stimulation.

Because studies examining the effect of ethanol on K^+-stimulated calcium uptake were undertaken using relatively long incubation times, the results obtained may more likely reflect the slow phase of calcium uptake. In order to determine whether ethanol can modify the fast phase of calcium uptake, incubation times of 1–60 sec were tested (Leslie, Barr, Chandler, & Farrar, 1983). Ethanol in concentrations of 80 mM (368 mg/dl) could inhibit K^+-stimulated calcium uptake into synaptosomes from the cerebral cortex of rats only with incubation times of 1 and 3 sec. At these times the rates of calcium uptake were significantly greater than those obtained at later incubation times. Using 3-sec incubations, concentrations of ethanol of 25–150 mM (115–690 mg/dl) inhibited uptake from 9–31%. Ethanol generally inhibited calcium uptake in midbrain, cerebellum, and brain stem only when incubations times did not exceed 5 sec.

K^+-stimulated calcium uptake has been measured in animals chronically treated with ethanol in a liquid diet for 7–10 days (Friedman *et al.*, 1980; Harris & Hood, 1980). When the animals were killed without allowing for the elimination of ethanol from the body, a significant reduction in calcium uptake was observed, as well as a diminished effect of added ethanol *in vitro* on uptake. No measurements were made in animals undergoing a withdrawal syndrome. No alteration on the fast phase of calcium uptake was observed in rats after 8 weeks on a liquid diet containing ethanol (Lesslie *et al.*, 1983). However, tolerance to the inhibitory effect of ethanol added *in vitro* was obtained.

The ability of lysed synaptosomes from mice to sequester calcium intracellularly was examined in the presence of ethanol (Garrett & Ross, 1983; Harris, 1981). This would provide information on whether neurons can maintain low intracellular calcium concentrations. Ethanol *in vitro* was capable of inhibiting this nonmitochondrial, ATP-dependent process with concentrations of at least 50 mM (230 mg/dl) (Harris, 1981). However, concentrations in excess of 400 mM (1840 mg/dl) ethanol were required to obtain a marked effect. Administration of a single dose of ethanol (4 g/kg, intraperitoneally) also reduced calcium uptake (Garrett & Ross, 1983). In mice given ethanol in a liquid diet for 7 days, ATP-dependent calcium uptake was slightly reduced in the absence of added ethanol *in vitro* (Harris, 1981). Also, tolerance developed to the effect of added ethanol after both acute and chronic administration of ethanol.

The effect of ethanol on the calcium–sodium exchange mechanism has recently been examined (Michaelis & Michaelis, 1983; Michaelis, Michaelis, & Tehan, 1983). This was approached by loading resealed synaptic membrane vesicles with sodium chloride and then determining the rate of calcium uptake. Ethanol was found to be generally inhibitory of Na^+-dependent calcium uptake. However, changes in incubating temperatures had variable effects on the ability of ethanol to exert this action, especially at concentrations less than 50 mM (230 mg/dl). At 35°C, ethanol was inhibitory, but at 23°C, it was stimulatory. No effect of ethanol on calcium uptake was observed at 16°C.

In another approach to calcium efflux, ^{45}Ca outflow from prelabeled erythrocytes and Ca^{2+}-ATPase activity in synaptic plasma membranes were measured in the presence of ethanol *in vitro* (Yamamoto & Harris, 1983b). Concentrations of ethanol as low as 50 mM (230 mg/dl) were effective in stimulating both processes. The elevated activity of Ca^{2+}-ATPase was further enhanced as the concentration of calcium in the medium was increased. In another study, administration of a single dose of ethanol (4 g/kg, intraperitoneally) inhibited Ca^{2+}-ATPase activity (Garrett & Ross, 1983).

Reports concerning the effects of ethanol on calcium binding have been fairly consistent in their findings. An early study using erythrocyte ghost membranes demonstrated that ethanol and other alcohols in a homologous series significantly enhanced calcium binding (Seeman, Chau, Goldberg, Sauks, & Sax, 1971). Ethanol was effective at concentrations as low as 20 mM (92 mg/dl). The potencies of other alcohols were proportional to their lipid solubilities.

In more recent studies in which synaptosomal calcium binding was measured, ethanol was again found to increase binding (Harris & Fenner, 1982; Michaelis & Myers, 1979). This effect was apparent at concentrations of ethanol as low as 5 mM (23 mg/dl). In addition, the increased calcium binding appears to be onto the internal surface of synaptosomes (Harris & Fenner, 1982). This was determined by promoting influx of calcium using the calcium ionophore A23187 and removing external calcium by washing the synaptosomes with sodium chloride-EGTA solutions. Ethanol did not alter calcium binding to the external surface unless concentrations of 800 mM (3680 mg/dl) were incubated with the tissue preparations.

An effort has been made to determine the nature of the binding site to which calcium binding is enhanced by ethanol (Chweh & Leslie, 1981). Calcium binding to a number of acidic lipids was measured, including phosphatidic acid, phosphatidylinositol, phosphatidylserine, cardiolipin, and sulfatide. The largest effect of ethanol [80 mM (368 mg/dl)] was an increase of about 22% in calcium binding to sulfatide.

Chronic ethanol treatment has not produced consistent results on calcium binding. In one study, mice were treated for 7 days with ethanol in a liquid diet (Harris & Fenner, 1982). Synaptosomal calcium binding was unaffected, as well as the ability of ethanol *in vitro* to enhance binding. In another study, in which rats were treated for 16 days with ethanol in a liquid diet, calcium binding was reduced (Michaelis & Myers, 1979). Ethanol added *in vitro* was less effective in increasing calcium binding. The duration of ethanol ingestion may therefore play a role in the results obtained.

If calcium movements in the brain are altered after acute and chronic treatment with ethanol, then some of the behavioral manifestations of these treatments in animals might be altered by the administration of calcium or calcium antagonists. This possibility has been tested by injecting calcium and other suitably related compounds into the brain prior to the measurement of ethanol intoxication or signs of physical dependence.

Calcium as well as other divalent cations, such as manganese and cadmium, increased the times animals slept after a given dose of ethanol (Erickson, Tyler, & Harris, 1978; Harris, 1979). Combinations of calcium ionophores and doses of calcium that were by themselves ineffective in augmenting ethanol-induced depression also increased sleeping times. Calcium antagonists, such as verapamil and lanthanum chloride, did not alter sleeping times, but EDTA and EGTA, calcium chelators, effectively reduced sleeping times.

The effect of calcium and calcium antagonists was tested in ethanol-dependent mice by measuring convulsions on handling (Harris, 1979). Convulsions on handling have been shown to be a useful endpoint for assessing the intensity of an ethanol withdrawal syndrome (Goldstein, 1972). A dose of calcium chloride, 0.4 μmol/mouse, intraventricularly, significantly suppressed withdrawal convulsions. Conversely, the lethality of EGTA was elevated in ethanol-dependent animals.

These results appear to be just opposite of what would be predicted, especially after a single of ethanol. If ethanol inhibits calcium uptake and other calcium-mediated processes, then administration of calcium might have been expected to be an ethanol antagonist. The ethanol-augmenting effect of calcium might be a reflection of its membrane-stabilizing properties and may involve mechanisms different than those related to calcium uptake. This might be the case especially if intracellular calcium is important in the depressant effect of ethanol. Little injected calcium would enter the neuron.

Ethanol apears to alter calcium movements in organs in addition to the brain. Most directly, ethanol in concentrations of 25–200 mM (115–920 mg/dl) reduced calcium uptake into liver microsomes in a concentration-dependent manner (Ponnappa *et al.*, 1982). After chronic ethanol treatment for 35–40 days in a liquid diet, uptake was enhanced and the inhibitory effect of ethanol *in vitro* was reduced, indicating the development of tolerance. Calcium uptake and retention in liver mitochondria were reduced after 5–7 weeks of ethanol administration (Korsten, Gordon, Kingenstein, & Lieber, 1983). In the heart, ethanol inhibited both calcium uptake and binding to microsomes enriched with sarcoplasmic reticulum, but only at very high concentrations (Swartz, Tepke, Katz, & Rubin, 1974). Both processes were inhibited in dogs chronically treated for 6 months (Bing, Tillmanns, Fauvel, Seeler, & Mao, 1974). Calcium uptake in sarcoplasmic reticulum from skeletal muscle was unaffected after 8–12 weeks of ethanol consumption in a liquid diet (Mrak, 1983). Finally, chronic treatment with ethanol for 12 days has been reported to inhibit intestinal absorption of calcium (Krawitt, 1973).

In a more indirect study, the role of calcium in the effect of ethanol on electrically evoked contractions of the ileum longitudinal muscle/myenteric plexus preparation has been examined (Mayer, Khanna, & Kalant, 1980). Concentrations of ethanol of 40–160 mM (184–736 mg/dl) inhibited contractions in a concentration-dependent manner. The addition of higher concentrations of calcium to the medium partially antagonized this effect. After 4 weeks of ethanol injections (3 g/kg, intraperitoneally) every 12 hr, tolerance developed to the inhibitory effect of ethanol on contractions. Under these conditions, higher calcium concentrations exerted a greater antagonism to the actions of ethanol. These data were interpreted to suggest that less calcium was available for the excitation–secretion coupling mechanism and that chronic ethanol treatment leads to an increased responsiveness to calcium.

Commentary

An action of alcohols on ion movements seems to conform to most of the criteria for a possible mechanism of action as outlined in Chapter 1. Physiologically relevant concentrations of ethanol can inhibit stimulus-induced uptake of both sodium and calcium into synaptosomes and can stimulate calcium-mediated potassium efflux out of synaptosomes. The effect is reversible on sodium uptake, the only system on which this property was examined. The potencies of different alcohols relate directly to their lipid solubilities in all of the systems studied. Finally, all of these events are involved with neuroexcitability.

Based on the evidence presented, some of the ethanol-induced alterations in calcium uptake may be a consequence of changes in sodium uptake. In most instances in which calcium uptake was affected, the stimuli, such as veratridine and glutamate, also promote sodium movements. Although K^+-stimulated calcium uptake is not accompanied by enhanced sodium uptake, ethanol inhibits this process. On the other hand, calcium uptake stimulated by phosphatidic acid, a calcium ionophore, was not affected by ethanol in physiologically compatible concentrations. This suggests that an inhibition of stimulus-induced sodium uptake may represent in some cases an initial action of ethanol and that the inhibition of stimulus-induced calcium uptake may represent the consequence of such an action. The comparison of the effect of ethanol on sodium uptake and on the fast phase of calcium uptake make this possibility particularly viable. The reduction of calcium uptake, in turn, could modulate some of the other more secondary actions of ethanol, such as those on neurotransmitter release (Hunt & Majchrowicz, 1979).

A more direct involvement of calcium cannot be ruled out. For example, the stimulation by ethanol of calcium binding and calcium-mediated potassium efflux may represent different mechanisms than those responsible for the inhibition of calcium uptake. In fact, enhanced calcium binding by ethanol has been suggested to be the stimulus for accelerated calcium-mediated potassium efflux (Yamamoto & Harris, 1983a). A combination of all of these events may in some way contribute to ethanol-induced depression.

By what mechanism could ethanol alter the normal movements of ions? Based on evidence presented in Chapter 2, indicating that alcohols can increase the mobility of lipids in membranes, the two actions of alcohols could be related. For example, it has been demonstrated that the lipid environment surrounding sodium channels is important to express some of their properties (Baumgold, 1980; Catterall, 1980; Villegas, Barnola, & Camejo, 1970). In fact, tetrodotoxin binds strongly to cholesterol (Villegas et al., 1970), a lipid that has been suggested to be important in the development of ethanol tolerance (Chin et al., 1978). This may mean that cholesterol is a constituent of the sodium channel. In addition, lipids may be important components in membranes to which calcium binds (Hemminki, 1974; Kimizuka & Koketsu, 1962).

Alterations in the fluidity of the membrane might be able to alter the ability of ion channels to function normally. Unsaturated fatty acid methyl esters can disorder membranes (Fontaine, Matsumoto, Goodman, & Rasmussen, 1980) and were found to inhibit veratridine-stimulated sodium and calcium uptake, but not potassium-stimulated calcium uptake (Harris, 1984; Stokes & Harris, 1982). It is interesting to note at this point that veratridine-stimulated calcium uptake is inhibited by tetrodotoxin, while potassium-stimulated uptake is not (Blaustein, 1975), indicating that the former process is more closely aligned with the function of the sodium channel. Ethanol-induced fluidization might sufficiently perturb the lipid environment so that normal interaction between lipids and the channel is impaired. Also, an increased fluidity could result in the exposure of a greater number of calcium binding sites and in that manner facilitate calcium-induced potassium movements.

The data provide some tantalizing sepculations. However, more research needs to be done to assess in more detail the relationships between membrane lipids and ion channels. Furthermore, a convincing relationship between the ability of ethanol to fluidize membranes and to inhibit ion flux is lacking. More direct studies to correlate these changes need to be attempted. In addition, when assessing the relevance of the effect of ethanol on stimulated ion uptake, research needs to be focused more on the physiological processes involved *in vivo*. This will help in determining to what extent some of the effects of ethanol are interrelated. Finally, the possible role of ion movements in the development or expression of tolerance and physical dependence should be explored in detail.

5. Membrane-bound enzymes

Many of the functions of membranes are performed by complex enzyme systems embedded within them. As with the electrical properties of neurons and their concomitant ion movements, as discussed in Chapters 3 and 4, respectively, alterations in the microenvironment in which enzyme systems reside may have profound consequences on their ability to function properly. Since alcohols probably interact with membranes in ways that may alter this microenvironment, it is important to examine what effects alcohols may have on these systems and whether there are possible consequences on cellular activity.

In this chapter, we shall review the evidence suggesting that alcohols may disrupt enzymatic activity in membranes predominantly in the brain, whether such changes could adversely influence normal cell function, and whether the major effects of alcohols can be explained by them. Mainly two enzymes will be discussed in this chapter, the sodium- and potassium-activated adenosine triphosphatase and adenylate cyclase. This approach is taken mostly because these enzymes have been extensively studied after ethanol exposure. Other enzymes will be examined where appropriate. Initially, we shall discuss some general considerations applicable to the study of enzymes.

Methodological considerations

Enzymes are proteins that catalyze chemical reactions. These reactions involve the conversion of a substrate to a product and can occur in soluble and particulate fractions of cells. Often the reactions will not proceed without enzymatic catalysis because of unfavorable thermodynamic conditions. In order for many enzymatic reactions to take place additional substances, called cofactors, are involved. Some cofactors, such as ions, remain in their original form after the reaction, while others, such as those involved in oxidation and reduction reactions, are metabolized.

Enzymatic reactions are generally studied *in vitro*, where the conditions, such as substrate and cofactor concentrations, pH, and temperature can be precisely defined. The source of the enzymes can be either crude tissue preparations or preparations at various levels of purification.

Although it is beyond the scope of this chapter to provide a detailed treatise of enzymology, a few properties of enzymes will occasionally be presented. These properties include equilibria constants and rates of reactions and how ethanol might change them.

In enzymatic reactions, there is first a reversible reaction between the enzyme (E) and the substrate (S) to form an enzyme–substrate complex (ES) (White, Handler, & Smith, 1968). The product (p) is then formed with the enzyme reverting to its original state. This relationship can be expressed by the following reactions:

$$E + S \underset{k_{-1}}{\overset{k_1}{\rightleftharpoons}} ES \underset{k_{-2}}{\overset{k_2}{\rightleftharpoons}} P + E \tag{1}$$

where k_1, k_{-1}, k_2, and k_{-2} are the reaction rate constants. Since the rate for formation of ES is dependent on the concentrations of E and S, the rates of formation (V_f) and disappearance (V_d) of P can be expressed as

$$V_f = k_1([E_T] - [ES])[S] \tag{2}$$

$$V_d = k_{-1}[ES] + k_2[ES] \tag{3}$$

where $[E_T]$ is the total concentration of the enzyme and $[E_T] - [ES]$ the concentration of the unassociated enzyme. (Since at the beginning of the reaction, the concentration of P is negligible, k_{-2} in Equation 1 can be ignored.) At equilibrium, $V_f = V_d$ and Equations 2 and 3 can be equated and rearranged to give

$$([E_T] - [ES])[S]/[ES] = (k_{-1} + k_2)/k_1 = K_m \tag{4}$$

K_m, the Michaelis–Menten constant, is a complex equilibrium constant incorporating the three reactions indicated in Equation 1 and has been used an index of the affinity of the substrate for the enzyme.

Since there is a finite concentration of the enzyme, there is a point at which raising the concentration of the substrate will saturate the enzyme and the reaction will reach a maximum rate (V_{max}), expressed as

$$V_{max} = k_2[E_T] \tag{5}$$

The K_m and V_{max} of a reaction are the most common properties measured in biological experiments.

The values for K_m and V_{max} cannot readily be calculated from Equations 4 and 5 because [ES] and [E] are difficult to measure. This can be overcome by measuring the initial rate of reaction, expressed as

$$V = k_2[ES] \tag{6}$$

If the concentration of the substrate is high relative to the concentration of the enzyme, all of the enzyme will be present as ES. Consequently, if Equation 4 is solved for [ES], the value of [ES] substituted from Equation 6, the result divided by Equation 5, and the subsequent equation rearranged, the following equation is obtained:

$$V = \frac{V_{max}}{1 + K_m/[S]}$$
(7)

The reciprocal and rearrangement of Equation 7 yields

$$1/V = 1/V_{max} + (K_m/V_{max})(1/[S])$$
(8)

which is a linear expression where, when plotted, $1/V_{max}$ is the Y-intercept and K_m/V_{max} the slope of the line. When $1/V = 0$, the negative of the X-intercept is equal to K_m. An example of such a plot can be found in Figure 5-1 and is called the Lineweaver–Burke plot.

Alterations in enzymatic activity are often correlated to changes in K_m or V_{max} of the reaction. K_m is inversely related to the affinity of the substrate for the active site on the enzyme. In one sense, the affinity indicates how much substrate is necessary to induce a given rate of reaction, that is, how much of the ES is formed. In fact, K_m is equal to the concentration of substrate needed to attain one-half of V_{max}. In other words, the higher the affinity of the substrate is for the active site, the smaller the concentration of substrate required to induce the given reaction rate. At

Figure 5-1. Example of Lineweaver–Burke plot. A, normal plot; B, competitive inhibition; C, noncompetitive inhibition.

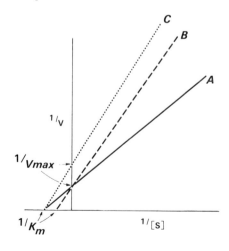

saturating concentrations of the substrate, all of the sites are occupied with maximum concentrations of ES formed. Therefore, the affinity does not contribute to the maximum rate of reaction.

When K_m is changed by a treatment, this means that the concentration of substrate needed to induce a given reaction rate is altered. A major circumstance under which this will occur is when a compound other than the substrate also has affinity for the active site. In the presence of such a substance, K_m for the substrate will be increased. This is called competitive inhibition. Another way K_m can be altered is when access to the active site is restricted or enhanced without a change in the total number of active sites available for reaction.

V_{max} is related to the number of active sites on the enzyme available for the reaction and is not influenced by K_m. If enough substrate is added to the reaction mixture, all the active sites will be occupied and V_{max} will be achieved. Consequently, when V_{max} is changed, this reflects an alteration in the number of these sites. This could result from changes in the concentration of the enzyme or a conformational change in the structure of the enzyme, thereby altering the number of available active sites. When a compound other than the substrate reduces V_{max}, this is known as noncompetitive inhibition.

Whether a treatment alters K_m or V_{max} of an enzymatic reaction can be determined from a Lineweaver–Burke plot. With a change in K_m, the slope of the line is changed and the Y-intercept ($1/V_{max}$) remains the same. With a change in V_{max}, the slope of the line is also changed, but now the X-intercept remains the same. Examples of competitive and noncompetitive inhibition are shown in Figure 5-1.

Sodium- and potassium-activated adenosine triphosphatase

As discussed in Chapters 3 and 4, maintaining proper ionic gradients for sodium and potassium across neuronal membranes is important for maintaining electrical excitability of neurons and is an active process requiring energy. The enzymatic complex that mediates the transport of these ions across membranes is the sodium- and potassium-activated adenosine triphosphatase (Na-K-ATPase).

The Na-K-ATPase transports sodium and potassium through a series of reactions, involving the phosphorylation of the enzyme by ATP (DeWeer, 1975; Hobbs & Albers, 1980; Schwartz, Lindenmayer, & Allen, 1975). These reactions can be represented as follows:

$$E + ATP \xrightarrow{Na^+} E_1 \sim P + ADP \tag{9}$$

$$E_1 \sim P \xrightarrow{Mg^{2+}} E_2 - P \tag{10}$$

$$E_2 - P + H_2O \xrightarrow{K^+} E + P_i \tag{11}$$

It is believed that the Na-K-ATPase is phosphorylated by ATP, and intracellular sodium binds to the "activated" enzyme (9). A conformational change is catalyzed by magnesium and the sodium is transported through the membrane to the outside (10). The enzyme is then dephosphorylated by hydrolysis and extracellular potassium is transported into the cell (11).

The Na-K-ATPase appears to be a large protein, consisting of two main subunits, the α and β subunits. The β subunit has the properties of a glycoprotein. The enzyme also has a small proteolipid subunit. The presence of phospholipids is essential to Na-K-ATPase activity. Phosphorylation and the binding of ouabain, a cardiac glycoside that inhibits the Na-K-ATPase, occurs on the inner and outer surfaces of the membrane, respectively, through which the α subunit traverses.

Stoichiometrically, the bulk of the evidence suggests that for every three sodium ions transported out of the neuron, two potassium ions are transported into the neuron. This net movement of charge across the membrane is the basis of an electrogenic pump that can contribute to the resting membrane potential.

Ethanol has been shown to inhibit microsomal Na-K-ATPase activity *in vitro* in a concentration-dependent manner in the brains of rats, guinea pigs, and mice, and in the electroplaque of the electric eel (Goldstein & Israel, 1972; Israel, Kalant, & Laufer, 1965; Israel & Salazar, 1967; Järnefelt, 1961). Although concentrations of ethanol as low as 54 mM (250 mg/dl) were tested, convincing effects were not observed until concentrations reached 109 mM (500 mg/dl) (Israel et al., 1965). The effectiveness of other aliphatic alcohols to inhibit the Na-K-ATPase was proportional to their lipid solubilities (Israel et al., 1966; Sun & Samorajski, 1970).

Using a kinetic analysis, the effect of ethanol on the Na-K-ATPase was competitive with respect to potassium ion (Israel et al., 1965, 1966). When the potassium concentration in the medium was increased, the degree of inhibition of the Na-K-ATPase by ethanol was reduced. Other alkali metals, such as rubidium and cesium, were also effective in reducing the effects of ethanol (Kalant, Woo, & Endrenyi, 1978). However, considering the physiological concentrations of potassium in the brain, which are equivalent to those that reduce this inhibition, it may be difficult for ethanol to have an inhibitory effect on the Na-K-ATPase *in vivo* at a dose that would not be lethal (Akera, Rech, Marquis, Tobin, & Brody, 1973).

With an Arrhenius analysis (see Chapter 2), ethanol at a concentration of 500 mM (2300 mg/dl) altered the transition temperature for the Na-K-ATPase, indicating that ethanol alters the temperature at which the membrane transforms from the gel to liquid states (Levental & Tabakoff,

1980). When the ethanol was added to mouse synaptosomal membranes, the transition temperature was reduced.

The effectiveness of ethanol on the Na-K-ATPase appears also to depend on the age of the animal (Sun & Samorajski, 1975). Na-K-ATPase activity was measured in synaptosomal fractions of mice and human brains. The mice ranged in age from 3 to 29 months old, and the humans ranged in age from 19 to 84 years old. Ethanol was more effective on Na-K-ATPase activity in the older animals. Mice older than 26 months and humans older than 65 years were the most sensitive.

In some recent studies, the possible interaction of ethanol, the Na-K-ATPase, and catecholamines was examined. Some time ago, catecholamines were shown to stimulate Na-K-ATPase activity (Yoshimura, 1973). The inhibitory effect of ethanol on Na-K-ATPase activity *in vitro* was found to be considerably enhanced in the presence of low concentrations of catecholamines and was competitive with respect to potassium (Kalant & Rangaraj, 1981; Rangaraj & Kalant, 1979). The effect of ethanol was significant at concentrations as low as 6.25 mM (28.7 mg/dl). Concentrations as little as 1 pM of l-norepinephrine, but not of d-norepinephrine nor of 100 nM dopamine, were effective. In fact, stimulation of the Na-K-ATPase by catecholamines was not a prerequisite for the enhanced inhibitory effect of ethanol. Catecholamines merely needed to be present in the incubation medium.

The enhanced inhibitory effect of ethanol in the presence of catecholamines appears to be receptor-mediated. α-Adrenergic but not β-adrenergic antagonists were effective in blocking this action of catecholamines (Rangaraj & Kalant, 1979, 1980). The data presented suggested that catecholamines can sensitize the Na-K-ATPase, so that ethanol can be inhibitory at concentrations of potassium found *in vivo*.

To evaluate the possible role of the Na-K-ATPase in ethanol intoxication, ions that affect Na-K-ATPase activity *in vitro* were injected into animals to determine if the signs of intoxication could be altered. Potassium, which was shown earlier to antagonize the inhibition of the Na-K-ATPase by ethanol, was administered in intraperitoneal doses of 5 mmol/kg. This treatment reduced the degree of intoxication induced by a 2-g/kg intraperitoneal dose of ethanol by about 15% (Israel *et al.*, 1965). This dose of potassium elevated serum potassium concentrations from 6.6 to 9.4 mEq/liter. Potassium concentrations in brain were not measured.

In another experiment, animals were injected with cadmium, a noncompetitive inhibitor of Na-K-ATPase activity with respect to ATP (Magour, Kristof, Baumann, & Assmann, 1981; Yamamoto, Sutoo, & Misawa, 1981). When intraperitoneal doses of 0.56–1.68 mg/kg were administered along with ethanol (3–4.5 g/kg), ethanol sleeping times were elevated up to 300%. Ethanol-induced hypothermia was also enhanced. Blood ethanol concentrations were not altered by cadmium. The highest dose of cadmium elevated brain cadmium concentrations four-fold and $4\mu M$ cadmium incubated with a synaptosomal or microsomal preparation inhibited Na-K-ATPase activity by 50%.

A number of reports have explored the possibility that if ethanol inhibits the Na-K-ATPase, chronic ethanol administration might result not only in the development of behavioral tolerance, but of tolerance to the inhibitory effect of ethanol on the Na-K-ATPase. Also, a compensatory increase in the activity of the enzyme might occur. The first such study measured Na-K-ATPase activity in homogenates of cerebral cortex from rats given single daily doses of ethanol for 21–26 days, a dosing regimen that induced behavioral tolerance (Israel, Kalant, LeBlanc, Bernstein, & Salazar, 1970). Na-K-ATPase activity in these preparations was elevated by 65%. Other studies in which ethanol was administered by inhalation for 7 days (Roach, Khan, Coffman, Pennington, & Davis, 1973), by liquid diet for 2 and 7 weeks (Guerri, Wallace, & Grisola, 1978; Israel & Kuriyama, 1971), or by oral intubation for 7 days (Cowan, Cardeal & Cavalheiro, 1980) obtained similar results. Regional distribution studies suggested that the elevated Na-K-ATPase activity was confined to the cerebral cortex and hippocampus (Knox, Perrin, & Sen, 1972). In a recent study, an increase in Na-K-ATPase activity correlated with an equivalent increase in phosphatidylcholine, which activates the enzyme (Sun & Sun, 1983). This change might be the basis for the observed increase in Na-K-ATPase activity.

[³H]Ouabain binding was also reported to be elevated by 47–100% in cats given ethanol intragastrically for 5 weeks (Sharma & Banerjee, 1979). Scatchard analysis (see Chapter 6) indicated that chronic ethanol treatment increased the number of available ouabain binding sites, possibly indicating an increased content of the Na-K-ATPase in the membrane. The effect was observed only in the cerebral cortex, cerebellum, amygdala, and hippocampus.

The effectiveness of chronic ethanol treatment to elevate Na-K-ATPase activity has been disputed by several laboratories. In rats treated identically to those in the study of Israel et al. (1970), no effect on Na-K-ATPase activity or [³H]ouabain binding was observed even though the animals were behaviorally tolerant (Akera et al., 1973). Similar negative results were observed in mice administered ethanol by inhalation for 3 days (Goldstein & Israel, 1972), mice treated for 7 days in a liquid diet (Levental & Tabakoff, 1980), and rats treated for 21 days on a liquid diet (Westcott & Weiner, 1983). Using Arrhenius analysis, either the transition temperature for the Na-K-ATPase was lower and ethanol added *in vitro* had no effect on activity (Levental & Tabakoff, 1980; Rangaraj & Kalant, 1982) or no effect at all was observed after chronic ethanol treatment (Westcott & Weiner, 1983). Catecholamine sensitization of the Na-K-ATPase to ethanol was not altered by chronic ethanol treatment in whole-brain preparations (Rangaraj & Kalant, 1982). However, in another study do-pamine-stimulated Na-K-ATPase activity was elevated in the hippocampus and midbrain 24 hr after withdrawal (Keane & Leonard, 1983).

One report may shed some light on these inconsistencies. Rats were administered ethanol in a liquid diet for 4 weeks and Na-K-ATPase was measured at different times after withdrawal (Rangaraj & Kalant, 1978). While still on the diet, Na-K-ATPase activity was not altered. However, 12–48 hr after withdrawal, enzymatic activity was accelerated in brain homogenates by 13–15%. In lysed synaptosomes, activity was increased by 28% at 24 hr and 16% at 48 hr. Although no withdrawal signs were reported, the changes roughly correlate with the time course of such signs in rats rendered ethanol dependent by chronic gastric intubation of ethanol (Majchrowicz, 1975).

In additional experiments, rats were injected with amphetamine or were forced to swim, with Na-K-ATPase activity being measured thereafter (Rangaraj & Kalant, 1978). Both treatments elevated Na-K-ATPase activity. Also, the addition of 0.1 mM norepinephrine to preparations from un-treated animals increased activity. When 50 mM (230-mg/dl) ethanol was included with the norepinephrine in the incubation medium, Na-K-ATPase activity was reduced. Ethanol alone had no effect on the enzyme. These data were interpreted to suggest that the accelerated norepinephrine turn-over observed after ethanol withdrawal by a number of investigators (see Hunt, 1979) might play a role in the elevated Na-K-ATPase activity ob-served under similar conditions. Unfortunately, norepinephrine turnover is also elevated while ethanol is present in the body, a time when no effect of Na-K-ATPase activity is found.

Finally, a study has been reported that used cultured cells to examine the effect of acute and chronic ethanol exposure on Na-K-ATPase activity (Syapin, Stefanovic, Mandel, & Noble, 1976). Hamster astroblasts and mouse neuroblastoma cell lines were used. Incubation of the cells with ethanol in a concentration of 100 mM (460 mg/dl) inhibited Na-K-ATPase activity only in the astroblasts. No effect was observed in the neuronal cell lines. Cells that were chronically incubated with the same concentration of ethanol for up to 68 days showed a different response. Na-K-ATPase activity in one of the neuroblastoma cell lines was significantly elevated with no change observed in activity in other neuroblastoma and astro-blastoma cell lines. No tolerance to the acute effect of ethanol on Na-K-ATPase activity was seen in the astroblasts. In other experiments, ethanol concentrations of up to 43.4 mM (200 mg/dl) were incubated for 5 days with HeLa cells derived from human cervix or L-cells from mouse fibro-blasts (Lindsay, 1974). Na-K-ATPase activity was elevated in the HeLa cells but not in the L-cells. These data suggest that the effects of both acute and chronic administration of ethanol on the Na-K-ATPase may depend on the characteristics of the cells under study and do not support the idea that chronic depression of Na-K-ATPase activity should necessarily lead in time to compensatory increases in activity.

From the data presented, it is not clear whether the Na-K-ATPase plays a significant role in the actions of ethanol. Inhibition of this enzyme *in vitro* has been observed in a number of laboratories and is competitive with respect to potassium. However, unphysiologically low concentrations of potassium were generally required in the assay media in order for ethanol to have much of an inhibitory effect on the Na-K-ATPase. On the other hand, the observation that the inhibition was reversible and could be found with other alcohols with potencies correlating with their lipid solubilities is consistent with a role of the Na-K-ATPase in the mechanism of action of ethanol (see Chapter 1). The possible interaction of the Na-K-ATPase with catecholamines *in vivo* might be an interesting way in which the Na-K-ATPase might be sensitized to ethanol.

The differences in the results obtained from experiments in which ethanol was chronically administered are difficult to reconcile. When variables such as length of treatment and mode of administration are taken into account, no clear reasons for the different results among laboratories are apparent. The assay conditions seemed to be identical.

In the final analysis, the important question is whether alterations in the activity of the Na-K-ATPase can explain the effects of ethanol in the living animal. This is by no means clear. For example, would inhibition of the Na-K-ATPase explain the depressant effects of ethanol?

Since more sodium is transported out of a neuron than potassium is transported into the neuron by the Na-K-ATPase, this electrogenic pump could contribute to the resting membrane potential (DeWeer, 1975). Since this would reflect a net movement of positive charges to the extracellular fluid, this would exert a hyperpolarizing influence on the neuron. Hence, inhibition of the Na-K-ATPase might lead to depolarization of a neuron, making it more likely to fire when an excitatory stimulus was applied.

In many published reports, inhibition of the Na-K-ATPase is associated with excitation, not depression. For example, ouabain when directly injected into the brain or perfused through the ventricular system induces convulsions (Bignami & Palladini, 1966). In addition, aluminum ions, competitive inhibitors of the Na-K-ATPase, induce a chronic state of epilepsy when applied as a cream to the surface of the cerebral cortex (Harmony, Urba-Holmgren, Urbay, & Szava, 1968).

Convulsants and anticonvulsants have had consistent effects on ion movements, but not on Na-K-ATPase activity. Pentylenetetrazole, a convulsant, enhances the accumulation of intracellular sodium and extracellular potassium (Colfer & Essex, 1947), while diphenylhydantoin, an anticonvulsant, has the opposite effect (Woodbury, 1955). However, no agreement on the effects of these drugs on Na-K-ATPase activity is available (Bignami, Palladini, & Venturini, 1966; Brown & Stone, 1973; Festoff & Appel, 1968; Formby, 1970; Lewin & Bleck, 1971; Rawson & Pincus, 1968).

In summary, there is no conclusive evidence that ethanol-induced alterations in Na-K-ATPase activity *in vitro* in any way contribute to the depressant actions of ethanol. If changes in Na-K-ATPase activity occur *in vivo* after ethanol administration, in all likelihood, the changes in activity observed are secondary to changes in neuronal activity rather than a cause of them.

Adenylate cyclase and other enzymes related to cyclic nucleotides

It is now believed that the cyclic nucleotides, cyclic adenosine 3′,5′-monophosphate (cAMP) and cyclic guanosine 3′,5′-monophosphate (cGMP) play an important role as second messengers in the actions of hormones. They are involved in the processing of hormonal input into appropriate physiological responses through reactions in membranes, especially in the nervous system (Greengard, 1978; Nathanson, 1977). Key components are the enzyme complexes that synthesize these cyclic nucleotides. The basic metabolic reactions associated with their synthesis and degradation are as follows:

$$ATP \xrightarrow{Mg^{2+}} cAMP \longrightarrow 5'\text{-AMP}$$

$$GTP \xrightarrow{Mn^{2+}} cGMP \longrightarrow 5'\text{-GMP}$$

Adenylate and guanylate cyclase catalyze the synthesis of cAMP and cGMP, respectively. Adenylate cyclase requires magnesium for its activity and guanylate cyclase requires manganese. The cyclic nucleotides are hydrolyzed by phosphodiesterases to their respective 5′-monophosphates.

Adenylate cyclase is a receptor-coupled system traversing the cell membrane and is composed of three components. The first component, the receptor, is responsive to stimulation by a number of neurotransmitters, including dopamine, norepinephrine, serotonin, and histamine (Nathanson, 1977). Each transmitter has its own, separate receptor. The second component involves the coupling of the receptor on the outer surface of the cell membrane to adenylate cyclase and is believed to involve a guanine nucleotide-stimulated regulatory protein (Minocherhomjee & Roufogalis, 1982). Guanine nucleotides, such as GTP, not only enhance adenylate cyclase activity, but reduce the affinity of agonists for their receptors. Both stimulatory and inhibitory regulatory proteins may exist. The stimulatory regulatory protein can be activated by cholera toxin by inhibiting GTP degradation. Finally, the third component is the catalytic unit of adenylate cyclase located in the inner leaflet on the membrane. The catalytic unit can be stimulated by sodium fluoride (NaF) via the stimulatory regulatory protein. It is on the inner surface of the membrane that cAMP is synthesized. To what extent these various components are attached to each other and how exactly they interact is not known.

Guanylate cyclase is less understood, both with respect to how it works and to its physiological role in cellular function (Nathanson, 1977). Subcellular distribution studies have found guanylate cyclase mostly in soluble fractions. However, this could reflect a loosely bound enzyme. Like adenylate cyclase, it appears to be responsive to neurotransmitters, including acetylcholine, histamine, norepinephrine, and glutamate (Greengard, 1978).

Both adenylate cyclase and guanylate cyclase are stimulated by calcium (Nathanson, 1977), which may play a role in the actions of cyclic nucleotides (Berridge, 1975; Rasmussen & Goodman, 1977). Calcium movements could regulate the activities of these enzymes under different physiological conditions, including modulation of neurotransmission.

Cyclic nucleotides exert their biological actions through specific protein kinases in membranes that promote protein phosphorylation (Greengard, 1978; Williams & Rodnight, 1977). The proteins are subsequently dephosphorylated by phosphoprotein phosphatases. Protein phosphorylation is believed to be involved in a number of biological functions, including regulating enzymatic activity and ion permeability. In this latter case, protein phosphorylation might change the conformation of the protein in a manner allowing for an increased passage of certain ions. An illustration of the relationship of the cyclases with protein kinases is found in Figure 5-2.

Acute effects of ethanol on adenylate cyclase in the brain

The action of alcohols on the enzymes associated with cyclic nucleotide metabolism has been studied in earnest only recently. Although acute ethanol administration *in vivo* had been previously shown to have no effect on adenylate cyclase nor phosphodiesterase activities (Kuriyama & Israel, 1973), experiments in which ethanol was added *in vitro* to brain homogenates have indicated that ethanol can stimulate adenylate cyclase. Ethanol in concentrations as low as 68 mM (313 mg/dl) increased dopamine-sensitive adenylate cyclase activity in mouse striatum in a concentration-dependent manner and was fully reversible (Rabin & Molinoff, 1981). Basal adenylate cyclase activity was also increased by ethanol, but a minimum concentration of 168 mM (773 mg/dl) was required. These effects were due to an increase in the maximum activity of the enzyme (V_{max}) and were not mediated through the release of catecholamines acting

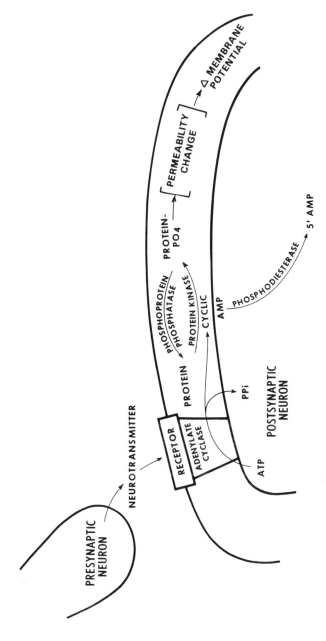

Figure 5-2. Diagram of synapse, including the relationship between the presynaptic terminal, adenylate cyclase, protein kinase, and physiological responses. From P. Greengard, *Cyclic nucleotides, phosphorylated proteins, and neuronal function.* New York: Raven Press, 1978. Reprinted by permission.

on their receptors, since dopaminergic, α-adrenergic, and β-adrenergic antagonists could not block the stimulation of adenylate cyclase activity by ethanol. Maximum activity was increased 26 and 71% with concentrations of ethanol of 100 and 300 mM (460 and 1380 mg/dl), respectively.

In another study, ethanol stimulated striatal adenylate cyclase activity in a concentration-dependent manner when guanine nucleotides were included in the assay medium (Luthin & Tabakoff, 1984). A significant effect of slightly less than 10% could be observed with a concentration of ethanol of 50 mM (230 mg/dl). Kinetic analysis revealed that this stimulation reflected an increase in V_{max} similar to that observed with dopamine-stimulated adenylate cyclase without added guanine nucleotides. NaF-stimulated adenylate cyclase activity was also enhanced by ethanol. Finally, the transition temperatures from an Arrhenius analysis of basal, dopamine-, and NaF-stimulated adenylate cyclase activities were not altered by ethanol in concentrations of 75–750 mM (345–3450 mg/dl) (Hoffman & Tabakoff, 1982). However, in the presence of guanine nucleotides, the transition temperature was reduced in the presence of benzyl alcohol (Needham & Houslay, 1982). These data suggested that ethanol acts on the guanine nucleotide, regulatory protein and facilitates the activity of the catalytic unit, thereby enhancing cAMP synthesis.

Basal, isoproterenol-, and NaF–adenylate activities in the presence of GTP in the cerebral cortex and cerebellum were also stimulated by ethanol (Rabin & Molinoff, 1981). The lowest concentration used was 300 mM (1380 mg/dl).

In order to gain further information on the role of the regulatory and catalytic subunits in the effect of ethanol on adenylate cyclase, variants of the S49 lymphoma cell line were employed (Rabin & Molinoff, 1983). The variants differ in the completeness of the components of the receptor-adenylate cyclase complex. Ethanol increased adenylate cyclase in all the variants, except the CYC$^-$ line that does not contain a regulatory subunit. In brain tissue from the caudate nucleus, ethanol increased V_{max} of adenylate cyclase in the presence of GTP, consistent with that reported by Luthin and Tabakoff (1984). In the presence of dopamine and GTP, ethanol did not activate the enzyme any further than dopamine or GTP alone. Inclusion in the medium of cholera toxin, which enhances adenylate cyclase activity by preventing the hydrolysis of GTP, did not alter the stimulatory effect of ethanol on the enzyme, suggesting that ethanol does not inhibit inactivation. Taken together, the data further support an action of ethanol on the regulatory subunit of adenylate cyclase.

Prostaglandins can also stimulate adenylate cyclase (Nathanson, 1977). Ethanol was tested for its ability to alter this stimulation (Rotrosen, Mandio, Segarnick, Traficante, & Gershon, 1980). Ethanol elevated prostaglandin-stimulated cAMP formation in striatal slices, but only at concentrations of at least 100 mM (460 mg/dl). Guanine nucleotides were not included in the assays.

Ethanol stimulates or has no effect on adenylate cyclase in other tissues besides the brain, except for the stomach (discussed in a later section). These include the liver, kidney, intestine, fat, and skin (Gorman & Bitensky, 1970; Greene, Herman, & Kraemer, 1971; Mashiter, Mashiter, & Field, 1974; Stock & Schmidt, 1978; Vesely, Lehotay, & Levey, 1978; Yoshikawa, Adachi, Halprin, & Levine, 1976). However, unphysiologically high concentrations of ethanol were required in most cases to induce an effect.

Chronic effects of ethanol on adenylate cyclase in the brain

The effect of chronic ethanol treatment on the adenylate cyclase system was studied in a number of laboratories, using a variety of approaches. Using the most direct methods, adenylate cyclase was measured in homogenates with and without transmitter stimulation. An early study indicated that basal adenylate cyclase activity in the cerebral cortex from mice was significantly elevated after 1–3 weeks of ethanol administration in a liquid diet (Israel, Kimura, & Kuriyama, 1972; Kuriyama & Israel, 1973). Sodium fluoride stimulation was unaffected.

In mice treated with ethanol in a liquid diet for 7 days, dopamine-sensitive adenylate cyclase was slightly reduced by about 15% of the corpus striatum, but only at 24 hr after withdrawal (Tabakoff & Hoffman, 1979). No effect was observed at 8 hr, 3 days, and 7 days after withdrawal. Addition of 50 mM (230 mg/dl) ethanol to the assay medium reversed the inhibition of 24 hr. A replication of this study in another laboratory did not find any effect of chronic ethanol treatment on dopamine-sensitive adenylate cyclase activity (Rabin, Wolfe, Dibner, Zahniser, Melchoir, & Molinoff, 1980). Also, no effect on activity was reported in rats treated for 4 or 8 days with ethanol by intragastric intubation (Hunt, Majchrowicz, Dalton, Swartzwelder, & Wixon, 1979; Seeber & Kuschinsky, 1976). Adenylate cyclase activity in the caudate nucleus in the presence of guanine nucleotides after chronic ethanol administration has not been reported.

Finally, the ability of calcium to stimulate adenylate cyclase after ethanol administration has been examined (von Hungen & Baxter, 1982). This stimulation was not altered after 3 weeks of ethanol consumption in a liquid diet.

Another approach taken in chronic studies involving adenylate cyclase has been the measurement of [³H]cAMP formation from [³H]adenine in brain slices *in vitro*. This cAMP generating system can be stimulated by neurotransmitters. In one study, mice were given ethanol in a liquid diet for 2 weeks and basal cAMP formation in slices from the cerebral cortex was elevated two-fold (Israel *et al.*, 1972). Addition of norepinephrine to the incubation medium did not further enhance activity. It was not clear whether the animals had been withdrawn from ethanol or what the blood ethanol concentrations were at the time the animals were killed.

More recently, rats were given ethanol for up to 4 days by intragastric intubation (Smith, Jacobyansky, Shen, Pathman, & Thurman, 1981). Both cerebral basal and norepinephrine-stimulated cAMP formation was elevated, but only after 4 days of treatment. However, after only 3 days of treatment, increased cAMP formation could be observed, if the animals were withdrawn from ethanol. This effect was maximal 16–18 hr after withdrawal, at a time when withdrawal syndrome scores were highest. By 24 hr after withdrawal, cAMP formation returned to control levels. The stimulation of cAMP formation by chronic ethanol treatment is probably mediated by β-adrenergic receptors, since addition of propranolol to the incubation medium blocked this effect (Smith, 1981).

One particular set of experiments has provided some very interesting information concerning the effect of long-term chronic ethanol treatment on the cAMP generating system. In these studies, rats consumed ethanol in the drinking fluid for 16 weeks. Two hours after ethanol was withdrawn, cerebral norepinephrine-stimulated cAMP formation was considerably reduced as shown by a 4.3-fold shift to the right in the norepinephrine concentration–response curves (French, Palmer, Narod, Reid, & Ramey, 1975; French, Reid, Palmer, Narod, & Ramey, 1974). However, 3 days after withdrawal the opposite response was obtained. Norepinephrine-stimulated cAMP formation was significantly elevated with the concentration–response curves for norepinephrine shifted to the left 2.4-fold (French & Palmer, 1973; French et al., 1975). No changes in the maximum response to norepinephrine were observed in any of the studies. Also, the adrenergic supersensitivity appeared relatively nonspecific, since both α- and β-adrenergic antagonists only partially reduced the enhanced activity, which was also apparent with other agonists including histamine and serotonin (French, Palmer, & Narod, 1975). A similar subsensitivity was observed in the liver after chronic ethanol administration, but no supersensitivity was found 3 days after withdrawal (French, Palmer, & Narod, 1976).

Effects of ethanol on protein kinases in the brain

Since cyclic nucleotides induce their biological effects on protein kinases, a study of whether ethanol could exert an action on the cAMP-dependent protein kinase in mouse brain was undertaken (Kuriyama, Nakagawa, Muramatsu, & Kakita, 1976). Sixty minutes after a single 4-g/kg intraperitoneal dose of ethanol, no effect on either basal or cAMP-dependent protein kinase activity in the cerebral cortex was observed. However, 2 weeks after ethanol administration in a liquid diet, synaptosomal cAMP-dependent protein kinase activity was elevated four-fold. By 7 days after withdrawal, activity had returned to control values.

Effects of ethanol on guanylate cyclase in the brain

Guanylate cyclase activity has been examined in a number of tissues, including the brain, heart, liver, pancreas, intestine, stomach, spleen, lung, and kidney. Ethanol added to tissue homogenates had an inhibitory effect. In all cases, however, unphysiologically high concentrations of ethanol were generally required to observe any effect on the enzyme *in vitro* (Hunt, Redos, Dalton, & Catravas, 1977; Vesely *et al.*, 1978; Vesely & Levey, 1977).

After chronic ethanol administration, guanylate cyclase activity was reported to be elevated, but this depended on how long the animals were treated. If animals received ethanol for only 24 hr, no change in activity was observed in mouse cerebral cortex (Kuriyama, 1977). However, when mice were treated for up to 8 weeks with ethanol in a liquid diet, guanylate cyclase activity in the vestibular nuclei slowly increased over the first 10 days (Eliasson, Kiessling, & Scarpellini, 1981). But after 8 weeks of treatment, activity had returned to control levels.

Effects of ethanol on cyclic nucleotide content in the brain

The effectiveness of cyclic nucleotides as second messengers in the process of synaptic transmission depends, in part, on the concentration of cyclic nucleotides in contact with the protein kinases. Consequently, it would be reasonable to determine whether changes in cyclic nucleotide concentrations are altered by ethanol as a possible result of changes in adenylate or guanylate cyclase activities.

Numerous studies have appeared over the last 10 years studying the effects of acute and chronic administration of ethanol on cyclic nucleotide concentrations in various parts of the brain (see review of Hunt, 1979). The effect of acute ethanol treatment on cAMP levels has been controversial. Both increases and decreases, depending on the area of the brain examined, and no effect at all have been reported (Breese, Lundberg, Mailman, Frye, & Mueller, 1979; Orenberg, Renson, & Barchas, 1976; Redos, Hunt, & Catravas, 1976; Volicer & Gold, 1973). Since there is a significant postmortem accumulation of cAMP (Schmidt, Schmidt, & Robinson, 1971), the issues associated with these studies related to how fast adenylate cyclase and phosphodiesterase were inactivated. When the enzymes were inactivated by focusing a high-intensity microwave beam on the head of the animal, no change in cAMP levels was observed (Breese *et al.*, 1979; Redos, Hunt, & Catravas, 1976). With slower methods of inactivation cAMP levels were generally reduced (Orenberg *et al.*, 1976; Volicer & Gold, 1973). This might result from a depressed rate of postmortem elevation of cAMP after ethanol treatment (Volicer & Gold, 1973).

Single doses of ethanol have consistently reduced cGMP in most areas of the brain examined (e.g., Hunt et al., 1977; Volicer & Hurter, 1977). The effect was dose dependent and was most pronounced in the cerebellum. In fact, a 6-g/kg oral dose of ethanol could deplete cerebellar cGMP by as much as 95% within 2 hr (Redos, Catravas, & Hunt, 1976). Since guanylate cyclase activity is stimulated by calcium, the effect of ethanol on cerebellar cGMP levels was examined when ethanol was administered concurrently with the calcium ionophore A23187 (Dodson & Johnson, 1980). Although A23187 could itself raise cGMP levels, it had no effect on the ability of ethanol to deplete cGMP.

In spite of the dramatic effects of ethanol administration on cGMP levels, the significance of the observations has been questioned because of possible involvement of altered motor and respiratory function after ethanol treatment (Lundberg, Breese, Mailman, Frye, & Mueller, 1979). Paralyzing animals or altering arterial carbon dioxide and oxygen tensions significantly reduced control cerebellar cGMP levels and the effectiveness of ethanol to deplete cGMP. Therefore, this effect of ethanol might be secondary to other physiological responses. Also, the data presented do not demonstrate a correlation between cyclic nucleotide levels and enzymatic activity responsible for synthesizing the cyclic nucleotides.

Chronic ethanol treatment has generally resulted in increases in cyclic nucleotide levels. This has depended on how long the animals had been treated. After oral administration of ethanol for only 4 days, no alterations in either cAMP or cGMP concentrations were found in any of the areas of the brain examined (Hunt et al., 1977). However, with treatments of 6 days to 4 weeks, elevations in both nucleotides have been reported (Eliasson et al., 1981; Kuriyama & Israel, 1973; Shen, Jacobyansky, Pathman, & Thurman, 1983; Volicer & Hurter, 1977). In some cases, these changes have occurred at times when adenylate and guanylate cyclase activities or cAMP synthesis in brain slices were also elevated (Eliasson et al., 1981; Kuriyama & Israel, 1973; Shen et al., 1983; Smith et al., 1981). However, comparative time course studies have not tended to demonstrate a direct relationship between cyclic nucleotide synthetic activity and corresponding tissue concentrations.

Two studies have attempted to modify ethanol tolerance and dependence by administering to animals cyclic nucleotides or their dibutyryl derivatives. In one study, the ability of ethanol to induce acute tolerance was examined in rats using the hexobarbital anesthesia threshold (Wahlström, 1975). Acute tolerance can develop within a few hours after a single dose of ethanol. Fifteen minutes after an intraperitoneal dose of ethanol, less hexobarbital was needed to induce anesthesia than when ethanol was given 3 hr before the test, even though the blood ethanol concentrations were similar. Brain ethanol concentrations were not determined. Pretreatment with an intravenous dose of cAMP of 10 mg/kg, 6 hr before the test, enhanced the acute tolerance induced by ethanol. The significance of the data is unclear because it is unlikely that much cAMP would get into the brain, in part because of esterases in blood that would metabolize cAMP and because cAMP does not cross the blood–brain barrier.

In another study, the dibutyryl derivatives of cAMP and cGMP were tested for their efficacy in altering ethanol withdrawal-induced head twitches in mice (Collier, Hammond, & Schneider, 1976). When injected into the ventricular system of the brain, dibutyryl cAMP reduced the head twitches, while dibutyryl cGMP enhanced them.

Effects of ethanol on the stomach

Another organ in which the effect of ethanol has been studied to some extent is the stomach. Ethanol alters gastric acid secretion, a process thought to be mediated by cAMP (Amer, 1972; Kimberg, 1974), depending on the species (Lorber, Vincente, & Chey, 1974). To study the role of cAMP in the action of ethanol, ethanol was applied directly onto the gastric mucosa from a number of species. Concentrations of 217–10,900 mM (1000–50,000 mg/dl) were used. These concentrations are not unlike those obtained from drinking commercial alcoholic beverages (3–50% ethanol).

In the rat, increasing concentrations of ethanol depressed both acid secretion and cAMP levels (Puurunen & Karppanen, 1975). A biphasic effect on both acid secretion and cAMP levels was observed in the dog (Beazell & Ivy, 1940; Puurunen, Karppanen, Kairaluoma, & Larmi, 1976). At concentrations of ethanol below 4350 mM (20,000 mg/dl), both acid secretion and cAMP levels were increased. However, above these concentrations ethanol reduced both factors. Finally, in humans, ethanol stimulated both acid secretion and mucosal cAMP levels (Karppanen, Puurunen, Kairaluoma, & Larmi, 1976).

In attempting to determine the mechanism underlying the effect of ethanol on mucosal cAMP levels, adenylate cyclase activity was measured in the presence of ethanol. Ethanol tended to modify enzymatic activity in a manner analogous to the ethanol-induced changes in cAMP levels. In humans, adenylate cyclase activity was stimulated (Karppanen *et al.*, 1976), whereas in the rat, it was inhibited (Puurunen & Karppanen, 1975). In the dog, adenylate cyclase was increased at concentrations of ethanol associated with elevated cAMP concentrations (Puurunen *et al.*, 1976). At the higher concentrations of ethanol associated with reduced cAMP content, no effect of ethanol on adenylate cyclase was observed.

In another approach, the concentration of the synthetic precursor of cAMP, ATP, was measured in the gastric mucosa after ethanol application. In both rats and dogs, ATP and cAMP levels were reduced, suggesting that the availability of ATP for the synthesis of cAMP may be an important determinant in the action of ethanol on cAMP levels in these species (Puurunen, Hiltunen, & Karppanen, 1977; Tague & Shanbour, 1977).

Since prostaglandins inhibit gastric acid secretion (Bennett & Fleshler, 1970; Wilson, 1972), the possible role of these substances in the action of ethanol on acid secretion was examined. Rats were pretreated with inhibitors of prostaglandin synthesis and the ability of ethanol to depress acid secretion in this species was measured (Karppanen & Puurunen, 1976; Puurunen, 1978). Ethanol could reduce acid secretion in control animals. However, in those animals pretreated with prostaglandin synthesis inhibitors, this effect was antagonized. No measurements of cAMP levels or adenylate cyclase activity were reported in these experiments. These data suggested that ethanol may stimulate prostaglandin synthesis.

Commentary

From the available evidence, ethanol can stimulate adenylate cyclase, but not guanylate cyclase activities *in vitro* using brain preparations. In the caudate nucleus, the efficacy of this stimulation of adenylate cyclase depends on the presence of dopamine or guanine nucleotides. Even in the presence of guanine nucleotides, the effect of ethanol in physiologically compatible concentrations on adenylate cyclase activity tends to be small. In addition, the role of guanine nucleotides in the physiological function of adenylate cyclase *in vivo* has not been demonstrated. There is yet no information to support a role of adenylate cyclase stimulation by ethanol in its intoxicating properties.

In the stomach, the possibility that adenylate cyclase might play a role in ethanol-induced alterations in gastric acid secretion is more compelling. Most studies generally indicate that a correlation exists between acid secretion and adenylate cyclase activity with accompanying changes in cAMP concentrations after ethanol exposure. Both increases and decreases in these parameters have been observed, depending on the species and concentration of ethanol used. Although the concentrations of ethanol necessary to induce these effects are quite high, they are similar to those found in alcoholic beverages. Consequently, the local effect of ethanol on the stomach in these concentrations is quite possible after drinking such beverages.

How ethanol exerts its effect on adenylate cyclase is unknown. Because of its apparently direct interaction with membranes (see Chapter 2), ethanol may alter the environment of the enzyme complex in such a manner as to change enzymatic activity.

Lipids appear to play a role in adenylate cyclase activity, since removing lipids from membranes destroys activity (Lefkowitz, Limbird, Mukherjee, & Caron, 1976). An interaction of ethanol with membrane lipids could be a factor in altered enzymatic activity. A number of agents in addition to alcohols exist that can either increase or decrease the intrinsic order of membranes. A few studies measured both membrane order and adenylate cyclase activity after exposure to these agents. For example, cis-vaccenic acid and benzyl alcohol can disorder membranes and stimulate adenylate cyclase from turkey erythrocytes and hepatic plasma membranes, respectively (Gordon, Sauerheber, Esgate, Dipple, Marchmont, & Houslay, 1980; Hanski, Rimon, & Levitzki, 1979). It was suggested that the increased fluidity facilitated the coupling of the regulatory protein with the catalytic unit. On the other hand, increasing the cholesterol content of Chinese hamster ovary cells resulted in a more rigid membrane and an enhanced adenylate cyclase activity (Sinensky, Minnenan, & Molinoff, 1979). Elevated adenylate cyclase activity associated with either increased or decreased order of the membrane could be a function of how the treatments alter membrane order or the preparation under study. It would appear that a systematic study that would attempt to correlate membrane order with adenylate cyclase activity after ethanol exposure in the same tissue would be warranted.

Chronic treatment with ethanol alters adenylate cyclase activity or cAMP synthesis in brain slices, especially if the duration of treatment was long. In most cases, there appears to be a biphasic effect depending on the state of the animal after ethanol withdrawal. If intoxication is present, neurotransmitter-stimulated cAMP synthesis is depressed. However, during the days after withdrawal, neurotransmitter-stimulated cAMP synthesis is accelerated. There is no clear relationship between the two effects on cAMP synthesis, since the enhanced enzymatic activity can be observed after shorter ethanol exposures than can the depressed activity. On the other hand, both effects have been associated with parallel changes in β-adrenergic ligand binding after 60 days of ethanol treatment (see Chapter 6).

To what extent changes in adenylate cyclase activity or cAMP synthesis in brain slices are related to tolerance or physical dependence is not clear. No consistent correlations have been found between these phenomena.

It cannot be determined from the reported data whether the changes in synthetic activity observed after chronic ethanol administration are a result of adaptation to a constant interaction between ethanol and the receptor–adenylate cyclase complex or a response to changes in presynaptic input (Dismukes & Daly, 1976). The first possibility is feasible to account for the depressed synthetic activity observed after chronic ethanol administration. Such an adaptation could occur over a long period of time even with the low-level stimulatory effect of ethanol. Also, if membranes become more rigid with chronic ethanol administration (Lyon & Goldstein, 1983), it might be more difficult for the components of the receptor-adenylate cyclase complex to couple (Tabakoff & Hoffman, 1979).

The rather rapid reversal from depression to stimulation of synthetic activity after ethanol withdrawal might suggest a response to altered presynaptic input. For example, norepinephrine turnover is increased after ethanol withdrawal (Hunt & Majchrowicz, 1974; Pohorecky, Jaffe, & Berkeley, 1974; Thadani, Kulig, Brown, & Beard, 1976). This may demand a greater cAMP synthetic activity to mediate the enhanced stimulation of adrenergic receptors. It is interesting to note that in one laboratory in which mice were treated with ethanol for 2 weeks, increased adenylate cyclase activity, cAMP levels, and cAMP-dependent protein kinase activity were all observed (Kuriyama & Israel, 1973; Kuriyama *et al.*, 1976).

Other enzymes

A number of reports have appeared that study several other enzymes in membranes. One area of interest relates to phospholipid metabolism. In Chapter 2, evidence suggesting that chronic ethanol administration may alter lipid composition in membranes was discussed. Consequently, changes in the enzymatic machinery involved in the synthesis or degradation of lipids would be of interest to study after ethanol treatment. Unfortunately, few studies have appeared on this subject.

Phospholipid metabolism has been examined after both acute and chronic ethanol treatment involving measurements of the turnover of various phospholipids in membranes. In one report, phospholipid turnover was measured in synaptosomal and microsomal fractions by determining the rate of incorporation *in vivo* of intraventricularly injected [^{3}H]glycerol and [^{32}P]phosphoric acid into phosphatidylcholine (PC), phosphatidylinositol plus phosphatidylserine (PI + PS), and phosphatidylethanolamine (PE) (Lee, Friedman, & Loh, 1980). After a single, 3.5-g/kg intraperitoneal dose of ethanol, incorporation of [^{3}H]glycerol, but not [^{32}P]phosphoric acid, was accelerated into PC and PI + PS fractions, 1 hr after treatment. When rats were rendered tolerant by intragastric intubation of 3 g/kg of ethanol, twice a day for 3 days, there was no tolerance to the acute effect of ethanol on phospholipid turnover. In fact, increases in incorporation of ^{32}P-labeled synaptosomal and microsomal PI + PS and microsomal PC fractions were observed over that obtained with an acute dose of ethanol. Finally, in ethanol-dependent rats, which received up to 6 g/kg, three times a day for 3 days, only the ^{32}P-labeled microsomal PE fractions were increased when the animals were still intoxicated. During the ethanol withdrawal syndrome, the ^{3}H-labeled synaptosomal PI + PS fraction was elevated and the ^{32}P-labeled microsomal PI + PS fraction was reduced. In the heart, the incorporation of [^{3}H-methyl]methionine, but not [^{3}H]choline into PC was accelerated after chronic ethanol administration (Prasad & Edwards, 1983). This effect was due to an increase in phospholipid methyltransferase activity.

In another study, 7% ethanol was administered in a liquid diet for 8 days and the incorporation of ^{32}P into PI and phosphoric acid in synaptosomes was measured (Smith, 1981). No effect was observed on incorporation with or without stimulation with carbamylcholine, a cholinergic agonist. Addition of 100-mM (460-mg/dl) ethanol to synaptosomal preparations from untreated animals reduced carbamylcholine-induced increases of ^{32}P incorporation into phosphatidic acid with no effect on unstimulated incorporation.

The turnover of acyl groups on phospholipids has been studied after chronic ethanol administration (Sun, Creech, Corbin, & Sun, 1977). This was done by measuring the rate of incorporation of [$1-^{14}C$]arachidonic acid into 1-acyl-glycerophosphorylcholine (GPC). When rats were treated with two daily 4-g/kg oral doses of ethanol for 21 days, ^{14}C-labeled GPC was elevated 8–24 hr after withdrawal. A greater increase was observed when the animals drank ethanol in the drinking water for 13 months.

Ecto-5'-nucleotidase, an outer-surface enzyme, has been studied after ethanol exposure in the cell membranes of glial C6 cell lines grown in culture. This enzyme is believed to catalyze the conversion of membrane-impermeable nucleotides to membrane-permeable nucleosides, such as adenosine. Acute ethanol exposure in concentrations of 10–100 mM (46–460 mg/dl) increased the activity of ecto-5'-nucleotidase in a concentration-dependent manner up to 42% (Syapin, Stefanovic, Mandel, & Noble, 1980a). Higher concentrations of ethanol had no further effect. If the ethanol was removed from the medium the activity returned to control values.

Stimulation of ecto-5'-nucleotidase activity was also observed after exposure of the cells to 100-mM (460-mg/dl) ethanol for 6–8 days and the subsequent removal of the ethanol (Syapin et al., 1980a). The addition of ethanol at concentrations below 150 mM (690 mg/dl) did not further increase enzymatic activity, suggesting the development of tolerance to the acute effects of ethanol. A kinetic analysis of activity without added ethanol indicated that K_m of the enzyme for 5'-AMP was increased without an effect on V_{max} (Syapin, Stefanovic, Mandel, & Noble, 1980b). The data were interpreted to suggest that the membrane had undergone a structural rearrangement thereby increasing the availability of the active site of the enzyme.

Protein phosphorylation has been studied in erythrocyte ghosts after acute and chronic ethanol treatment (Pant, Virmani, & Majchrowicz, 1982). A single 6-g/kg oral dose of ethanol was without effect. However, after 4 days of chronic ethanol treatment administered by gastric intubation, protein phosphorylation was elevated. Calcium which normally inhibited phosphorylation was less effective.

Uptake mechanisms

A number of substances are actively transported into cells by energy-mediated carrier systems. After being released into the synaptic cleft, many neurotransmitters are inactivated by being taken up by nerve endings or glial cells (Cooper, Bloom, & Roth, 1982). These uptake mechanisms are energy dependent and may derive this energy from the Na-K-ATPase (Bogdanski, Tissari, & Brodie, 1968).

Several studies have attempted to determine whether ethanol can alter these uptake systems. In general, ethanol in nonlethal concentrations did not change the uptake of catecholamines, serotonin, GABA, and glutamate into synaptosomes *in vitro* or after administration of a single dose of ethanol (Mullin & Ferko, 1983; Roach, Davis, Pennington, & Nordyke, 1973; Thadani & Truitt, 1977). In ethanol-dependent rats treated for 7 days by inhalation, only glutamate uptake was altered and was increased (Roach *et al.*, 1973).

In other experiments, the effect of ethanol was examined on high-affinity choline uptake (Hunt, Majchrowicz, & Dalton, 1979; Jope & Jenden, 1981). Measurements of high-affinity choline uptake have been used as an index of acetylcholine synthesis and release (Murrin, DeHaven, & Kuhar, 1977). Although ethanol had no direct effect on high-affinity choline uptake in concentrations up to 200 mM (920 mg/dl), ethanol either elevated or reduced uptake in rats given a single dose of ethanol, depending on the area of the brain studied. In the striatum, ethanol increased choline uptake in a dose-dependent manner, but only at blood ethanol concentrations above 43.5 mM (200 mg/dl). In the hippocampus, uptake was reduced only when blood ethanol concentrations exceeded 87.0 mM (400 mg/dl). In rats chronically treated for 4 days by intragastric intubation, high-affinity choline uptake was not altered when the animals were intoxicated or during overt withdrawal signs (Hunt *et al.*, 1979). However, 24 hr after withdrawal, choline uptake was elevated only in the striatum, returning to control values after 7 days.

High-affinity choline uptake has also been studied in cultured cells exposed to ethanol (Massarelli, Syapin, & Noble, 1976). The cell lines included hamster NN astroblasts, rat C6 glioblasts, mouse neuroblastoma c1300 adrenergic clone M1, and S21 cholinergic clone. Ethanol in a concentration of 100 mM (460 mg/dl) had no effect on choline uptake in any of the cell lines exposed for 15 min. Chronic exposure of the cells to the same concentration of ethanol, however, in most cases resulted in transient increases in high-affinity choline uptake. The duration of exposure required to induce this effect was an important variable. The S21 cholinergic neuroblasts needed to be exposed to ethanol for only 7 days to obtain a 40% increase in activity. The glial cell lines required exposure time of 15–34 days. With further exposure, the elevated uptake disappeared. Withdrawal of ethanol did not alter activity in any of the cell lines.

Commentary

From the evidence presented, there is no conclusive evidence to suggest that there is a direct action of ethanol *in vivo* on membrane-bound enzymes after a single dose nor that such action could mediate any of the physiological responses that are described as intoxication. In most cases, the concentrations of ethanol required to elicit a significant effect are generally too high to be compatible with life. In instances where concentrations of ethanol below 100 mM (460 mg/dl) were able to alter enzymatic activity, the conditions under which it would occur were not clearly analogous to a physiological condition found *in vivo*. Indeed, this is a major problem in interpreting enzymatic activities *in vitro*.

In most cases, enzymes are studied under optimal conditions, that is, conditions under which activity is maximal at given substrate and cofactor concentrations. In general, measurements of enzymatic activity *in vitro* reflect the total capacity and properties of an enzyme to catalyze a chemical reaction. Under *in vivo* conditions, the influence of such factors as substrate availability and/or the interactive properties of various possible modulators or enzymatic activity are often difficult to determine.

In the case of substrate availability with respect to the two major enzyme systems discussed, the Na-K-ATPase and adenylate cyclase, ATP is the substrate for both of them. There has not always been agreement on the effect of ethanol on tissue ATP concentrations, but when an alteration has been observed, ATP concentrations were decreased, such as in the brain and stomach (Puurunen *et al.*, 1977; Tague & Shanbour, 1977; Veloso, Passaneau, & Veech, 1972). It would be difficult to reconcile an inhibition in the brain of Na-K-ATPase activity on the one hand, and stimulation of adenylate cyclase on the other, if ATP availability were an important factor in the reported changes.

One way in which the role of enzymes can be examined *in vivo* is with the use of activators and inhibitors of the enzymes. Measuring a physiological endpoint and correlating it to changes in enzymatic activity after drug pretreatment can provide indirect evidence for or against the possible involvement of the enzyme in expressing the endpoint. Unfortunately, such drugs that act on the Na-K-ATPase and adenylate cyclase are either nonspecific or induce other actions that makes the interpretation of the information obtained difficult.

The responses of membrane-bound enzymes to chronic ethanol administration suggest that the properties of membranes may change as a result of constant perturbation. This would be consistent with information described in other chapters of this book, such as alterations in membrane composition (see Chapter 2) and in the properties of neurotransmitter receptors (see Chapter 6). It is interesting to note instances of parallel changes in several related parameters under similar experimental circumstances, as has been observed with noradrenergic receptor binding and cAMP synthesis. However, it is difficult to relate these changes to such manifestations of chronic ethanol treatment as tolerance and physical dependence. The biggest problem of interpretation is whether these changes are the cause or a result of the physiological phenomena.

In summary, ethanol may exert some of its actions on membranes through enzymes embedded in it. However, it remains to be determined whether significant and sufficient alterations exist *in vivo* that can account for some of the complex actions of ethanol.

6. Neuroreceptors

As discussed in Chapter 5, an ethanol-induced change in the microenvironment of a membrane may have profound effects on the ability of functional entities within membranes to perform their normal actions. Since neurotransmitters transfer electrical information from neuron to neuron by interacting with appropriate receptors on the surface of postsynaptic neurons, an action of ethanol on membranes may result in a disruption of the normal translation of transmitter–receptor derived information into electrical impulses. In this chapter, we shall examine the reports addressing this issue and attempt to put into perspective the relevance of the observations.

Over the last decade, the general approach to studying the properties of receptors has involved the binding characteristics of radioligands that interact specifically with a given receptor. To understand the significance and potential limitations in the interpretation of generated data, we shall begin with a discussion of the basis of such measurements.

Methodological considerations

In all binding studies, the two parameters that are most often determined are the affinity of the ligand for the receptor and the maximum number of binding sites, that is, the number of receptors, in the tissue. Both the affinity and the maximum number of binding sites are indexes of the efficiency of neurotransmitter–receptor interactions and, therefore, of the proper transmission of electrical information from one neuron to another.

The basic premise of binding studies is that a radioligand interacts with a receptor with a certain affinity and this interaction is defined by the following equation:

$$[L] + [R] \underset{k_{-1}}{\overset{k_1}{\rightleftharpoons}} [LR] \tag{1}$$

where [L] is the concentration of the ligand, [R] the concentration of the receptor, [LR] the concentration of the ligand–receptor complex, and k_{-1} and k_1 the dissociation and association rate constants, respectively. Since there is only a finite concentration of receptors, the maximum number of binding sites (B_{max}) can be defined as

$$B_{max} = [LR] + [R] \tag{2}$$

Since [LR] depends on the affinity of the ligand for the receptor, as measured by the equilibrium dissociation constant (K_D),

$$K_D = k_{-1}/k_1 = [L][R]/[LR] \tag{3}$$

By substituting Equation 3 into Equation 2 and rearranging, [LR] can be expressed as

$$[LR] = B_{max}[L]/([L] + K_D) \tag{4}$$

If [LR] is considered the amount of ligand bound (B) to the receptor and [L] the free, unbound concentration of ligand (F), then substituting B for [LR] and F for [L] yields

$$B = B_{max}F/(F + K_D) \tag{5}$$

Rearranging Equation 5,

$$B/F = (B_{max} - B)/K_D \tag{6}$$

Equation 6 is the classic Scatchard equation from which standard calculations of affinity (K_D) and maximum number of binding sites (B_{max}) are computed. When a single population of binding sites exists, a linear function is obtained, where

$$K_D = -1/\text{slope} \quad \text{and} \quad B_{max} = B \quad \text{when } B/F = 0 \tag{7}$$

For a more complete derivation of these equations, the reader should consult Bennett (1978).

In practice, K_D and B_{max} are determined experimentally by measuring the amount of radioligand specifically bound (B) to receptors at different radioligand concentrations after equilibrium has been attained. The tissue is incubated with the radioligand in a suitable medium for an appropriate period of time and then the bound and unbound ligands are separated from one another by rapid filtration or centrifugation. Specific binding is considered binding actually to receptors and is saturable. Nonspecific binding, which is unsaturable, generally represents nonreceptor interactions with tissue, the incubation vessel, or the glass fiber filters normally used. Nonspecific binding is determined by measuring binding in the presence of a specific inhibitor of radioligand binding. The difference between total binding and nonspecific binding represents specific binding.

The specific binding (B) determined at each radioligand concentration is plotted against B/F. From the linear relationship obtained, K_D and B_{max} can be calculated from Equation 7. B_{max} is considered the apparent number of binding sites, since the maximum number of sites cannot always be determined. Some sites may be embedded deep in a membrane where the ligand cannot react with it. An example of such a plot, the Scatchard plot, is given in Figure 6-1. Changes in these two parameters indicate how a particular treatment can alter receptor function.

The knowledge of the properties of neuroreceptors has advanced considerably over the last decade. Using radioligand techniques, receptors for a variety of neurotransmitters have been described, including various subtypes with selective functions of their own (Snyder, Bruns, Daly, & Innes, 1981). Based on tissue distributions of these subtypes, opportunities for selective actions by specially designed drugs have been pursued. In the remainder of this chapter, we shall examine the responses of various transmitter receptors to ethanol exposure and relate them to presynaptic actions of ethanol.

Catecholamine receptors

The properties of the receptors for dopamine and norepinephrine have been extensively characterized and a number of subtypes have been identified for both receptor systems (Creese, Sibley, Leff, & Hamblin, 1981; Hoffman & Lefkowitz, 1980; Kebabian & Calne, 1979; Minneman & Molinoff, 1980; Seeman, 1980).

The existence of up to four dopamine receptors or subtypes, as indicated by different binding sites, has been postulated. This is based primarily

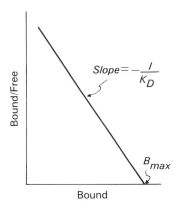

Figure 6-1. Example of a Scatchard plot, which allows for the calculation of affinity (K_D) of the ligand for the receptor and the maximum number of binding sites (B_{max}).

on their relative affinities for dopamine and dopaminergic antagonists, as summarized by Seeman (1980). Dopamine receptors have also been distinguished on the basis of whether they are linked to adenylate cyclase (Kebabian & Calne, 1979).

D-1 binding sites are related to those receptors associated with adenylate cyclase, and their stimulation leads to an increase in cAMP synthesis. They also have low affinities for dopamine and dopaminergic antagonists, such as haloperidol and spiroperidol. D-2 binding sites, on the other hand, are not linked to adenylate cyclase, and have a low affinity for dopamine but a high affinity for the antagonists. D-3 binding sites have a high affinity for dopamine but a low affinity for the antagonists. Finally, D-4 binding sites have a high affinity for both dopamine and the antagonists.

D-1 and D-2 receptors are the ones best characterized (Creese et al., 1981; Seeman, 1980). They differ not only on the basis of ligand affinity, but on cellular localizations. For example, in the caudate nucleus, where dopaminergic receptors have been studied extensively, D-1 receptors are predominantly localized on nondopaminergic cell bodies (Fuxe, Hall, & Köhler, 1979). Only about 50–60% of the D-2 binding sites are found on these cell bodies (Murrin, Gale, & Kuhar, 1979); the rest are located on corticostriatal fibers (Schwartz, Creese, Coyle, & Snyder, 1978).

D-3 and D-4 receptors and their significance are less understood. Some evidence suggests that D-3 receptors might represent, in part, dopaminergic autoreceptors located on presynaptic nerve terminals (Nagy, Lee, Seeman, & Fibiger, 1978). Autoreceptors are postulated to reduce transmitter release from these terminals when they are stimulated (Langer, 1977, 1980). D-4 receptors might represent only a conformational state of one of the other receptors sites, such as the D-2 receptor (Seeman, 1980).

Dopamine receptor binding can be regulated by guanine nucleotides. The binding of radioligands to D-1 receptors, linked to adenylate cyclase, is reduced by GTP (Creese et al., 1981). This is analogous to the absolute requirement of guanine nucleotides for optimal adenylate cyclase activity, as discussed in Chapter 5.

Finally, it should be mentioned that some of the radioligands that bind to dopaminergic receptors also bind to other receptors as well. [^{3}H]Spiroperidol, used extensively to study D-2 receptors, will bind to α-1 adrenergic and serotonin-2 receptors (these will be defined later), especially in the cerebral cortex (Leysen, Niemegeers, Tollenaere, & Laduron, 1978; Peroutka, U'Prichard, Greenberg, & Snyder, 1977). The different receptors can be distinguished with the use of specific inhibitors for these receptors in the incubation medium (Seeman, 1980).

A variety of noradrenergic receptors and subtypes have also been identified (Hoffman & Lefkowitz, 1980; Minneman & Molinoff, 1980). These receptors are broadly grouped as α- and β-adrenergic, each with its own two subtypes. The existence of α- and β-adrenergic receptors has been known for some time (Ahlquist, 1948). The β-adrenergic receptor subtypes were identified subsequently (Lands, Arnold, McAuliff, Luduena, & Brown, 1967), and then the α-adrenergic receptor subtypes (Starke, 1977). The β-adrenergic receptor subtypes β-1 and β-2, were first differentiated on the basis of their relative affinities for norepinephrine and epinephrine. β-1 receptors have about the same affinity for both norepinephrine and epinephrine, while β-2 receptors have a greater affinity for epinephrine. With radioligand binding assays, the subtypes can be characterized, using inhibitors relatively selective for each subtype (Minneman & Molinoff, 1980). Differentiating the α-receptor subtypes can also be accomplished using inhibitors selective for each subtype (Hoffman & Lefkowitz, 1980). In addition, radioligands that are subtype specific have been successfully employed.

As with dopaminergic receptors, some of the noradrenergic receptor subtypes are linked to adenylate cyclase (Lefkowitz *et al.*, 1976). Stimulation of β-receptors, both β-1 and β-2 subtypes, leads to an activation of adenylate cyclase (Williams & Lefkowitz, 1977). On the other hand, α-receptor stimulation leads to an inhibition of adenylate cyclase (Jakobs, Saur, & Schultz, 1978). Guanine nucleotides are required for a maximal effect of stimulation of both α- and β-receptors (Creese, Usdin, & Snyder, 1979).

It is well known that the long-term disruption of receptor activity, either resulting from changes in presynaptic input or from direct actions on the receptors themselves, can lead to the development of super- and subsensitivity (Schwartz, Costentin, Martres, Protais, & Baudry, 1978). Super- or subsensitivity is expressed by enhanced or reduced responses, respectively, to a normal stimulus. Receptor binding methods have been applied in an attempt to determine the mechanism by which these changes in sensitivity occur. In a number of instances, the properties of catecholamine receptors have been altered. For example, depletion of catecholamines or chronic blockade of receptors leads to an elevation in the number of catecholamine binding sites (Burt, Creese, & Snyder, 1976; Skolnick, Stalvey, Daly, Hoyler, & Davis, 1978). Conversely, long-term treatment with stimulants of receptors reduces the number of receptors (Mukherjee, Caron, & Lefkowitz, 1975).

Radioligand binding assays have been used extensively over the last 5 years to determine whether acute or chronic ethanol administration can affect receptor function. Studies of catecholamine receptors have examined a number of aspects of ethanol treatment. These have included their role in acute intoxication and in the development of tolerance and physical dependence and of brain damage. Also, the importance of various receptor subtypes has been addressed.

In general, few reports have examined whether ethanol added *in vitro* or the administration of a single dose of ethanol alters catecholamine receptor function. [³H]Spiroperidol, a dopaminergic antagonist, has been used to determine what effect ethanol has on dopaminergic receptors in the rat caudate nucleus. When ethanol was incubated *in vitro* with striatal homogenates, little effect could be convincingly demonstrated at concentrations of ethanol below 50–100 mM (230–460 mg/dl) (Hruska & Silbergeld, 1980; Reggiani, Barbaccia, Spano, & Trabucchi, 1980b). At higher concentrations, ethanol exerted a dose-dependent reduction in [³H]spiroperidol binding (Hruska & Silbergeld, 1980). Using a Scatchard analysis, ethanol reduced the affinity of the radioligand for the dopaminergic receptor without influencing the apparent number of binding sites. Upon further analysis, the decreased affinity was due to a depressed rate of association of the ligand with the receptor, while the rate of dissociation was elevated. In another study, no effect on binding could be observed at ethanol concentrations below 750 mM (3450 mg/dl) (Rabin & Molinoff, 1981).

After a single, 3-g/kg oral dose of ethanol, no change in [³H]spiroperidol binding could be detected (Barbaccia, Reggiani, Spano, & Trabucchi, 1980; Lai, Carino, & Horita, 1980). This is not surprising if it is presumed that ethanol must be in contact with the dopaminergic receptor at the time the binding determinations are made. Ethanol is washed out of the tissue during the preparation of the homogenates.

Chronic ethanol treatment has produced varying results on the binding of different radioligands for catecholamine receptors. Most of the studies examining dopaminergic receptors have used [³H]spiroperidol or [³H]haloperidol, both dopaminergic antagonists, as radioligands. The results obtained from these studies seem to depend on the duration of ethanol administration. With only 4–7 days of treatment, binding was unaffected in the caudate nucleus (Hunt & Dalton, 1981; Rabin et al., 1980; Tabakoff & Hoffman, 1979). After 14 days of treatment with daily 6-g/kg oral doses of ethanol, binding was elevated (Lai et al., 1980), while after 13 months of ethanol treatment, binding was reduced 4 weeks after withdrawal, a finding related to a decrease in apparent number of binding sites (Pelham, Marquis, Kugelmann, & Munsat, 1980).

Studies examining the effect of chronic ethanol administration on noradrenergic receptor binding have been relatively consistent and have depended on the length of treatment. After 4 days of continuous intoxication, no effect was observed on either α- or β-receptor binding (Hunt & Dalton, 1981). When the treatment period was extended to 7–60 days, a reduction in the apparent number of β receptors was detected without an effect on α receptors (Banerjee, Sharma, & Khanna, 1978; Muller, Britton, & Seeman, 1980; Rabin et al., 1980). The β-2 receptor was selectively modified (Rabin et al., 1980). After 60 days of ethanol treatment, β-receptor binding was measured either while the animals were intoxicated or 3 days after withdrawal (Banerjee et al., 1978). β-Receptor binding was reduced during intoxication, but elevated 3 days after withdrawal. These changes correlated with reported alterations in catecholamine-stimulated adenylate cyclase (see Chapter 5). One study reported an increase in β-receptor binding after 10 days of ethanol inhalation, but only during the withdrawal syndrome (Kuriyama, Muramatsu, Aiso, & Ueno, 1981).

Several indirect pharmacological studies have addressed the involvement of dopaminergic receptors in the consequences of chronic ethanol administration. Using mice treated with an ethanol-containing liquid diet for 7 days, a number of biochemical, behavioral, and physiological endpoints were examined. These endpoints related to actions of dopaminergic agonists and antagonists. Dopaminergic agonists can reduce striatal dopamine synthesis and induce locomotor excitation and hypothermia. On the other hand, dopamine antagonists can elevate striatal dopamine synthesis. When these drugs were administered to mice 24 hr after withdrawal, in all cases they were less effective in inducing their usual actions (Black, Hoffman, & Tabakoff, 1980; Hoffman & Tabakoff, 1977; Tabakoff & Hoffman, 1978; Tabakoff, Hoffman, & Ritzman, 1978). These results suggested that dopaminergic subsensitivity developed after chronic ethanol treatment and withdrawal. In another experiment, in which rats were administered ethanol at a daily oral dose of 6 g/kg for 14 days, the dopaminergic agonist apomorphine elicited a greater degree of stereotyped behavior and enhanced locomotor activity than did control animals 15 hr after the last dose of ethanol (Lai et al., 1980).

Other studies of dopaminergic sensitivity were undertaken in rats treated for 210 days. The withdrawal syndrome observed after the cessation of treatment exhibited two separate overt phases (Liljequist & Engel, 1979). During the first 24 hr after withdrawal, the signs of the ensuing syndrome were similar to those described after shorter treatments with ethanol (see Chapter 1). However, 3–5 days after withdrawal, coordinated behavioral activation was obtained, characterized by increased forward locomotion, rearing, grooming, and sniffing. This phase developed only if the animals were treated for at least 5 months. During the later phase of withdrawal, dopaminergic sensitivity was increased (Engel & Liljequist, 1976; Liljequist, 1978). This was demonstrated by enhanced locomotor activity, induced by local application of dopamine in the nucleus accumbens.

From the data presented, it does not appear that ethanol has any significant direct effect on catecholamine receptors. However, there is substantial evidence that after chronic ethanol treatment, these receptors become progressively desensitized the longer the animals are treated. After about a week of treatment, dopamine receptors become less responsive to a number of stimuli that normally exert their effects through these receptors. It is only after considerably longer treatment that this desensitization is manifested as a reduction in the number of receptors. It has been suggested that receptors initially uncouple from their effectors (Tabakoff & Hoffman, 1979).

Since subsensitivity develops to both dopaminergic agonists and antagonists, uncoupling might occur with the other receptor systems as well. In fact, dopamine neurons in the caudate nucleus react after chronic ethanol withdrawal in a manner similar to that obtained after chronic treatment with dopaminergic agonists. After chronic treatment with apomorphine or amphetamine, dopamine turnover and release are reduced (Riffee & Gerald, 1977). The same effect is observed after ethanol withdrawal (Darden & Hunt, 1977; Hunt & Majchrowicz, 1974). A concomitant reduction in [³H]apomorphine binding is observed after chronic apomorphine or amphetamine treatment (Muller & Seeman, 1979), but not after chronic ethanol treatment (Hunt & Dalton, 1981). This might suggest the uncoupling of presynaptic dopaminergic receptors from their effectors, with no alteration in receptor binding.

Another mechanism to explain alterations in catecholamine receptor function might be based, in part, on chronic changes in presynaptic input. For example, a number of studies have indicated that chronic ethanol treatment results in an acceleration of norepinephrine turnover (Hunt & Majchrowicz, 1974; Pohorecky et al., 1974; Thadani et al., 1976). The effects of dopamine turnover and release are less clear and may depend on whether measurements are obtained while animals are still intoxicated or are undergoing an ethanol withdrawal syndrome. Several reports have indicated that dopamine turnover and release are elevated during chronic intoxication (Darden & Hunt, 1977; Karoum, Wyatt, & Majchrowicz, 1976), but reduced during the withdrawal syndrome (Darden & Hunt, 1977; Hunt & Majchrowicz, 1974). Such alterations in catecholamine activity could lead to receptor desensitization.

Serotonin receptors

Serotonin binding sites have been identified in the brain using [³H] serotonin and [³H]lysergic acid diethylamide (LSD) as radioligands (Bennett & Snyder, 1976). These ligands have high affinity and specificity for the serotonergic receptor that appears to be on postsynaptic sites.

Some recent evidence suggests that there may be at least two distinct receptor subtypes, based on the ability of typically nonserotonergic drugs to bind to serotonergic receptors. [³H]Spiroperidol, a dopaminergic antagonist, has been postulated to bind to a subtype of serotonergic receptors by virtue of its ability to displace [³H]serotonin and [³H]LSD with different affinities (Peroutka & Snyder, 1979). Thus, the binding site for [³H]serotonin is designated as the serotonin-1 receptor and the binding site for [³H]spiroperidol is designated as the serotonin-2 receptor. LSD has a higher affinity for the serotonin-2 receptor. These subtypes have other differences. Serotonin-1 receptors are regulated by guanine nucleotides and are linked to adenylate cyclase, while serotonin-2 receptors are not (Peroutka, Lebovitz, & Snyder, 1979). In addition, they have different distributions in the brain (Peroutka & Snyder, 1981).

Functionally, the two serotonin receptors may mediate different actions of serotonin. Drugs that stimulate serotonergic transmission can induce behavioral hyperactivity. This is opposed to the well-known inhibitory properties of serotonin, especially as they relate to sleep. The behavioral hyperactivity is characterized by resting tremor, hindlimb abduction, splayed hindlimbs, snake tail, side-to-side head weaving, and head twitching (Corne, Pickering, & Warner, 1963; Graham-Smith, 1971; Jacobs, 1976; Sloviter, Drust, & Connor, 1978). Through comparisons of the potencies of various serotonergic antagonists to inhibit 5-hydroxytryptophan-induced head twitches, serotonin-sensitive adenylate cyclase, and [^{3}H]serotonin and [^{3}H]spiroperidol bindings, the inhibitory effects of serotonin appear to reflect interactions with the serotonin-1 receptor, while its excitatory effects appear to reflect interactions with the serotonin-2 receptor (Peroutka, Lebovitz, & Snyder, 1981).

Very few studies have been published dealing with the effect of ethanol on serotonin receptors. One report discusses experiments in which ethanol was added *in vitro* to mouse brain membranes (Hirsch, 1981). Ethanol inhibited the binding of both [^{3}H]serotonin and [^{3}H]LSD, with the effect on LSD binding being three times greater. Scatchard analysis showed that the apparent number of binding sites was reduced, but the affinity was increased by ethanol. Since LSD binding to membranes showed a greater sensitivity to ethanol, ethanol may have a more specific effect on serotonin-2 receptors. This idea has not been addressed. It should be mentioned that the concentrations of ethanol capable of inducing a significant inhibition of [^{3}H]LSD binding exceeded 200 mM (920 mg/dl), above those concentrations compatible with life.

One study examined the role of serotonergic receptors by determining whether the serotonergic antagonist methysergide could influence the duration of ethanol-induced sleeping times (Blum, Wallace, Calhoun, Tabor, & Eubanks, 1974). This treatment was found to increase sleeping times.

[^{3}H]Serotonin binding was measured after chronic ethanol treatment in only two studies, which differed in their length of ethanol treatment. When rats were treated with two daily 4-g/kg oral doses of ethanol for 11–15 days and killed 10 hr after the last dose, [^{3}H]serotonin binding was not significantly elevated in the caudate nucleus and brainstem, but was reduced in the hippocampus (Muller *et al.*, 1980). Continuous intoxication for 4 days had no effect on serotonin binding (Hunt & Dalton, 1981).

The ability of a serotonergic antagonist to modify an ethanol withdrawal syndrome has been examined (Blum, Wallace, Schwertner, & Eubanks, 1976). Ethanol was administered by inhalation for 3 days, accompanied by daily pyrazole injections to stabilize the blood ethanol concentrations.

After withdrawal of the ethanol, methysergide was administered intracerebrally, 5 and 13 hr later and withdrawal convulsions on handling were measured. This treatment increased the incidence of such convulsions. Other studies in which animals were treated with serotonergic drugs that either enhance or reduce serotonergic activity presynaptically were without effect (Goldstein, 1973; Griffiths, Littleton, & Ortiz, 1974).

Given the limited number of studies addressing whether serotonergic receptors are affected by the addition of ethanol *in vitro*, or by acute or chronic ethanol treatment, few firm conclusions can be drawn. There appears to be no significant direct action of ethanol on serotonergic receptors. On the other hand, there have been a variety of reports concerning the effect of ethanol on serotonin turnover in whole-brain preparations after chronic ethanol treatment (Hunt, 1979). However, by and large they have been inconclusive because of so many different reported results. Localized changes in specific brain structures in serotonin turnover and release have not been studied and may account for some of the regional changes in serotonin binding reported in one study (Muller *et al.*, 1980).

One interesting speculation might relate one of the serotonin receptor subtypes to some of the signs of the ethanol withdrawal syndrome. As mentioned earlier, behavioral hyperactivity has been associated with stimulation of serotonin-2 receptors. Such signs as tremor, hindlimb abnormalities, and aberrant head movements have been observed, not only after serotonin-2 receptor stimulation, but also during an ethanol withdrawal syndrome in experimental animals (Collier, Hammond, & Schneider, 1976; Majchrowicz, 1975). Head twitches seen after ethanol withdrawal are antagonized by serotonin antagonists (Collier *et al.*, 1976). If supersensitivity of serotonin-2 receptors occurs after chronic ethanol administration, it would be interesting to determine if it correlates with the expression of some of the ethanol withdrawal signs.

Acetylcholine receptors

Acetylcholine receptors exist in two general forms, nicotinic and muscarinic receptors. In brain, muscarinic receptors predominate (Krnjevic, 1974). The properties of muscarinic receptors and the biological results of their stimulation have been extensively examined (Heilbronn & Bartfai, 1978). Physiologically, muscarinic receptors mediate slow responses with relatively long latencies and durations.

Using radioligand techniques, muscarinic receptors have been characterized in detail. The most widely used ligand has been [³H]quinuclidinyl benzylate (QNB) (Yamamura & Snyder, 1974). With this ligand, one receptor with up to three possible configurations has been identified (Ehlert, Roeske, & Yamamura, 1981). This conclusion was drawn from the observation that muscarinic antagonists produce monophasic displacement curves of [³H]QNB binding, while agonists do not. Agonist binding is regulated by guanine nucleotides (Berrie, Birdsall, Burgen, & Hulme, 1979; Ehlert, Roeske, Rosenberger, & Yamamura, 1980; Ehlert, *et al.*, 1981).

Presynaptic muscarinic receptors may also exist in the brain. Acetylcholine release from brain slices *in vitro* has been reported to be reduced by cholinergic agonists and stimulated by antagonists (Hadházy & Szerb, 1977; Polak & Meeuws, 1966).

Muscarinic receptors can be desensitized with long-term cholinergic stimulation. Chronic treatment with cholinesterase inhibitors, for example, leads to a reduction in the number of muscarinic binding sites (Ehlert, Kokka, & Fairhurst, 1980).

In all of the studies involving ethanol treatment reported to date, muscarinic cholinergic receptors were studied with [³H]QNB as the radioligand. Although ethanol in concentrations up to 200 mM (920 mg/dl) does not alter QNB binding to membranes *in vitro* (Hunt, Majchrowicz, Dalton, Swartzwelder, & Wixon, 1979), there have been reports suggesting that chronic ethanol administration can induce changes in binding. As with the other receptor systems previously discussed, the length of chronic ethanol treatment has been the major difference among the various reports. With short-term chronic treatment for 4 days, no change of [³H]QNB binding could be observed in any of the brain areas studied (Hunt & Dalton, 1981). After 7–8 days of treatment, binding was elevated in the hippocampus and cerebral cortex and whole-brain synaptosomes, an effect reflecting an increase in the apparent number of binding sites (Rabin *et al.*, 1980; Tabakoff, Munoz-Marcus, & Fields, 1979). This response was reversible within 24 hr (Tabakoff *et al.*, 1979). No change was detected after 11–15 days of ethanol treatment, two daily 4-g/kg oral doses (Muller *et al.*, 1980).

An effort was undertaken to assess cholinergic receptor function under conditions more analogous to human drinking patterns than those previously described. When rats were permitted to consume ethanol in their drinking fluid for 18–75 weeks, striatal [³H]QNB binding was significantly elevated (Pelham *et al.*, 1980; Nordberg & Wahlström, 1982). This response could be observed only if the animals had been withdrawn from ethanol for up to 8 days and was correlated with a reduction in choline acetyltransferase activity. No other brain area was affected.

As with the previous receptor systems discussed, there appears to be no direct effect of ethanol on acetylcholine receptors. However, with long-term treatment with ethanol, an elevation in the number of muscarinic receptor binding sites has been observed. Presynaptic changes in acetylcholine release have been detected, at least after a single dose of ethanol. Under these conditions, cholinergic activity appears to be reduced in a number of areas (Erickson & Graham, 1973; Hunt, Majchrowicz, & Dalton, 1979). The effect of chronic ethanol administration on acetylcholine release has not been extensively studied. In fact, tolerance may rapidly develop to the acute effect of ethanol on release (Hunt, Majchrowicz, & Dalton, 1979). Consequently, at this time, there is no clear relationship between the reported presynaptic effects of ethanol and the receptor changes observed after chronic ethanol treatment.

GABA receptors

γ-Aminobutryic acid (GABA) receptors are believed to be part of a complex entity, characterized by three binding sites that bind three different classes of drugs (Olsen, 1981). The first of these binding sites binds GABA itself. There are two sites, a low-affinity and a high-affinity site, when [³H]GABA is used as the radioligand. These sites can be revealed by Scatchard analysis only if an endogenous inhibitor of binding is removed (Enna & Snyder, 1977; Toffano, Guidotti, & Costa, 1978). Investigators have eliminated this inhibitor either by solubilizing a membrane preparation with the detergent Triton X-100, or by extensively washing it with a buffer (Enna & Snyder, 1977; Ticku, 1980b). [³H]Muscimol, a GABA-ergic agonist, is also used as a radioligand and has only one binding site (Wang, Salvaterra, & Roberts, 1979). Presynaptic GABA autoreceptors may also exist on GABA terminals, based on the ability of GABA to inhibit GABA release from brain slices *in vitro* (Arbilla, Kamal, & Langer, 1979).

The second binding site selectively binds benzodiazepines, a class of drugs known for their anxiolytic properties. Benzodiazepines, such as diazepam, will bind to brain tissue with high affinity and to a single binding site, whose distribution roughly parallels that of the GABA binding site (Placheta & Karobath, 1979). More recent evidence has suggested that there may be two subtypes of the benzodiazepine receptor. One site appears to be coupled to the chloride ionophore and may mediate the sedative and ataxic properties of benzodiazepines (Lippa, Critchett, Sano, Klepner, Greenblatt, Coupet, & Beer, 1979; Squires, Benson, Braestrup, Coupet, Klepner, Myers, & Beer, 1979). The other site, not coupled to the chloride ionophore, may mediate the anxiolytic effects of benzodiazepines (Lippa *et al.*, 1979). As with GABA binding, there appears to be an endogenous inhibitor of benzodiazepine binding (Karobath, Sperk, & Schönbeck, 1978; Massotti & Guidotti, 1980). This inhibitor reduces the affinity and GABA stimulation of benzodiazepine binding.

The third binding site has been identified using a derivative of picotoxin, a convulsant that blocks GABA transmission without affecting the GABA receptor itself. (Olsen, Ticku, & Miller, 1978; Olsen, Ticku, Van Ness, & Greenlee, 1978). The radioligand used was [³H]α-dihydropicrotoxinin (DHP). Only one population of binding sites was detected, distinct from the GABA and benzodiazepine binding sites (Ticku, Ban, & Olsen,

1978). A variety of convulsants and depressants, including barbiturates, interact with this binding site (Ticku, 1980a).

These three binding sites form the GABA–benzodiazepine–chloride ionophore receptor complex, with much of the evidence to date supporting the theory that there is an interaction among these sites. For example, each of the three classes of ligands can modify the binding properties of the others, while the ligands bind only to their own specific receptors (Briley & Langer, 1978; Guidotti, Toffano, & Costa, 1978; Leeb-Lundberg, Snowden, & Olsen, 1980; Martin & Candy, 1978; Olsen *et al.*, 1978; Skolnick, Rice, Barker, & Paul, 1982; Ticku, 1980a). In addition, diazepam and pentobarbital can enhance GABA interactions with the chloride ionophore of voltage-clamped mouse spinal neurons grown in culture (Study & Barker, 1981).

As with the other receptors discussed, GABA receptors are sensitive to alterations in presynaptic input. When GABA neurons are destroyed using lesioning techniques, GABA binding is increased 7–15 days after the lesion, suggesting the development of supersensitivity (Campochiaro, Schwartz, & Coyle, 1977; Waddington & Cross, 1978).

Using the techniques of radioligand binding, a number of studies have appeared attempting to determine whether acute or chronic ethanol administration can alter the properties of the GABA–benzodiazepine–chloride ionophore receptor complex. After a 4-g/kg intraperitoneal dose of ethanol, GABA binding was reported to be elevated in both mice and rats, 30 min after injection (Ticku, 1980b; Ticku & Burch, 1980). This change, based on Scatchard analysis, was due to an increase in the apparent number of low-affinity binding sites. When a similar injection was administered and GABA binding determined 2–3 hr after injection, elevated binding was observed specifically in the cerebellum (Reggiani, Barbaccia, Spano, & Trabucchi, 1980a). This effect was due to an increase in the affinity of both high- and low-affinity binding sites. When a 4-g/kg oral dose was administered, no change in GABA binding was observed (Volicer & Biagioni, 1982b).

When animals have been treated with ethanol chronically, different results have been reported, depending on the manner and duration of treatment. A reduction in the apparent number of GABA binding sites in membranes derived from whole mouse brain was observed 14 days after consumption of a 10% ethanol solution (Ticku & Burch, 1980) or with increasing concentrations of ethanol in the drinking fluid (Unwin & Taberner, 1980). This effect was not present in rats treated for 21 days with a liquid diet containing 7% ethanol (Ticku, 1980b). However, when the ethanol was withdrawn, a reduced affinity of the low-affinity binding sites was revealed and correlated with an increased susceptibility to audiogenic seizures. Similar results were obtained when rats were treated for 7 days with 3 daily injections of ethanol, except a decrease in the affinity of the high-affinity binding site was also observed (Volicer, 1980; Volicer & Biaggioni, 1982b). Rats exposed to ethanol in an inhalation chamber for 4 days had a reduced number of [³H]muscimol binding sites in the cerebellum after withdrawal and correlated with an enhanced level of seizures (Linnoila, Stowell, Marganos, & Thurman, 1981). In yet another study, an elevation of the apparent number of both high- and low-affinity binding sites was obtained, specifically in the striatum, when rats were given a 6% ethanol solution to drink for 21 days (Reggiani *et al.*, 1980a). No effect on high-affinity GABA binding was observed after 4 days of continous intoxication (Hunt & Dalton, 1981). In human specimens derived from postmortem brains of alcoholics, the apparent number of GABA binding sites, as determined from [³H]muscimol binding, was increased over controls (Tran, Snyder, Major, & Hawley, 1981).

As one can see from the above discussion, a variety of results have been obtained on GABA binding and the results provide no clear picture concerning the effect ethanol actually has on the GABA receptor. One of the largest differences among the studies is the manner in which the endogenous inhibitor of GABA binding was removed, if at all. As discussed previously, this inhibitor is generally removed either by solubilizing the tissue in Triton X-100 or by extensive washing of the tissue. A possible interaction with or effect on this inhibitor by ethanol has not been examined. Such an effect could influence the results obtained. In support of this possibility, extensively washing the membrane preparation with Triton X-100 eliminated the reduced affinity of the GABA receptor observed during the ethanol withdrawal syndrome (Volicer & Biagioni, 1982b).

The effect of ethanol on the benzodiazepine receptor appears to be clearer than that for GABA binding. The degree to which the tissue is solubilized seems to influence the results obtained. When ethanol in concentrations of 10–100 mM (46–460 mg/dl) was incubated *in vitro* either with unwashed tissue or with tissue washed in Triton X-100, derived from animals given a single dose of ethanol, no effect on benzodiazepine binding could be demonstrated (Freund, 1980a; Volicer & Biagioni, 1982a). However, if tissue was solubilized with 1% Lubrol-Px, ethanol enhanced benzodiazepine binding in a dose-dependent manner in concentrations of 20–100 mM (92–460 mg/dl), an effect attributed to an increase in the affinity of the ligand for the receptor (Davis & Ticku, 1981; Ticku & Davis, 1981). The effect of ethanol was compared with other alcohols to determine whether their effectiveness to enhance binding was related to their lipid solubilties. No correlation was found (Davis & Ticku, 1981).

The effect of chronic ethanol treatment on benzodiazepine binding has depended on how the brain tissue from the animals was prepared and the length of ethanol treatment. When rats were exposed to ethanol by inhalation for 12–19 days, benzodiazepine binding to crude mitochondrial pellets was unaffected (Frye, Vogel, Mailman, Ondrusek, Wilson, Mueller,

& Breese, 1980; Karobath, Rogers, & Bloom, 1980). One study reported a reduction in benzodiazepine binding after 4.5 days of ethanol treatment, with daily 10-g/kg doses (Kochman, Hirsch, & Clay, 1981). When ethanol treatment was administered for 9 months, a small decrease in affinity and apparent number of binding sites was observed (Freund, 1980a).

Solubilization of membrane preparations with detergents may influence the observed effect of chronic ethanol treatment, similar to that observed for GABA binding. After 6 days of ethanol treatment and washing the membranes with Triton X-100, benzodiazepine binding was reduced (Volicer & Biagioni, 1982a). These data suggest that endogenous inhibitors may have to be removed in order for the effects of ethanol on benzodiazepine binding to be revealed. No studies of benzodiazepine binding using Lubrol-solubilized membranes in animals chronically treated with ethanol have been published.

Finally, the third binding site in the GABA–benzodiazepine–chloride ionophore receptor complex has been studied for possible interactions with ethanol. Ethanol in concentrations of 50–100 mM (230–460 mg/dl) was incubated with a Lubrol-solubilized membrane fraction and was found to inhibit DHP binding up to 22% (Davis & Ticku, 1981; Ticku & Davis, 1981). Since benzodiazepines enhance the ability of GABA to bind to its receptor (Guidotti *et al.*, 1978), and drugs that interact with the DHP receptor increase benzodiazepine binding (Leeb-Lundberg *et al.*, 1980; Skolnick *et al.*, 1982; Ticku, 1980a), an interaction by ethanol with the DHP binding site might indirectly facilitate the ability of benzodiazepine receptors to augment GABA transmission. No studies of the effect of chronic ethanol treatment on DHP binding have been reported.

Given the complexities and inconsistencies of the data discussed, the findings to date must be considered preliminary. A variety of methods and approaches to the study of the effects of ethanol on GABA receptors has been used. Making valid conclusions based on these data is difficult. The biggest impediment to evaluating chronic ethanol experiments has been differences in methods of chronic treatment, the duration of treatment, and the time after the last dose of ethanol when measurements of ligand binding were made. Some standardized approach to these studies is needed to allow for the reproducibility of data across various laboratories. Finally, the biological role of endogenous inhibitors of receptor binding needs to be explored further to determine their biological significance, what effect ethanol treatment might have on their activity, and how these inhibitors can be best removed from membrane preparations for binding studies, when needed.

Since ethanol can influence the binding of radioligands to the GABA–benzodiazepine–chloride ionophore receptor complex in concentrations that are physiologically tolerated, this effect of ethanol may be a candidate for a primary mechanism of action. Based on the criteria for proposed mechanisms of action for ethanol, discussed in Chapter 1, an action of ethanol on this receptor complex appears promising. Not only are the observed changes in receptor binding found with ethanol concentrations within the sublethal range, they are relevant to the behavioral consequences of ethanol, namely, depression. A number of aspects of the action of ethanol on this system need to be addressed. The reversibility of the ethanol-induced changes has not been determined nor have correlations of these changes with the development of and recovery from depression been reported. This latter point might be difficult to test, but determination of reversibility would be relatively straightforward. The lack of correlation between the effect of ethanol on benzodiazepine binding and lipid solubility is a bit troubling. However, ethanol may act more indirectly through the DHP binding site. The possible correlation of the effects of different alcohols with lipid solubility of alcohols with respect to this binding site has not been studied.

Pharmacological evidence exists indirectly supporting enhanced GABA transmission in the depressant effects of ethanol. If such actions were important, GABA agonists should augment the ethanol-induced depression and GABA antagonists should attenuate it. This has, in fact, been reported by several laboratories (Frye & Breese, 1982; Liljequist & Engel, 1982; Martz, Deitrich, & Harris, 1983).

The reported reductions in GABA and benzodiazepine binding after chronic ethanol treatment would be consistent with a role of GABA in the expression of at least one of the signs of the ethanol withdrawal syndrome, namely, seizures. A deficiency in GABA transmission has been implicated in the development of seizures (Wood, 1975). Various GABA agonists have been tested for their ability to modify withdrawal seizures. Irrespective of whether these drugs act directly on GABA receptors or increase the availability of GABA for receptor interactions, they were all effective in blocking withdrawal seizures (Cooper, Viik, Ferris, & White, 1979; Goldstein, 1973, 1979; Hillbom, 1975; Noble, Gillies, Vigran, & Mandel, 1976).

Taken together, the data suggest that some of the acute effects of ethanol may result from a facilitation of GABA transmission. This is based on the increased efficiency of GABA binding, through complex interactions of various components of the GABA–benzodiazepine–chloride ionophore receptor complex, and the possible enhancement of the inhibitory effect of GABA by ethanol at the electrophysiological level (see Chapter 3). These actions of ethanol were found at concentrations that induce overt behavior depression in animals.

Ethanol has a biphasic behavioral effect, with stimulation often seen at low blood ethanol concentrations and depression observed at high blood ethanol concentrations (Pohorecky, 1977). Recent studies have suggested that ethanol *in vivo* can reduce apparent GABA turnover at low blood ethanol concentrations (Supavilai & Karobath, 1980; Wixon & Hunt, 1980).

This reduced inhibitory input could be a contributing factor in behavioral stimulation under these conditions. Both the stimulatory and inhibitory effects of ethanol may be receptor mediated. There is some evidence that GABA receptors exist presynaptically on GABA neurons to regulate GABA release (Arbilla *et al.*, 1979). Conceivably, ethanol may be more effective in facilitating GABA receptor function at the presynaptic level. At lower concentrations of ethanol, presynaptic GABA receptors might be stimulated leading to a reduction in GABA release.

After chronic ethanol administration, GABA transmission appears to be reduced due to an inefficient interaction of GABA with its receptor. Again, this may result from a complex interaction among the various components of the GABA–benzodiazepine–chloride ionophore receptor system. To exacerbate this problem, presynaptic transmission may also be reduced (Wixon & Hunt, 1980). If both of these phenomena were to occur after chronic ethanol treatment, this would explain the efficacy of GABA agonists to suppress some of the signs of the withdrawal syndrome.

Glutamate receptors

In addition to GABA, another amino acid that has received some attention at the receptor level has been glutamate, a putative excitatory transmitter. Glutamate receptors have not been as extensively studied as other receptors systems, in part, because a role for glutamate as a transmitter has not been as well accepted as for other transmitter candidates (Peck, 1980). A discussion of glutamate receptors is being included in this volume because some studies have been reported addressing the possible role of these receptors in the actions of ethanol.

Glutamate had been found to bind specifically to sites on neural membrane fragments with high and low affinity. (Michaelis, Michaelis, & Boyarsky, 1974; Roberts, 1974). The high-affinity binding sites appear to be postsynaptic receptor sites, while the low-affinity sites are probably presynaptic uptake sites (Roberts, 1975). Binding to high-affinity sites may be regulated by guanine nucleotides (Sharif & Roberts, 1980).

[^{3}H]Glutamate binding has been measured in synaptosomes exposed to ethanol *in vitro* and in those obtained from rats after acute ethanol treatment (Michaelis, Mulvaney, & Freed, 1978). When brain tissue was incubated with ethanol in a concentration range *in vitro* of 10–50 mM (46–230 mg/dl), glutamate binding was elevated up to threefold. Elevated glutamate binding was also observed 2 hr after a 4-g/kg intraperitoneal injection of ethanol. These changes appeared to be due to an increase in the apparent number of binding sites.

More recently, the effect of ethanol *in vitro* on glutamate binding was examined further. Using synaptic membranes, ethanol was shown again to stimulate glutamate binding at concentrations below 50 mM (230 mg/dl) (Michaelis, Michaelis, Belieu, Grubbs, & Magruder, 1980; Michaelis, Chang, Roy, McFaul, & Zimbrick, 1983). Concentrations of ethanol above 50 mM were progressively less effective with no changes apparent at 100 mM (460 mg/dl). In addition, an endogenous inhibitor of glutamate binding was found with properties generally similar to gangliosides (Michaelis, Michaelis, Belieu, Grubbs, & Magruder, 1980). Ethanol antagonized this inhibitory effect of gangliosides on glutamate binding.

To determine whether the alterations in glutamate binding result from ethanol interactions with membranes, the temperature at which the rates of activation of binding change was determined by increasing the temperature of the incubating medium (Michaelis, Zimbrick, McFaul, Lampe, & Michaelis, 1980). Arrhenius-type plots (see Chapter 2) demonstrated a reduction of the transition temperature by ethanol exposure *in vitro*. The energy of activation above the transition temperature was reduced, but was unaffected below this temperature. This evidence indicated that ethanol may alter the microenvironment surrounding the glutamate receptor. In further support was the observation that ethanol had little effect on the binding of glutamate to a purified glutamate binding protein (Michaelis, Chang, Roy, McFaul, & Zimbrick, 1983). In addition, the biphasic effect of ethanol correlated with the biphasic effect of ethanol on lipid order observed by the same investigators (see Chapter 2).

Chronic treatment with ethanol in a liquid diet for 16 days also resulted in elevated glutamate binding, both when the measurements were made before withdrawal or 1 day after withdrawal (Michaelis *et al.*, 1978). This elevated glutamate binding dissipated over a 6-day period. The possibility that this elevated glutamate binding might mediate some of the signs of an ethanol withdrawal syndrome was tested with the use of the glutamate receptor inhibitor glutamate diethyl ester, which delays the onset of seizures induced by pentylenetetrazol (Abdul-Ghani, Bruce, & Bradford, 1982). Swiss–Webster mice were rendered ethanol dependent by ethanol inhalation for 3 days with daily injections of pyrazole to stabilize blood ethanol concentrations (Freed & Michaelis, 1978). The increased incidence of convulsions induced by handling and spontaneous locomotor behavior were both attenuated after the administration of the inhibitor. The drug itself induced no behavioral alterations of its own. In addition, the mice were more sensitive to kainic acid-induced convulsions than those induced by pentylenetetrazole. Because kainic acid is considered a glutamate agonist (Olney, Rhee, & Ho, 1974), these data suggest that the ethanol-treated mice may have developed supersensitivity to glutamate.

Glutamate receptor binding, like GABA binding, is one of the only systems that appears to be sensitive to acute ethanol treatment. Alterations are demonstrated even though the ethanol has been washed out of the membrane preparation. This suggests that the effect of ethanol on glutamate binding is indirect or is direct and not readily reversible with ethanol elimination. This is an interesting observation in light of recent findings that the apparent number of glutamate binding sites can be increased with as little as 30 min of electrical stimulation of identified pathways in the hippocampus (Baudry, Oliver, Creager, Wieraszko, & Lynch, 1980). Ethanol after low doses has been shown to have stimulatory effects in the hippocampus (see Chapter 3). Whether these last two observations are related and can be extrapolated to the whole brain is not clear. However, the idea that long-term stimulation of certain areas of the brain by ethanol could lead to a long-lasting effect on transmitter receptor function is intriguing.

Opiate receptors

Since the discovery of the endogenous opiates, interest in their biological function and the receptors on which they act has intensified (Beaumont & Hughes, 1979). It now appears that there are at least two opiate receptors. These have been designated the μ- and the δ-receptors in the brain (Chang, Hazum, & Cuatrecasas, 1980). The difference between these receptors has been described on the basis of the relative affinity of two classes of radioligands: the opiate alkaloids, such as dihydromorphine, and the opioid peptides, such as enkephalin. Other receptors have been postulated, including κ-, σ-, and recently λ-receptors (Gilbert & Martin, 1976; Grevel & Sadée, 1983). In addition, both pre- and postsynaptic receptors have been identified (Murrin, Coyle, & Kuhar, 1980).

Functionally, the μ- and δ-receptors are associated with different physiological and biochemical actions. The μ-receptor appears to mediate analgesia (Kosterlitz & Waterfield, 1975), while, on the other hand, the δ-receptors may mediate a number of behavioral and other physiological effects, including seizures, EEG changes, and satisfaction and reward (Chang *et al.*, 1980). The δ-receptor may be linked to adenylate cyclase, while GTP can inhibit opiate binding to both μ- and δ-receptors (Blume, 1978; Childers & Snyder, 1980; Pert, 1981). Sodium chloride can interfere with the ability of opiate agonists to bind to μ-receptors (Snyder & Innis, 1979). This property has been useful in screening various drugs for analgesic activity.

The κ-receptor is just beginning to be characterized. The ligand used as a prototype is [^{3}H]ethylketocyclazocine. Using computerized curve-fitting techniques, binding to the κ-receptor could be distinguished from that to the μ- and δ-receptors (Pfeiffer & Herz, 1982). In addition, there is evidence suggesting that the endogenous opioid peptide dynorphin is a natural ligand for the κ-receptor (Schulz, Wüster, & Herz, 1982).

The interaction of ethanol with opiate receptors has been studied both *in vitro* and *in vivo*, using [^{3}H]dihydromorphine and [^{3}H-D-Ala^2, D-Leu^5] enkephalin to examine μ- and δ-opiate receptors, respectively. When ethanol in concentrations of 100–1000 mM (460–4600 mg/dl) was incubated with membranes derived from whole rat brain or caudate nuclei from C57BL mice, δ-receptor binding was progressively decreased, an effect attributed to a reduced affinity of the ligand for the receptor (Hiller, Angel, & Simon, 1981, 1984; Tabakoff & Hoffman, 1983). This reduction of the affinity results from an increased rate of dissociation of the ligand from the receptor (Hiller *et al.*, 1984). Ethanol also lowered the affinity of the μ-receptor in mice, but not in rats. This difference appears to be due, in part, to different temperatures of incubation. Ethanol has a greater effect on the binding of the μ-receptor at higher incubating temperatures (Tabakoff & Hoffman, 1983). In fact, when rat membranes were incubated at higher temperatures, ethanol could reduce binding to μ-receptors in a concentration-dependent manner (LaBella, Pinsky, Havlicek, & Queen, 1979). Another possibility could be based on the concentration of the ligand used in the binding assay. In the study of Tabakoff & Hoffman (1983), the concentration of ligand was much less than that used by Hiller *et al.* (1981), increasing the likelihood of detecting a change in affinity of the ligand for the receptor. Finally, the ability of different alcohols to inhibit the binding to both μ- and δ-receptors under the appropriate conditions is increased with alcohols with higher lipid solubilities (Hiller *et al.*, 1981, 1984; Tabakoff & Hoffman, 1983). Alcohol had no effect on κ-receptor binding (Hiller *et al.*, 1984).

At lower, more physiologically compatible concentrations of ethanol, binding to the μ-receptor in the caudate nucleus was increased by slightly less that 20% (Tabakoff & Hoffman, 1983). This effect was due to an increase in the affinity of the μ-receptor binding sites and was reversible. In another study, the apparent number of μ-receptor binding sites was elevated with as little as 20 mM (92 mg/dl) ethanol (Levine, Hess, & Morley, 1983).

The effect of chronic ethanol treatment on opiate receptor binding has depended on the area of the brain studied and the manner and duration of treatment. After ethanol was administered for 7 days in a liquid diet, the affinity of the μ-receptor in the caudate nucleus was reduced 24 hr after withdrawal, but reverted to control levels within 72 hr after withdrawal (Hoffman, Urwyler, & Tabakoff, 1981). This altered affinity was due to an increased rate of dissociation of the ligand for the receptor. When sodium chloride was included in the assay, the affinity of the μ-receptor was decreased. This effect resulted from a higher dissociation rate constant and a lower associated rate constant. Chronic ethanol treatment perferentially depressed this effect of sodium chloride because of the general effect of ethanol on the dissociation rate constant. Binding to the δ-receptor was not affected in mice. When binding to the δ-receptor was measured in rats treated for 21–60 days with daily 9-g/kg oral doses of ethanol, the affinity of the ligand for this receptor was also decreased (Lucchi, Bosio, Spano,

& Trabucchi, 1981). On the other hand, when the binding to both μ- and δ-receptors was measured in rat forebrain after 21 days of treatment with 15% ethanol in the drinking water, the affinity for the δ-receptor was elevated with no effect on μ-receptor binding (Pfeiffer, Seizinger, & Herz, 1981). However, high concentrations of sodium chloride were included in the incubation medium, which might have lowered binding of the ligand to μ-receptors to an extent that the effect of chronic ethanol administration on those receptors may have been masked.

Other more indirect data have suggested that acute and chronic ethanol treatment exerts an action through opiate receptors. Acute ethanol treatment induces an increase in the acidic metabolites of dopamine in the brain (Bustos & Roth, 1976; Hunt & Majchrowicz, 1983; Karoum et al., 1976). Since opiates play a role in the regulation of striatal dopaminergic activity by stimulating the synthesis and release of dopamine (Urwyler & Tabakoff, 1981; Wood, Stotland, Richard, & Rackham, 1980), the stimulation of opiate receptors could be a causative factor in the elevation of the concentrations of dopamine metabolites. When animals were pretreated with an opiate antagonist, these metabolic changes induced by a single dose of ethanol were prevented (Reggiani et al., 1980b). In addition, the ability of morphine normally to induce dopaminergic hyperactivity was depressed in chronic ethanol-treated mice (Hoffman, Urwyler, & Tabakoff, 1982; Tabakoff, Urwyler, & Hoffman, 1981). These findings are consistent with the effects of ethanol on opiate binding.

Several behavioral studies have implicated the endogenous opiate system in some of the acute effects of ethanol. Ethanol has been presumed to be reinforcing and therefore to perpetuate drinking in humans. The possibility that endogenous opioids may mediate self-administration of ethanol by monkeys has been examined (Altshuler, Phillips, & Feinhandler, 1980). Monkeys were selected based on their ability to press a bar for intravenous infusions of ethanol and then were pretreated 30 min prior to a test session with naltrexone, an opiate antagonist. Test sessions lasted for 15 days. During the first 5 days, a small increase in the self-administration of ethanol was observed. After that point, however, self-administration was progressively reduced, as compared to control animals injected with saline.

The ability of opiate antagonists to modify the analgesic effect of ethanol has been examined. Using the tail-flick test, which determines the time required for a rodent to remove its tail from hot water, naloxone was reported consistently to abolish the analgesic effect of ethanol (Boada, Feria, & Sanz, 1981). When using the writhing response, naloxone was ineffective in antagonizing the analgesic effect of ethanol (Berkowitz, Finck, & Ngai, 1976). This lack of effect may be due, in part, to the very short 1-min time interval between naloxone pretreatment and the performance of the test.

Ethanol-induced changes in locomotor activity can be modified by opiate antagonists. The outcome of pretreatment with an opiate antagonist depends on the endpoint being measured and the species and strain of animal. Using three different strains of mice, the ability of naltrexone to block either the stimulatory or depressant effect of ethanol on locomotion was examined (Kiianmaa, Hoffman, & Tabakoff, 1983). Increased locomotor activity could be observed in DBA/2 and BALB/C mice, but not in C57BL/6 mice after ethanol treatment. Naltrexone could antagonize this stimulatory effect of ethanol in both strains. With respect to the depressive effects of ethanol, naltrexone had differential effects across the three strains, when measuring the duration of the loss of righting reflex. Depression was most effectively antagonized by naltrexone in the BALB mice. C57BL mice required 8 times the dose of naltrexone to obtain blockade of depression, and DBA mice were unresponsive to the drug. On the other hand, naloxone was unable to block several types of ethanol-induced behavioral decrements in rats (Jørgensen & Hole, 1981). Clinically, opiate antagonists have been reported to be effective in blocking ethanol overdoses (Barros & Rodreguez, 1981; Jeffreys, Flanagan, & Volans, 1980; Mackensie, 1979; Sørensen & Mattisson, 1978) and some of the psychomotor effects of low doses of ethanol (Jeffcoate, Herbert, Cullen, Hastlings, & Walder, 1979), but not ethanol-induced sensimotor impairment (Catley, Jordan, Frith, Lehane, Rhodes, & Jones, 1981). Other studies were unable to demonstrate any beneficial effect of naloxone on ethanol intoxication in humans (Catley, Lehane, & Jones, 1981; Kimball, Huang, Torget, & Houck, 1981; Mattila, Nuotto, & Seppala, 1981; Nuotto, Palva, & Lahdenranta, 1983; Whalley, Freeman, & Hunter, 1981). These data suggest that endogenous opiates may play a role in the actions of ethanol, but they may have genetic and endpoint-specific determinants.

Several attempts have been made to determine if stimulation of opiate receptors might play a role in the development of physical dependence on ethanol. These studies were based on the premise that ethanol and opiate dependence have a common mechanism (Blum, Briggs, Elston, Hirst, Hamilton, & Verebey, 1980). The approach taken was to ascertain whether an opiate antagonist could precipitate a withdrawal syndrome in ethanol-intoxicated animals or block one in progress. Naloxone treatment did not result in a withdrawal syndrome in the intoxicated animals (Goldstein & Judson, 1971). On the other hand, naloxone has been reported to suppress withdrawal seizures (Blum, Wallace, Schwertner, & Futterman, 1977). However, when further studied using appropriate blind techniques and evaluating several endpoints of withdrawal, these results were not confirmed (Hemmingsen & Sørensen, 1979).

The studies described up to this point begin to provide some consistent findings. At physiologically compatible doses of ethanol, it appears that opiate receptors, especially μ-receptors, are stimulated, at least in the caudate nucleus. Blockade of opiate receptors suppresses behavioral and neurochemical actions of ethanol. With chronic treatment with ethanol, adaptive changes may occur such that the opiate receptors are desensitized. Whether this effect is related to ethanol tolerance has not been determined.

No conclusive evidence supports the idea that opioids underlie the development and expression of ethanol dependence. However, the effects of ethanol seem to be consistent with the theory of Kosterlitz and Hughes (1975) concerning the mechanism for the development of opiate dependence. This theory suggests that exogenously administered opiates stimulate the opiate receptors and, in effect, displace the endogenously produced opioids. Through a negative feedback mechanism, the concentration of endogenous opioids would be reduced. When the exogenous drugs are removed, the usual inhibitory action of the endogenous opioids (Zieglänsberger, Fry, Moroder, Herz, & Wunsch, 1976) would not be present, thereby precipitating a withdrawal syndrome. This sort of mechanism may in some way be applicable to chronic ethanol treatment. Several studies have shown that both chronic opiate and ethanol treatments lead to a reduction in Met-enkephalin levels in several areas of the brain (Hong, Majchrowicz, Hunt, & Gillin, 1981; Przewlocki, Hollt, Duka, Kleber, Gramsch, Haarmann, & Herz, 1979; Schulz, Wüster, Duka, & Herz, 1980). With respect to chronic ethanol treatment, the observation that some of these effects may be apparent only during the withdrawal syndrome and not while the animals are still intoxicated (Hong et al., 1981) raises doubts about how applicable the above theory might be to ethanol dependence.

Commentary

The effect of ethanol on neurotransmitter receptors has received a fair amount of attention, but not enough to have a totally clear picture of whether and to what extent ethanol can disrupt receptor function. One point that should be raised relates to binding studies themselves. Although they are easy to perform and have been widely validated, there are many variables that have not yet been well defined. This especially relates to the mechanism of reported changes in binding. Using Scatchard analysis, an alteration in binding can be attributed to a change in the affinity for the receptor or a change in the apparent number of binding sites. As discussed previously, the properties of receptors can vary, depending on such factors as ionic composition and endogenous inhibitors of binding. The conditions encountered *in vivo* may be important in determining what effect ethanol treatment really has and the significance of that effect. Such considerations as the possible presence of yet undiscovered endogenous inhibitors and regulators must be considered for all receptor systems. Indeed, the actions of ethanol may be on these inhibitors and regulators, rather than on the receptors themselves.

In spite of the foregoing discussion, sufficient consistencies exist that allow for a few tentative conclusions to be made. On the whole, there is not much evidence to suggest that ethanol directly interacts with transmitter receptors, with a few exceptions. These exceptions are based on data derived from *in vitro* studies and indicate that ethanol might facilitate receptor function of several transmitters. Of the receptor systems studied, ethanol most likely exerts an effect on the GABA receptor complex. Most of the data accumulated so far indicate that ethanol disrupts this complex in such a manner as to enhance the binding of GABA to its receptor. This action would exert an inhibitory influence on neuronal function.

A direct effect of ethanol on glutamate and opiate receptors has also been observed. In these cases, receptor function is also enhanced. However, these systems have not been extensively studied and the data are still preliminary.

In spite of the multitude of experimental designs that have been used to study the effect of chronic treatment of ethanol on the transmitter receptors, a number of consistencies have emerged. In general, few studies have reported alterations in ligand binding during the first week of treatment. The longer the treatment continues, the greater the likelihood that changes will occur.

The effects that have been observed have depended on the length of treatment and the period after the last dose of ethanol that the measurements were made. When the binding of the ligand was determined while the animals were intoxicated, most studies have suggested that the receptors are desensitized. However, if withdrawal was permitted and the ethanol was eliminated from the body, the opposite effect was often observed. To what extent these alterations in sensitivity are reversible has generally not been studied. This biphasic effect was more likely to be observed with very long-term treatments with moderate doses of ethanol, and was longer lived than the responses observed after shorter treatment periods.

Can such alterations in receptor function explain any of the consequences of chronic ethanol administration? This is a question that has not been specifically addressed. The potential relevance, though, could possibly be inferred based on the time courses of receptor changes and other consequences of chronic ethanol treatment.

In Chapter 1, a number of considerations for interpreting results of chronic ethanol experiments were discussed. The major consequences of chronic ethanol administration are the development of physical dependence, tolerance, and brain damage. Their time courses for development and dissipation after ethanol withdrawal are considerably different. Physical dependence, as expressed by the presence of a withdrawal syndrome, lasts only a few days, tolerance can last a number of weeks, and brain damage is irreversible. Because the time courses of receptor alterations, when determined, vary, they may reflect an underlying mechanism of one of these processes.

In several instances, receptor binding was reported to be elevated, as in the case of β-adrenergic and cholinergic receptors, or reduced as in the case of GABA and opiate receptors, at a period when overt withdrawal reactions were observed. If these changes were to underlie the withdrawal syndrome, then appropriate drugs that interact with these receptors should be effective in blocking withdrawal signs. The studies reported using these drugs have been inconclusive or the drugs were ineffective (Goldstein, 1973; Hemmingsen & Sørensen, 1979; Hunt, 1979). An exception has been with the use of GABA-mimetics, as discussed earlier, for the suppression of withdrawal seizures. Finally, at a point when the development of physical dependence is maximal, receptor binding is unaffected, suggesting that changes in receptors are not necessary to evoke withdrawal signs (Hunt & Dalton, 1981).

Alterations in the properties of transmitter receptors have been suggested to mediate the tolerance developed after chronic treatment with a number of drugs (Overstreet & Yamamura, 1979). Reduction in the normal stimulation of receptors, either resulting from an impairment in synaptic input or by blockade of the receptor, can result in an elevation in the binding of a ligand to its receptor. Conversely, with chronic overstimulation of receptors, the binding of ligands has been reported to be reduced. The possibility that such changes could be involved in the development of ethanol tolerance is interesting. However, alterations in receptor properties should follow the development and dissipation of tolerance. This has not been well studied. In fact, under some conditions, the changes in binding totally reverse in the opposite direction within a few days, while under other conditions, the effects may not be reversible, independent of the presence of tolerance.

When ethanol has been administered for a long period of time, on the order of months, changes in receptor binding can last at least 1 month after withdrawal. This might reflect the development of brain damage. On the other hand, very long-term ethanol treatment may not always lead to any change in receptor binding at all. When miniature swine consumed about 4 g/kg for 3 years, no alterations in a variety of receptors were observed (Harris et al., 1983). The involvement of brain damage in the development of receptor alterations will be discussed further in Chapter 7.

How ethanol could produce these changes in the properties of receptors is unknown. Based on the discussion in Chapter 2, it would be tempting to assume that the fluidizing properties of acute treatment with ethanol on biological membranes somehow alter the configuration of a receptor in such a manner that enhanced functional interactions of the transmitter with its receptor occur. This possibility has some promise based on the involvement of lipids in receptor function (Loh & Law, 1980). With an increase in the fluidity of lipid layers in membranes, the receptor may have greater rotational mobility, thereby exposing more receptors to the ligand. Another possibility could be a direct action of ethanol on proteins associated with the receptor systems. A change in conformation might alter the availability of binding sites with which the ligand could interact.

Two presumed alternatives could explain the changes in receptor binding after long-term ethanol administration. These would include a chronic direct interaction of ethanol with receptors or their environment and a chronic alteration in presynaptic input, that is, transmitter release.

The effect of chronic ethanol administration on membrane fluidity may play a role in some of the effects on receptors. With the report that such treatment can make membranes more rigid (Lyon & Goldstein, 1983), the more restricted microenvironment in which the receptor might reside could reduce the exposure of binding sites to the ligands. This could be a possible mechanism for changes in the affinity of GABA and opiate receptors. If chronic fluidization of membranes stimulates a compensatory change, thereby making the membranes more rigid, then the influence of a changing microenvironment around receptors might account for the reversal in the changes in binding after ethanol withdrawal. When ethanol is present, its fluidizing effect would be balanced by the rigidifying effect of chronic ethanol treatment. After ethanol withdrawal, only membrane rigidity would be apparent. This could account for the rapid changes in receptor binding observed after ethanol withdrawal in some studies.

A number of alterations in transmitter activity at the presynaptic level have been reported and could possibly stimulate receptor changes, if they were to last long enough. Two examples, worth noting have been discussed in this chapter. They relate to noradrenergic and cholinergic activity. Norepinephrine turnover is accelerated with chronic ethanol treatment for at least a few weeks (Pohorecky et al., 1974). Choline acetyltransferase, the enzyme that catalyzes the synthesis of acetylcholine, is reduced after months of ethanol treatment. If these effects last long enough and precede the changes in receptor binding, then such alterations in presynaptic input could account for long-term changes in receptor function under some conditions.

Another possibility related to presynaptic input could be that the effect of transmitter input on one receptor system might modify the receptors in another receptor system. Although a role for this alternative has not been demonstrated in the effects of ethanol, such changes have been reported under other circumstances. For example, lesions of the substantia nigra with 6-hydroxydopamine or chronic treatment with haloperidol not only lead to dopaminergic supersensitivity in the caudate nucleus, they also lead to cholinergic subsensitivity as well (Gianutsos & Lal, 1976; Suga, 1980). Furthermore, chronic treatment with antidepressants, inhibitors of catecholamine uptake, not only reduces β-adrenergic and dopaminergic receptor binding, but also reduces opiate binding and enhances muscarinic cholinergic binding (Kolde & Matsushita, 1981; Reisine & Soubrie, 1982).

Whether there are physiological consequences of such interactions after ethanol treatment is poorly understood. It has been difficult to find studies that have been done with sufficiently similar experimental designs to make possible correlations between receptor systems. A few pharmacological studies have suggested that some of the biological changes observed after ethanol treatment might represent actions far removed from the primary interaction of ethanol with membranes, that is, actions far down the chain of events.

7. Brain damage

It is well known that chronic ethanol consumption can lead to brain damage. A variety of syndromes have been described in alcoholics and are believed to be caused either by malnutrition or by direct cytotoxicity (Dreyfus, 1974; Freund, 1973a). The two main syndromes associated with chronic ethanol consumption are Wernicke's encephalopathy and Korsakoff's psychosis. Wernicke's encephalopathy is characterized by mental confusion, ataxia, abnormal ocular mobility, and polyneuropathy. However, it is well accepted that this disorder results from a thiamine deficiency that develops from improper nutrition that can accompany chronic ethanol consumption. Patients with Korsakoff's psychosis develop learning and memory disabilities. According to Victor, Adams, and Collins (1971), these disabilities correlated best with lesions of the mammillary bodies, the medial dorsal nucleus of the thalamus, and the medial part of the pulvinar. This syndrome is not a result of a nutritional deficiency. Finally, cerebellar cortical degeneration has been reported in brain-damaged alcoholics and is characterized by spasticity, tremor, and ataxia. In severe cases, loss of cerebellar Purkinje and granular cells has been observed.

The mechanism responsible for the cytotoxicity of ethanol are unknown. If ethanol exerts its normal pharmacological effects through interactions with membranes, it is possible that such interactions may play a role in the development of brain damage. Although it is not clear whether alterations in membrane structure and function cause brain damage or are a result of it, there is value in examining biological systems related to membranes that may underlie some of the clinical manifestations of brain damage.

This chapter will not attempt to review comprehensively all that is known about brain damage. Such a treatment can be found elsewhere. Since this book is about the interactions of ethanol with membranes, emphasis will be placed on those studies which have examined membrane structure or function and on determining whether the evidence favors any putative mechanisms. In that sense, the approach taken will be along the lines of the first six chapters of this book.

Since studies involving the role of membranes in ethanol-induced brain damage require the use of experimental animals, an appropriate model is needed. In Chapter 1, the various considerations that should be taken into account when examining the chronic effects of an addictive drug were presented. On the basis of that discussion, when detecting a biological change after chronic administration of the drug, it is not always clear what this change represents. Since tolerance and physical dependence may be present in addition to cytotoxicity, care is required in designing experiments that allow for separation of these different responses to chronic ethanol administration.

One of the soundest approaches taken has been to measure biological endpoints after many months of ethanol administration and at a considerable time after ethanol withdrawal. This allows tolerance and physical dependence to dissipate. Experiments of this type will be the ones generally discussed because they are easiest to interpret. With this approach, animals have been found to have deficits in learning and memory long after ethanol withdrawal, suggesting the development of brain damage (Walker, Hunter, & Abraham, 1981).

In the remainder of this chapter, ethanol-induced brain damage will be examined from a number of perspectives, including direct morphological, physiological, and biochemical studies related to membrane structure and function. These studies have used both adult and pre- and neonatal animals. The aging process may provide clues about ethanol-induced brain damage. The similarities between these two processes, as well as various mechanisms that may underlie the development of brain damage will be discussed.

Morphological studies

One way to assess the consequences of chronic ethanol administration on membranes in the brain is to examine their structural integrity using histological techniques (Cox, 1982). A number of studies have been reported dealing with morphological alterations in the hippocampus and cerebellum. These areas of the brain were discussed in detail in Chapter 3 with respect to the electrophysiological effects of acute doses of ethanol. The anatomical features of these areas can be found there.

The structural integrity of the hippocampus was studied in mice that had been treated with ethanol in a liquid diet for 4 months followed by 2 months of abstinence (Riley & Walker, 1978). Blood ethanol concentrations ranged from 21.7 to 32.6 mM (100 to 150 mg/dl). Sections of the hippocampus and the dentate fascia associated with it were obtained and stained using the Golgi technique, a metal impregnation method that will stain black the whole neuron and its processes. The number of dendritic spines on which afferent fibers synapse was determined on 30-μm segments of dendrites. The number of these spines on the basilar dendrites of CA1 pyramidal cells in the hippocampus and on granule cells in the dentate fascia was significantly reduced by 50-60%. No gross alterations in dendritic morphology were observed.

In a recent study, comparisons of hippocampal morphology were made both before and after withdrawal from 4 months of chronic ethanol consumption (Phillips & Cragg, 1983). Blood ethanol concentrations were 2.1-14.9 mM (9.7-69 mg/dl). Histological examinations did not reveal any changes in cell numbers, based on the number of nucleoli present, before ethanol withdrawal. However, 4 months after withdrawal, cell numbers were slightly but significantly reduced, as were the control groups, when compared to the prewithdrawal groups. Using electron-microscopic analysis, no differences in the number of synapses were observed. However, the areas of the spine heads on basilar dendrites were reduced by 10%. The authors suggested that such an effect on spinal area would make spines more difficult to see under a light microscope and that the large decrease in the number of dendritic spines reported by Riley and Walker (1978) may have been overestimated. However, since the blood ethanol concentrations in the Phillips and Cragg (1983) study were much lower than those in the Riley and Walker (1978) study, comparisons may not be conclusive.

The effect on basilar dendritic spines may not be widespread on other dendritic trunks. Recently, the number of dendritic spines was determined on apical dendrites of CA1 neurons using electron-microscopic techniques (Lee et al., 1981). Rats were maintained on a 10% ethanol solution containing 1% saccharin for 18 weeks. The animals were not withdrawn from ethanol. Solid food was provided ad libitum. Blood ethanol concentrations ranged from 15.7 to 32.6 mM (72 to 150 mg/dl). In these studies, the number of spines on apical dendrites was unaltered.

Since the number of neurons in a tissue section cannot be easily determined with the Golgi technique because all cells are not impregnated by the dye, further experiments were undertaken using rats that were treated with ethanol for 5 months, then withdrawn for 2 months (Walker, Barnes, Zornetzer, Hunter, & Kubanis, 1980). The sections of the hippocampus were stained with cresyl violet or hematoxylin and eosin, dyes that allow visualization of all the neurons in a tissue section. The numbers of both pyramidal and granule cells were decreased. Since nutrition was maintained in these studies, the data provide evidence that nutritional deficits are not necessary prerequisites for the development of ethanol-induced brain damage.

Evidence of brain damage has been observed after shorter periods of ethanol consumption (West, Lind, Demuth, Parker, Alkana, Cassell, & Black, 1982). Unilateral lesions of the entorhinal cortex can lead to an increase in the density of acetylcholinesterase-stained sections of the dentate gyrus. This effect is believed to reflect lesion-induced sprouting of the remaining fibers to areas that have been deafferented by the lesion. When rats were maintained on ethanol in a liquid diet initially for 2 weeks, lesioned, then given ethanol for an additional 9 days, this lesion-induced increase in acetylcholinesterase was reduced. These data suggest that ethanol treatment retards the recovery function after brain injury.

A loss of cells has also been observed in the cerebellum. In rats that had been exposed to ethanol for 5 months, then withdrawn for 2 months, the number of Purkinje and granular cells, as well as the area of the molecular and granular layers, in each midsagittal section was reduced by 20–25% (Walker, Barnes, Riley, Hunter, & Zornetzer, 1980; Walker *et al.*, 1981). In another study in which rats were given ethanol in a 20% drinking solution for 1–18 months and apparently not withdrawn, the number of granular cells after at least 6 months of ethanol consumption was reduced (Tavares & Paula-Barbosa, 1982). Using ultrastructural analysis, degenerative changes in both granule cells and parallel fibers were found. Glial proliferation was also observed with the glial processes surrounding the degenerating cells.

Finally, the effect of long-term ethanol administration on cellular integrity may, in part, be dependent on age. In a recent study, two sets of rats were fed a liquid diet for 10 weeks (Pentley, 1982). One group was 3 months old at the start of the experiment and the other was 12 months old. The number of dendritic branches on cerebellar Purkinje cells after chronic ethanol consumption was reduced, but only in the older group of rats.

Electrophysiological studies

Several electrophysiological experiments have been reported that studied persistent changes in membrane properties that occur after withdrawal from long-term chronic ethanol treatment, and concurrent with the development of brain damage. As with the morphological studies, animals were administered ethanol for 5 months. All of the reports deal with functional changes in the hippocampus. (See Chapter 3 for discussion of basic concepts and methodology.)

Given the loss of pyramidal cells in the hippocampus, experiments were undertaken to determine whether afferent input to CA1 pyramidal cells was disrupted or whether the remaining pyramidal cells had an altered sensitivity to stimuli. In one study, field potentials elicited by stimulating Schaffer collateral and commissural fibers located in the stratum radiatum or originating in the ipilateral and contralateral CA3 regions, respectively (see Figure 3-2), were recorded from CA1 pyramidal cells (Abraham *et al.*, 1981). Neither the population EPSP nor the population spike was altered. With paired-pulse stimulation, the population spike elicited by the second pulse was elevated in the ethanol-treated animals. In addition, the inhibitory component of the field potential was reduced after low-frequency stimulation. The data suggested that the activity of intrinsic inhibitory neurons in the hippocampus was disrupted by chronic ethanol treatment.

Further support of an alternation in inhibitory mechanisms in the hippocampus comes from *in vitro* slice preparations obtained from rats chronically fed ethanol in a liquid diet for 20 weeks, then withdrawn for 3 more weeks (Durand & Carlen, 1984). In these experiments, intracellular recordings were obtained from CA1 pyramidal and granule cells after orthodromic stimulation of the stratum radiatum and perforant path, respectively. IPSPs and afterhyperpolarizations were significantly altered in the cells from ethanol-treated animals. The duration of both of these electrical events was reduced in both cell types. The maximum amplitudes were also reduced in the granule cells.

In other studies, a different approach was taken. In order to examine the distribution of synaptic currents in apical dendrites of CA1 pyramidal cells, a current-source density analysis of field potentials was employed. Current-source density analysis allows for a more precise localization of current sources and current sinks over shorter distances than can field potentials alone (Freeman & Nicholson, 1975). When recording from CA1 pyramidal cells, the current source refers to the passive flow of current out of the pyramidal cells and the current sink refers to the current flowing from the afferent fibers.

After rats were given ethanol for 5 months, then withdrawn for 2 more months, field potentials evoked by stimulation of the Schaffer collateral and commissural fibers in the stratum radiatum were recorded in 25-μm increments through the hippocampal CA1 region (Abraham, Manis, Hunter, Zornetzer, & Walker, 1982). Current source density analysis of control animals revealed two current sources, one at the pyramidal cell bodies and the other at the distal end of the apical dendrites. Two current sinks were found along the apical dendrites in the stratum radiatum. Ethanol treatment reduced the length of the current sink proximal to the pyramidal cell bodies and increased the amplitude of the distal sink. These data would suggest that chronic ethanol exposure can lead to alterations in the spatial distribution and efficiency of afferent input of the Schaffer collateral and commissural fibers onto CA1 pyramidal cells.

Current source analysis was also used to examine the afferent input to the dentate fascia (Abraham & Hunter, 1982). Afferent input to the granule cells of the dentate fascia arises from the lateral and medial entorhinal cortex, combines into the angular bundle, then synapses onto the dendrites of the granule cells in the molecular layer of the dentate fascia. Chronic ethanol treatment for 5 months followed by 2 months of withdrawal resulted in a reduction in the length of the current sink on the dendritic processes of the granule cells, suggesting a shrinkage of the field of afferent fibers from the entorhinal cortex.

Biochemical studies

Very few studies have appeared that demonstrate an apparently irreversible effect on membrane function using biochemical techniques. These studies used radioligand–receptor binding techniques. (See Chapter 6 for description.) Animals were treated with ethanol for at least 4 months and were withdrawn for up to 1 month when the measurements were made.

Ethanol was provided to rats in a liquid diet for 18–75 weeks and the binding of [^{3}H]QNB to muscarinic cholinergic receptors was measured in several areas of the brain (Nordberg & Wahlström, 1982; Pelham et al., 1980). QNB binding in the caudate nucleus and mammillary bodies was significantly elevated, reflecting an increase in the apparent number of receptors, based on Scatchard analysis (see Chapter 6). No effect was observed in the hippocampus or cerebral cortex. In addition, no alteration in binding was found after only 2 weeks of ethanol consumption. The increased QNB binding correlated with a reduction in the activity of choline acetyltransferase, the enzyme that catalyzes the synthesis of acetylcholine. These effects persisted for at least 4 weeks. When measuring [^{3}H]haloperidol binding to dopaminergic receptors, binding was significantly decreased after 13 months of ethanol treatment (Pelham et al., 1980).

The binding of [^{3}H]flunitrazepam to benzodiazepine receptors was measured in mice exposed to a liquid diet for 7 months, then withdrawn for 1 month (Freund, 1980a). A small decline in both the affinity of the ligand and number of receptors was observed. No effect was seen after only 2 weeks of ethanol consumption.

In Chapter 6, the effect of chronic ethanol administration on receptor binding was discussed at length with numerous changes in ligand binding being reported. These changes required a minimum duration of exposure to ethanol, usually at least 1 week. However, the effects were not long lasting, when time courses were determined, and often varied within the first few days after withdrawal. For example, in the case of β-adrenergic receptors, the binding of [^{3}H]dihydroalprenolol was reduced shortly after withdrawal from 60 days of ethanol consumption, when intoxication was still present in the animals, but was elevated 3 days after withdrawal (Banerjee et al., 1978).

The problem in determining the significance of the changes observed after chronic ethanol treatment is the inability to know whether the changes reflect tolerance, dependence, brain damage, or a combination of them. The few time courses that have been determined for the alterations in receptor binding after chronic ethanol treatment do not clearly correlate with any of these phenomena. If these alterations in receptor binding are relevant to the processes of tolerance and physical dependence, they should temporally correlate with their development and dissipation.

One possibility for which there is yet no supporting evidence is that many of the observed changes in biological endpoints related to membrane function might reflect the prodromal phases of brain damage. In the early stages of chronic ethanol administration, whatever cytotoxic effect ethanol may exert on membranes could be reversible. This would be dependent on the normal regenerative processes involving the synthesis of membrane constituents.

Similarities to aging

Considerable interest has been generated in the last several years into the possibility that ethanol-induced brain damage may have some similarity to the aging process or may be aggravated by old age. In this section, we shall examine the relationship between aging and brain damage with respect to membranes. A more global treatment of the subject can be found elsewhere (Freund, 1982; Wood & Armbrecht, 1982a).

One of the adverse consequences of aging is the development of dementia, one of the more devastating being Alzheimer's disease (Côté, 1981). Dementia is characterized by the loss of mental capabilities, such as memory, a reduction in brain weight, and a variety of histological changes. The memory disorders are believed to involve a lower activity of cholinergic neurons (Bartus, Dean, Beer, & Lippa, 1982; Davis & Yamamura, 1978). What may underlie this deficit is the impairment of the ability of the brain to synthesize neurotransmitters (Pradhan, 1980; Strong, Samorajski, & Gottesfeld, 1982). In the case of acetylcholine, choline acetyltransferase has been reported to be decreased, especially in the hippocampus.

Neurotransmitter receptors are also altered with age and in Alzheimer's disease. Aged laboratory animals have fewer cholinergic, dopaminergic, β-adrenergic, and GABA-ergic receptors (De Blasi, Cotecchia, & Mennini, 1982; Freund, 1980b; Kubanis, Zornetzer, & Freund, 1982; Maggi, Schmidt, Ghetti, & Enna, 1979; Makman, Ahn, Thai, Sharpless, Dvorkin, Horowitz, & Rosenfeld, 1979; Pradhan, 1980). The alterations in dopaminergic receptors were observed only for the antagonists and not for the agonists (De Blasi et al., 1982). The changes in β-adrenergic binding did not correlate temporally with decreases in norepinephrine-stimulated adenylate cyclase, which appeared much earlier (Maggi et al., 1979). Both elevated and reduced benzodiazepine binding have been reported in aged animals (De Blasi et al., 1982; Kubanis et al., 1982; Memo, Spano, & Trabucchi, 1981). Postmortem measurements in patients with Alzheimer's disease revealed that cholinergic, GABA-ergic, and dopaminergic receptors were reduced (Reisine, Yamamura, Bird, Spokes, & Enna, 1978). No changes in binding of ligands for α-adrenergic or serotonergic receptors were found (De Blasi et al., 1982).

Recently, reports have appeared addressing the question whether older animals are more sensitive to the actions of ethanol. These reports indicate that older mice become more intoxicated than younger mice with the same blood ethanol concentrations (Ritzmann & Springer, 1980; Wood et al., 1982). In addition, older mice that were rendered physically dependent on ethanol exhibited a more severe withdrawal syndrome than did younger mice. When comparing the hypothermic effect of ethanol to the duration of the ethanol-induced loss of the righting reflex, the hypothermic effect was less in older mice, even though the duration of the loss of the righting reflex in these animals was longer than in the younger mice (Wood & Armbrecht, 1982b). Blood ethanol concentrations between the older and younger mice were not significantly different.

A study was undertaken to determine whether the differences in sensitivity to ethanol as a function of age could be explained on the basis of the interactions of ethanol with membranes (Armbrecht et al., 1983). Synaptic plasma membranes, brain microsomal membranes, and erythrocyte membranes from mice ranging in age from 3 to 24 months were incubated with concentrations of ethanol in vitro from 250 to 500 mM (1150 to 2300 mg/dl). Membrane order was determined using EPR techniques and 5-doxylstearic acid as the free-radical probe. (See Chapter 2 for discussion of technique.) Ethanol had its greatest disordering effect on membranes derived from the youngest mice. Very little effect was observed with 500-mM (2300-mg/dl) ethanol in membranes from the oldest mice. Intrinsic membrane order did not significantly differ with age. Along with the reduced fluidizing effect of ethanol with age, there also were increases in the membrane concentrations of cholesterol and phospholipids.

The effect of ethanol on the Na-K-ATPase also differs with age. As discussed in Chapter 5, ethanol can inhibit this enzyme in vitro. When this action of ethanol was tested in older animals, Na-K-ATPase activity in synaptosomal membranes was much less sensitive than in younger animals (Sun & Samorajski, 1975).

Fetal alcohol syndrome

It is now accepted that consumption of alcoholic beverages by pregnant women can have adverse effects on the unborn child (Abel, Randall, & Riley, 1983; Colangelo & Jones, 1982; Rosett, 1979). Known as fetal alcohol syndrome, the abnormalities that occur include dysfunctions of the CNS, such as mental retardation, poor coordination, and hyperactive behavior, growth deficiencies, and characteristic facial features. In this section, we shall examine some of the evidence that neural consequences of fetal alcohol syndrome may involve actions of ethanol in utero on membranes.

In consideration of the mental and motor impairments in children with fetal alcohol syndrome, neuroanatomical studies have been undertaken in rats to determine whether fetal ethanol exposure has an adverse impact on cellular development in the hippocampus and cerebellum. In experiments in which the hippocampus was examined, pregnant rats were given ethanol in a liquid diet. In one report, ethanol was administered for the first 21 days of gestation with the daily consumption being about 12 g/kg (West, Hodges, & Black, 1981). The pups were reared by rats not given ethanol. When the neonates reached 60 days of age, hippocampal anatomy was assessed. The topography of the mossy fibers was found to be altered. Mossy fibers to the CA3 region of the hippocampus were hypertrophied. In another study with a similar experimental design in which pregnant rats ingested about 15 g/kg of ethanol during Days 10–21 of gestation, the number of pyramidal cells was reduced in the CA1 region (Barnes & Walker, 1981). No change in the number of granule cells was observed. Finally, when pregnant rats were administered oral doses of ethanol of 3 g/kg, twice daily, for the whole period of gestation, the number of dendritic spines on CA1 pyramidal cells was reduced (Abel, Jacobson, & Sherwin, 1983).

In other experiments, prenatal ethanol exposure influenced the degree of postnatal sprouting induced by lesions of the entorhinal cortex. As discussed earlier, chronic ethanol administration to adult animals can retard this process. When pregnant mothers received ethanol for the first 21 days of gestation, sprouting in the offspring after they reached adult age was significantly elevated (Dewey & West, 1984; West, Dewey, & Cassell, 1984). This effect was seen as an increase in the width, area, and acetylcholinesterase staining of the commissural/association fibers, but not of the mossy fibers of the dentate fascia. The data suggest that maternal drinking may have long-lasting consequences on neural plasticity of the offspring.

Abnormal development of the cerebellum has also been found in offspring of pregnant rats exposed to ethanol. When ethanol was administered to the mothers in a liquid diet between Days 3 and 20 of gestation and the pups examined 11 or 14 days after birth, cerebellar weight was reduced by 10% (Kornguth, Rutledge, Sunderland, Siegel, Carlson, Smollens, Juhl, & Young, 1979). The external granule cell layer was increased in these animals with no change observed in the thickness of the Purkinje cell layer. When neonates were exposed to ethanol by inhalation 3–20 days after birth, the number of Purkinje and granule cells was decreased (Bauer-Moffett & Altman, 1975, 1977). In other studies, rats exposed to 10% ethanol in the drinking water throughout gestation and lactation developed fewer granule cells at 21 days postpartum (Borges & Lewis, 1983b). With further analysis, this effect appeared to result from an increase in cell death and possibly to a loss of cell acquisition (Borges & Lewis, 1983a). These observations are consistent with the appearance of gross body tremors and poor motor coordination in animals treated under similar experimental conditions (Diaz & Samson, 1980).

Finally, a recent study examined the morphology of dendritic spines on pyramidal cells in the cerebral cortex from rats whose mothers were exposed to ethanol throughout pregnancy (Stoltenburg-Didinger & Spohr, 1983). As in the hippocampus (Abel *et al.*, 1983), the number of spines was reduced. In addition, the existing spines were long, thin, and entangled, rather than stubby and mushroom shaped.

Few reports have appeared on the effect of prenatal exposure of ethanol on the development of a functional endpoint of membrane function. In one report, the uptake of biogenic amines into synaptosomes or synaptic storage vesicles was determined in pregnant rats given ethanol in a liquid diet beginning on Day 13 of gestation and lasting until birth (Slotkin, Schanberg, & Kuhn, 1980). Uptake of catecholamines and indoleamines was measured in the neonates 2–19 days after birth. Little effect on synaptosomal uptake of norepinephrine, dopamine, and serotonin was observed. The uptake of norepinephrine into synaptic vesicles was slightly elevated. Little effect on basal or norepinephrine-stimulated adenylate cyclase and phosphodiesterase was observed in offspring from mothers given ethanol throughout gestation (Mena, Salinas, Martín del Río, & Herrera, 1982; Salinas & Fernández, 1983).

In recent studies with similar experimental designs, the binding of [³H]naloxone to rat striatum was measured in rats 4–25 days old whose mothers received 6% ethanol in a liquid diet beginning on Day 6 of gestation for the duration of pregnancy (Shah & West, 1983). Binding was found to be consistently reduced. The binding of ligands to cholinergic and serotonergic receptors was unaltered in the cerebral cortex, corpus striatum, and diencephalon (Chan & Abel, 1982).

Mechanisms of brain damage

The mechanisms by which chronic ethanol administration leads to the development of brain damage are unknown. However, two possible mechanisms can be considered. One suggests that chronic ethanol treatment stimulates lipid peroxidation and the other suggests that such treatment suppresses the normal turnover of membrane constituents by inhibiting protein synthesis.

Lipid peroxidation is the process of oxidation of polyunsaturated fatty acids by free radicals. As discussed in Chapter 2, free radicals contain an unpaired electron. Unlike the stable free radicals attached to spin-labeled molecular probes, free radicals produced in the body are very reactive and can interact with the double bonds of the fatty acids, initiating a chain reaction that results in the oxidation of the double bonds of many of the fatty acids, depending on the proximity of adjacent fatty acids (Mead, 1976). This process can lead to membrane damage, not only to lipids, but to proteins as well.

Free-radical reactions, including lipid peroxidation have been linked to the aging process (Harman, 1982). Progressive oxidation of polyunsaturated fatty acids is associated with the formation of fluorescent pigments called lipofuscin that are found in the form of granules in the cytoplasm of neurons (Côté, 1981). These pigments are believed to originate from the reaction products of peroxidized lipids and denatured proteins (Mead, 1976).

In an effort to determine whether lipid peroxidation occurring during the aging process might be accelerated by ethanol consumption and might be related to ethanol-induced learning impairment, mice that were 3 months old were fed an ethanol-containing liquid diet for 5 weeks and lipofuscin fluorescence was measured in preparations from whole brain (Freund, 1979). As the animals aged, lipofuscin fluorescence increased. However, ethanol consumption had no significant effect on this increased fluorescence, nor did it affect the nucleic acid and protein content. In animals that had received diets fortified with vitamin E, an antioxidant that inhibits lipid peroxidation, lipofuscin fluorescence was reduced equally in both ethanol-consuming and control mice. However, the learning deficits induced by chronic ethanol administration were not prevented. No measurements in the hippocampus were reported, where brain damage had been previously found under similar experimental conditions.

In the cerebellum, however, the number of lipofuscin granules in the cytoplasm of Purkinje cells increased after long-term ethanol consumption (Tavares & Paula-Barbosa, 1983). Eight-week-old rats were given 20% ethanol in the drinking water for 1–18 months. Histologically, a greater number of lipofuscin granules were apparent after 1 month of ethanol exposure, as compared to controls. With further ethanol treatment, an even greater increase in the number of lipofuscin granules was found, until the animals had received ethanol for 6 months. After that time, the number of granules increased considerably in the control animals, especially after 12 and 18 months of ethanol treatment. Although these observations might be related to the motor dysfunction associated with chronic ethanol consumption, such a conclusion would be difficult to make, since no measurements of motor capability were reported.

Lipid peroxidation-induced brain damage might be aggravated by a vitamin E deficiency that can occur in malnourished alcoholics. This possibility was tested by measuring plasma vitamin E concentrations in alcoholics (Majumdar, Shaw, & Thompson, 1983). Of the patients examined, 32% of them had subnormal concentrations of vitamin E.

Superoxide dismutase is an enzyme involved with the removal of oxygen radicals that are formed during the reduction of oxygen to water in many biological reactions (Fridovich, 1976). The activity of this enzyme has been measured in a variety of cultured neural cells in the presence of ethanol (Ledig, M'Paria, Louis, Freid, & Mandel, 1980). Acute exposure of cells to 100 mM (460 mg/dl) ethanol led to a rapid inhibition of superoxide dismutase in both neuronal and glial cell lines. However, when the same concentration of ethanol was included in the growth medium of the cells, inhibition of the enzyme did not occur for three days and only in glial cell lines. When the ethanol was removed from the growth medium, superoxide dismutase activity returned to control values within 2 days.

Rats exposed to acute or chronic ethanol administration also exhibited a reduced superoxide dismutase activity in the brain (Ledig, M'Paria, & Mandel, 1981). Single doses of ethanol inhibited superoxide dismutase activity in a dose-dependent manner. Three daily 2-g/kg doses of ethanol or consumption of a 20% ethanol solution also resulted in lower superoxide dismutase activity. In the latter case, activity decreased slowly until reaching a plateau at 35% inhibition. Similar results were obtained in 3-week-old animals born to mothers drinking 10% ethanol for 4 months. It was suggested from the data presented that ethanol exposure may lead to an accumulation of oxygen radicals through inhibition of superoxide dismutase and may underlie some of the toxic effects of ethanol.

The possibility that superoxide dismutase activity may be reduced in human alcoholics has been tested by measuring the activity of the enzyme in postmortem brain tissue derived from alcoholics (Marklund, Oreland, Perdahl, & Winblad, 1983). Small changes were observed in the hypothalamus, hippocampus, and corpus striatum. However, the changes depended on whether the values were normalized to brain weight or to the amount of protein. In any event, it does not appear in the opinion of the authors that alterations in superoxide dismutase activity would be related to any possible brain damage in the patients. The presence or absence of brain damage was not reported, however.

Since membrane integrity depends, in part, on the resynthesis of normally degraded constituents, it is necessary that the required enzymatic apparatus be fully operational. Obviously, protein synthesis is extremely important to maintain this process. Chronic ethanol administration has been shown to inhibit protein synthesis in the brain, an effect recently reviewed (Tewari & Noble, 1979).

The observation that ethanol both *in vitro* and *in vivo* inhibits the incorporation of [³H]leucine into proteins in the brain was made in the early 1970s (Jarlstedt, 1972; Jarlstedt & Hamberger, 1972; Khawaja, Lindholm, & Niittylä, 1978; Kuriyama, Sze, & Rauscher, 1971; Tewari & Noble, 1971). The effect continues with prolonged ethanol administration. Similar results have been found in fetal and neonatal animals born to ethanol-drinking mothers (Rawat, 1975). It is not clear what the exact mechanism of this inhibition is, but two prominent and important reactions in the process of protein synthesis have been reported to be reduced by ethanol treatment:

the aminoacylation of transfer ribonucleic acid (tRNA) and the association of ribosomal subunits (Fleming, Tewari, & Noble, 1975; Tewari, Murray, & Nobel, 1978). In order for protein synthesis to occur, amino acids are first combined with specific tRNA molecules, which in turn allows for the proper sequencing of amino acids into proteins, as determined by the sequence of nucleotides in messenger RNA (mRNA) (Watson, 1976). The formation of peptide bonds occurs on the ribosomes, which properly orient the aminoacyl–tRNA molecules with the mRNA and support the growing polypeptide chain. Therefore, ethanol appears to interfere with the complex reactions necessary for successful protein synthesis.

There may also be defects in the ability of the brain to synthesize RNA after prolonged ethanol consumption (Tewari, Fleming, & Noble, 1975). The incorporation of [5-^{3}H]orotic acid into all types of RNA, except for nuclear RNA (nRNA), is significantly reduced in mice administered ethanol in the drinking water for 10 weeks. Orotic acid incorporation into nRNA was slightly elevated shortly after injection but was reduced thereafter. No alteration was observed in the availability of nucleotides for RNA synthesis.

The rationale that a defect in protein synthesis could contribute to brain damage is obvious. If a cell cannot replenish its constituents when they are metabolized, the cell will ultimately die. To what extent suppression of protein synthesis is involved in the destruction of membranes or in the apparently irreversible alterations in membrane function after chronic ethanol exposure is not known, since all studies have dealt with protein synthesis in general, and not in membranes. Also, the protein content of the tissue in the studies presented was not reported. Thus, it is not clear whether prolonged suppression of protein synthesis leads to a reduced protein concentration in membranes.

The reduced ability of the brain to synthesize proteins seems relatively nonspecific and may involve alterations in RNA metabolism. Whether this latter process is the cause of the decreased protein synthesis or whether ethanol independently interferes with many stages of the process is not known. In any event, it is not unreasonable to suspect that such a process could have untoward effects on membrane structure and function.

Commentary

On the basis of what has been presented in this chapter, it is apparent that little has been published on ethanol-induced brain damage at the level of the membrane. Since cells die after suitably long periods of ethanol consumption, it is not unreasonable to assume that alterations in membrane structure or function might somehow play a role in the cell's demise. This could result from direct and continuous toxic effects of ethanol on membranes from which the cell ultimately cannot recover, or from some indirect, possibly metabolic alterations that prevent cells from synthesizing membrane constituents that are normally metabolized and are then replenished.

The studies described here are largely descriptive, but demonstrate conclusively that brain damage can be induced by ethanol in spite of a sufficient nutritional state. The morphological changes observed are relatively specific to the hippocampus and cerebellum. These changes include the loss of dendritic spines to which afferent fibers attach in order to transmit information to other neurons, and the reduction of certain cell types, such as CA1 pyramidal cells and cerebellar Purkinje and granule cells. This is significant because two of the major problems associated with ethanol-induced brain damage are learning and motor disabilities. However, a systematic undertaking to examine other areas of the brain has not been reported. This, of course, would be a laborious, time-consuming endeavor.

Other morphological, electrophysiological, and biochemical studies indicate that in some cases afferent input to cells that are lost become more or less numerous depending on the areas of the brain examined. Also, receptors for neurotransmitters can in some cases proliferate or decline depending again on the brain area, and the transmitter itself. It is not clear whether proliferating receptors reflect temporary supersensitivity resulting from the loss of afferent input, such as possibly in the case of hippocampal cholinergic fibers or whether the cholinergic receptors could be completely lost, if ethanol consumption were long enough. This would have some parallel to the aging process.

It is interesting to note that some of the morphological effects observed after chronic ethanol administration to adult animals are also observed in fetal animals, except that the period of ethanol exposure in this case is considerably less, days versus months. The most prominent similarities are the reduction in the number of dendritic spines on hippocampal CA1 pyramidal cells and the actual number of hippocampal pyramidal cells and cerebellar Purkinje cells.

Why the brain of fetal animals is more sensitive to the effects of ethanol is not entirely clear, but it could be related to at least two factors. One, the enzymes needed to metabolize ethanol are not well developed in fetal livers (Seppälä, Räihä, & Tamminen, 1971; Waltman & Iniquez, 1972). This would increase the amount of ethanol in contact with the brain, thereby increasing the likelihood of toxic actions. The other factor relates to the developing nervous system in fetal animals. Cells in the brain are rapidly dividing, and it is crucial that the synthetic mechanisms to form and to maintain cellular integrity be functioning properly. Since protein synthesis has been reported to be reduced in fetal animals, this may contribute to cell loss.

Ethanol-induced brain damage might be more likely with advancing age. However, it is not clear whether the similarities in the descriptive profiles of aging and ethanol-induced brain damage suggest that either common mechanisms exist between them or that unrelated actions result in similar abnormalities. No clear connection between aging and ethanol-induced brain damage with respect to membrane function is yet apparent.

In fact, a distinctive difference is found between chronic ethanol administration and the effect of a single dose of ethanol on older animals. As discussed earlier, older animals are more sensitive to the intoxicating effect of ethanol, but less sensitive to the hypothermic and membrane-disordering effects. Also, when animals are chronically treated with ethanol, it has been reported that tolerance dissipates for both the intoxicating and hypothermic effects (Khanna, Kalant, Lê, & LeBlanc, 1980).

The responses of neurotransmitter receptors to aging and chronic ethanol administration have in some cases been similar. However, changes in the density of receptors in themselves may not be very revealing about functional deficits. Freund (1982) points this out by indicating that under normal physiological conditions, the properties of the receptors can vary widely.

Clearly, there is a need for more comprehensive studies of possible relationships between the membrane effects of aging and ethanol. The mechanism of ethanol-induced brain damage is not at all understood. There is so little known that it is difficult to propose viable explanations for brain damage. Unfortunately, evidence is lacking that convincingly supports any possible mechanism. Any mechanism, though, will have to explain cell destruction.

8. Therapeutic approaches

One of the ultimate purposes of biological research is to find ways to treat people inflicted with diseases. Alcoholism in this context is the consumption of ethanol to the extent that it causes several diseases. Currently, the pharmacological treatment of many of the diverse causes and consequences of excessive use of ethanol is unsatisfactory. A better understanding of the effects of ethanol on membrane structure and function could contribute to the development of more effective treatment. From the various effects of ethanol on biological membranes described throughout this book, several such approaches can be explored.

There are aspects of the consequences of ethanol ingestion that might be subject to modification by an antagonist. These include acute depression of the CNS, especially in the case of ethanol overdoses, and the withdrawal syndrome that can develop after abrupt withdrawal from chronic ethanol ingestion.

In order to put into perspective the issues involved in treating ethanol-related problems, a short review of the clinical signs associated with ethanol consumption will be presented. In an acute situation, the effects of ethanol depend on the concentration of ethanol in the blood and, therefore, the brain (Barry, 1979). At low blood ethanol concentrations, a stimulatory phase occurs, characterized by euphoria and a release of inhibitions. This is believed to result from inhibitory influences of ethanol on inhibitory neurons in the brain. With increasing concentrations of ethanol, motor dysfunction develops, characterized by disturbances of gait and balance. At the highest concentrations, ethanol induces anesthesia and respiratory depression, that can be fatal in cases of clinical overdoses. It is for this latter condition that effective treatment is needed.

Physical dependence on ethanol is a complex phenomenon. Clinically, it is expressed as an ethanol withdrawal syndrome that develops as a result of the abrupt cessation of long-term drinking. The withdrawal syndrome is displayed in two phases (Gross, Lewis, & Hasty, 1974; Victor & Adams, 1953). During the first 2 days after withdrawal, patients can exhibit tremors, hallucinations, and convulsions. During the next few days in severe cases, delirium tremens can develop. Patients with delirium tremens have an altered sense of perception, suffer from hallucinations, and have an overactive autonomic nervous system, characterized by fever, tachycardia, and profuse perspiration. Delirium tremens can be life-threatening and constitutes a medical emergency.

In the remainder of this chapter, a number of therapeutic approaches will be considered that utilize the various effects of ethanol on membranes. Extensive reviews of pharmacological treatment of ethanol-related problems can be found elsewhere (Alkana & Noble, 1979; Gessner, 1979; Sellers & Kalant, 1976; Thompson, 1978). The approaches to be discussed here include the use of hyperbaric environments (high pressure) and hypothermia, membrane stabilizers, drugs that interact with neurotransmitter receptors, and drug replacement therapy to counteract ethanol overdose and the signs and symptoms of the ethanol withdrawal syndrome.

Hyperbaric environments and hypothermia

Considerable evidence has been accumulated that supports the hypothesis that ethanol expands and disorders membranes and that these actions may reflect the primary mechanism of action of ethanol (see Chapters 1 and 2). By virtue of its physical and chemical properties, ethanol probably dissolves in membranes, distorting their normal structural integrity. If the increased mobility of molecules within the membrane contributes to the biological consequences of ethanol, a mechanism that might reduce this mobility could be a means by which the biological consequences of ethanol could be attenuated.

One approach that has been investigated is the use of hyperbaric environments. The logic for using hyperbaric environments is based on the idea that if membranes are expanded by ethanol, then creating a condition whereby the membrane could be contracted and, therefore, the mobility of membrane lipids could be reduced, the treatment of ethanol overdoses should be facilitated (see Chapter 1). As an initial test of this hypothesis, the membrane-disordering effect of ethanol was examined in hyperbaric environments. In this study, 100 atm of helium was able to antagonize the disordering effect of ethanol concentrations of 1087–2174 mM (5000–10,000 mg/dl) in spin-labeled (see Chapter 2) membranes derived from the claw nerves of the crayfish (Mastrangelo, *et al.*, 1979).

Hyperbaric environments have been successfully used to antagonize the effects of anesthetics (Halsey, 1982). With this as a basis, the ability of high pressure to reduce the depressant effect of ethanol has been examined. Initial studies demonstrated that air or oxygen under pressure could antagonize ethanol intoxication and that the effectiveness was dependent on the intensity of the pressure (Halsey & Wardley-Smith, 1975; Alkana & Syapin, 1979). However, pressures of 30–68 atm were used, which in themselves are toxic.

The use of different atmospheric compositions has been further refined. In order to eliminate a number of difficulties of using air or oxygen alone, including oxygen toxicity and nitrogen narcosis, mixtures of helium and oxygen have been tested. In experiments where the partial pressure of oxygen was kept constant, helium–oxygen mixtures were quite effective in reducing ethanol sleep-times without altering the blood ethanol concentration at which animals awakened (Alkana & Malcolm, 1981, 1982a; Malcolm & Alkana, 1982). It is interesting to note that hyperbaric helium-oxygen was more effective at lower doses of ethanol, that is, at lower levels of depression.

The intrinsic fluidity of membranes can be altered by changing the temperature of their environment. Elevating the temperature makes the membrane more fluid, while reducing the temperature makes the membrane more rigid. If ethanol disorders membranes, as would be observed with an increase in temperature, then reducing the body temperature should counteract the actions of ethanol. Reducing the temperature of membranes *in vitro* can partially reverse the disordering effect of ethanol (Chin & Goldstein, 1981).

Changing the ambient temperature to which animals are exposed can alter their sensitivity to ethanol intoxication. Depression and lethality were enhanced in rodents when the environmental temperature was elevated (Dinh & Gailis, 1979; Pohorecky & Rizek, 1981). Conversely, lowering the environmental temperature had the opposite effect. With body temperatures as low as 32°C, sleeping times were reduced 43% (Malcolm & Alkana, 1981). Hypothermia did not accelerate ethanol metabolism. In fact, blood ethanol concentrations at the time the animals awoke were higher than at normal temperatures. In addition, the lethal dose of ethanol was elevated with lowered environmental temperatures (Malcolm & Alkana, 1983).

The foregoing data suggest that hyperbaric environments and induced hypothermia should have a beneficial effect in reversing ethanol intoxication in humans. The circumstances most suited for such a treatment would be acute ethanol overdoses. At present, treatment to reduce the life-threatening consequences of such conditions is inadequate. With the availability of small hyperbaric chambers and standard means of controlling body temperature in hospitals, this approach is worth further study and possible clinical trials. At present, no such trials have been reported.

Membrane stabilizers

The electrical excitability of neurons is determined by a number of factors, including the distribution of ions, the concentration gradients of these ions, the permeability of the neuronal membrane to these ions, and the functional activity of ion channels and ion pumps (see Chapters 3 and

4). Manipulating any of these parameters can either increase or decrease the ability of a neuron to develop and propagate action potentials. Stabilizing membranes could have value in the treatment of hyperexcitable conditions, such as those present during an ethanol withdrawal syndrome. In this section, we shall examine the effectiveness of membrane stabilizers in treating withdrawal signs and symptoms.

A few drugs that stabilize membranes have been tested for their ability to suppress the ethanol withdrawal syndrome, including anticonvulsants and local anesthetics. These drugs have the capability of blocking the voltage-dependent increases in sodium current involved in the initiation of an action potential (Lipicky, Gilbert, & Stillman, 1972; Pincus, 1972; Ritchie & Greengard, 1966; Schwartz & Vogel, 1977). These drugs may exert this effect through a direct interaction with sodium channels (Creveling, McNeal, Daly, & Brown, 1983; Willow & Catterall, 1982).

The usefulness of phenytoin (Dilantin) in the management of withdrawal seizures has been controversial. When patients were given 100 mg of phenytoin three times a day, in combination with chlordiazepoxide, they developed fewer seizures, especially when they had a history of seizures (Sampliner & Iber, 1974). In another study, combined therapy with chlordiazepoxide and phenytoin was no more effective in reducing seizures than chlordiazepoxide alone (Rothstein, 1973). Clinical studies such as these are difficult to evaluate because of the lack of proper controls and of sufficient patient histories (Gessner, 1979).

In animal experiments, phenytoin was tested for its ability to prevent withdrawal seizures. In mice rendered physically dependent by ethanol inhalation for three days, 12-mg/kg intraperitoneal or 50-mg/kg oral doses of phenytoin, when administered 3.5 hr after withdrawal, were ineffective in reducing the intensity of seizures induced when the mouse was elevated by the tail (Gessner, 1974). A 100-mg/kg intraperitoneal dose of phenytoin initially reduced seizures, but elevated them thereafter.

A more recent study has suggested that phenytoin may have been ineffective in previous studies because of its slow accumulation in the blood (Chu, 1981). Blood concentrations of phenytoin that are therapeutically effective in blocking grand mal seizures were not obtained for 4–8 hr after administration and required higher doses than used in previous studies. When rats that had been treated with ethanol orally for 2 weeks were administered 250 mg/kg of phenytoin along with the last dose of ethanol and again 12 hr later, few seizures were observed after an auditory stimulus. The incidence of seizures seemed to relate to the blood phenytoin concentrations. Blood phenytoin concentrations in those animals that had no seizures were 15 μg/ml, but in those that did, they were only 4 μg/ml.

The use of lidocaine (Lidocaine), a local anesthetic, to treat withdrawal seizures has received little attention. Its use was suggested by Freund (1973c) based on experiments with mice. Mice that drank ethanol in a liquid diet for 6 days, received multiple, subcutaneous, 2.5- to 20-mg/kg doses of lidocaine every 20 min after the ethanol was withdrawn. None of the doses of lidocaine in themselves altered the overt behavior of control mice. However, the incidence and severity of spontaneous and audiogenic seizures were reduced in a dose-dependent manner. Clinical trials using lidocaine to treat the ethanol withdrawal syndrome have been reported.

In a different study, d-propranolol, another local anesthetic, was examined for its possible effectiveness in suppressing an ethanol withdrawal syndrome (Freund, 1977). Nonsedative doses suppressed both tremors and seizures. However, the effect was relatively short-lived, with successive doses needed every 90 min to maintained the drug's therapeutic benefit.

Pharmacological manipulation of neuroreceptors

Acute and chronic administration of ethanol can alter the interaction of a neurotransmitter with its receptor in a number of complex ways. Ethanol can either influence the properties of the receptor itself (see Chapter 6) or modify the synaptic input, that is, the amount of transmitter available to interact with its receptor. In the context of possible therapeutic approaches, it does not matter whether the ethanol-induced changes in receptor function are presynaptic or postsynaptic. What is important is how the interaction of the transmitter with its receptor can be modified in order to obtain the desired therapeutic benefit. In this section, we shall examine the pharmacological studies that manipulate transmitter function after ethanol administration to see whether the drugs being studied have any value in treating the adverse effects of ethanol exposure.

The most useful drugs that modify transmitter function for the treatment of the adverse effects of ethanol have been those that interfere with GABA-ergic transmission. As discussed in Chapter 6, the GABA receptor appears to be a complex system that is characterized by its ability to bind three different classes of ligands. These include GABA and GABA-like drugs, benzodiazepines, and dihydropicrotoxinin, the last of which can be displaced from its binding sites by barbiturates.

In experimental animals, both GABA and benzodiazepine receptors have been reported to be reduced after chronic ethanol administration (see review of Hunt, 1983). This information suggests that the use of drugs that stimulate either type of receptor would be effective in suppressing the ethanol withdrawal syndrome.

The benzodiazepines have been used for some time for the clinical management of the ethanol withdrawal syndrome and are considered the drugs of choice (Sellers & Kalant, 1976). In most cases, chlordiazepoxide (Librium) is used. However, other benzodiazepines, such as diazepam (Valium), are equally effective. These drugs can control anxiety, restlessness, tremor, seizures, and delirium tremens associated with the ethanol withdrawal syndrome.

The use of benzodiazepines does have some drawbacks. The major ones include sedation and enhancement of the actions of ethanol (Guerrero-Figueroa, Merrill, & Rye, 1970). In addition, benzodiazepines appear to disturb sleep during recovery from ethanol withdrawal (Funderburk, Allen, & Wagman, 1978) and may maintain ethanol consumption (Deutsch & Walton, 1977). Possibly because chronic ethanol consumption can reduce the apparent number of benzodiazepine binding sites (Freund, 1980a; Volicer & Biagioni, 1982a), large doses of benzodiazepines are often required to obtain the desirable clinical results (Woo & Greenblatt, 1979).

Benzodiazepines exert their action on at least two receptor subtypes. One subtype appears to be coupled to the chloride ionophore and mediates the sedative and ataxic effects of ethanol, while the other one, not coupled to the chloride ionophore, mediates the anxiolytic and anticonvulsant effects (Lippa et al., 1979; Squires et al., 1979). These subtypes have been exploited pharmacologically and a new class of drugs has been developed that acts preferentially on the receptor subtype involved with the anxiolytic and anticonvulsant effects of benzodiazepines (Klepner, Lippa, Benson, Sano, & Beer, 1979). These drugs, called the triazolopyridazines, are not benzodiazepines. Because they are devoid of the undesirable side effects of benzodiazepines, the triazolopyridazines might be worthwhile compounds to test as a possible improved treatment of the ethanol withdrawal syndrome. Any improvement, however, would probably be small.

Drugs that more directly alter the interaction of GABA with its receptors have shown some efficacy in reducing the frequency and severity of seizures during an ethanol withdrawal syndrome in experimental animals. In these cases, drugs have been used that directly act on GABA receptors (e.g., GABA and muscimol) or that increase the amount of GABA that can interact with its receptor by inhibiting its metabolism (e.g., aminooxyacetic acid and n-dipropylacetate) or uptake (e.g., l-2,4-diaminobutyric acid), thereby inducing its accumulation at receptor sites (Cooper et al., 1979; Goldstein, 1973, 1979; Hillbom, 1975; Noble, Gillies, Vigran, & Mandel, 1976). None of these drugs have been tested clinically.

Antagonists of the GABA-ergic receptor have been tested for their ability to decrease the depressant effects of ethanol. For example, bicuculline reduces the sleeping time of animals injected with ethanol (Frye & Breese, 1982; Liljequist & Engel, 1982; Martz et al., 1983). Such antagonists probably have no clinical usefulness because they are also convulsants.

Considerable evidence has been accumulated to suggest that catecholamines play some role in the acute and chronic effects of ethanol (Hunt & Majchrowicz, 1979). One of the therapeutic approaches that has been explored is the possibility that altering the activity of catecholamines through their receptors might prove beneficial in treating some of the consequences of ethanol ingestion. In experimental animals, the effects of such drugs in modifying the response to a single dose of ethanol have depended, in part, on the endpoint being measured. Ethanol can have either stimulatory or depressant actions depending on the dose used, as discussed earlier in this chapter.

The stimulatory effects in experimental animals are expressed as an increase in locomotor activity. Initial studies in which catecholamine synthesis was inhibited indicated that the release of catecholamines may play an underlying role in ethanol-induced hyperactivity (Carlsson, Engel, & Svensson, 1972). However, when drugs that act directly on catecholamine receptors were tested for their ability to modify this response, various results were obtained. Dopaminergic agonists inhibited ethanol-induced locomotion (Carlsson, Engel, Ströbom, Svensson, & Waldeck, 1974) and dopaminergic antagonists enhanced it (Matchett & Erickson, 1977), suggesting the possible involvement of presynaptic dopaminergic receptors (Carlsson *et al.*, 1974). α-adrenergic antagonists blocked the locomotor stimulation, but β-adrenergic antagonists did not (Matchett & Erickson, 1977).

The depressant actions of ethanol were also altered by drugs that interact with catecholaminergic systems. In experimental animals, dopaminergic agonists have been reported to reduce the depressive effects of ethanol, while dopaminergic antagonists enhanced them (Bacopoulos, Bize, Levine, & Van Orden, 1979); Messiha, 1978). Another study found that a dopaminergic agonist increases narcosis (Blum, Calhoun, Merritt, & Wallace, 1973). β-Adrenergic antagonists have been reported to reduce or enhance the depressive effects of ethanol (Matchett & Erickson, 1977; Muñoz & Guivernau, 1980; Smith, Hayashida, & Kim, 1970; Wimbish, Martz, & Forney, 1977). α-Adrenergic antagonists and amphetamine were ineffective (Abdallah & Roby, 1975; Matchett & Erickson, 1977).

Several clinical studies have been initiated to determine whether drugs that alter catecholaminergic function might have efficacy in treating ethanol-related problems in humans. Propranolol, a β-adrenergic antagonist, has been tested, but no clear benefit has been suggested by the data. In one study, a battery of tests that assess the cognitive, perceptual, and motor skills of the patient was used (Mendelson, Rossi, Berstein, & Kuehnlie, 1974). The effects of doses of ethanol that resulted in peak blood ethanol concentrations of 10.9–30.4 mM (50–140 mg/dl) were not altered by propranolol pretreatment. In another study, propranolol enhanced the actions of ethanol (Alkana, Parker, Cohen, Birch, & Noble, 1976). On the other hand, when human subjects were given L-dopa, aminophylline, or ephedrine, drugs that would enhance catecholamine–receptor reactions, the effects of ethanol were reduced (Alkana *et al.*, 1977). Apomorphine and amantadine, dopaminergic agonists, were not effective antagonists of ethanol (Alkana, Parker, Cohen, Birch, & Noble, 1982).

Drugs that alter the interactions of catecholamines with their receptors have also been tested for their ability to modify the signs and symptoms of the ethanol withdrawal syndrome. In studies with experimental animals, drugs that reduced the concentration of either norepinephrine or dopamine at their receptors or directly interact with the receptors had relatively consistent effects on the withdrawal syndrome, when measuring convulsions induced by handling or the incidence of head twitches. Drugs that reduced catecholamine–receptor interactions exacerbated the severity of withdrawal (Blum & Wallace, 1974; Collier et al., 1976; Goldstein, 1973; Yamanaka, 1982). On the other hand, drugs that increased catecholamine–receptor interactions suppressed the withdrawal signs (Björkqvist, 1975; Blum, Eubanks, Wallace, & Schwertner, 1976; Collier et al., 1976).

In light of these results, it is interesting to note that dopaminergic antagonists, specifically phenothiazines and butyrophenones, have been used clinically to treat the ethanol withdrawal syndrome (Gessner, 1979; Sellers & Kalant, 1976). They have proven to be less than satisfactory because of their many side effects, including hypotension, motor disturbances, and enhanced susceptibility to seizures. The antipsychotic activity of these drugs has some value in treating withdrawal-related hallucinosis as long as they are given after the convulsive phase of ethanol withdrawal (Sellers & Kalant, 1976).

With the observation that ethanol may enhance the binding of endogenous opiates to their receptors in vitro (Levine, Hess, & Morley, 1983; Tabakoff & Hoffman, 1983), the possibility that antagonists of opiates might be useful in blocking the actions of ethanol has been examined. In animal studies, there are reports indicating that such antagonists can reduce a number of the effects of ethanol, including the stimulatory, depressive, anticonflict, and analgesic effects of ethanol (Boada, Feria, & Sanz, 1981; Kiianmaa, Hoffman, & Tabakoff, 1983; Middaugh, Read, & Boggan, 1978; Vogel, Frye, Koepke, Mailman, Mueller, & Breese, 1981). However, the drugs were not always effective (Jørgensen & Hole, 1981).

Several recent clinical studies have appeared that have indicated that naloxone, an opiate antagonist, could reverse the effects of ethanol (Barros & Rodriquez, 1981; Jeffcoate et al., 1979; Jeffreys et al., 1980; Mackensie, 1979; Sørensen & Mattison, 1978). Other studies reported that naloxone was ineffective (Catley, Lehane, & Jones, 1981; Ewing & McCarty, 1983; Kimbal et al., 1980; Mattila, Nuotto, & Seppala, 1981; Nuotto, Palva, & Lahdenranta, 1983; Whalley, Freeman, & Hunter, 1981). The lack of consistency among these reports has been attributed to poorly controlled studies and other confounding factors, such as the presence of other drugs, head injuries, and shock (Dole, Fishman, Goldfrank, Khanna, & McGivern, 1982). A naloxone-induced elevation of ethanol elimination may also play a role (Badawy & Evans, 1981).

No clinical studies have been reported that attempted to suppress an ethanol withdrawal syndrome with opiate antagonists. The efficacy of these drugs has been inconsistent in laboratory animals. In one study, naloxone was found to suppress withdrawal seizures (Blum, Wallace, Schwertner, & Futterman, 1977). However, in a controlled, single-blind study assessing a number of signs of withdrawal, this finding was not confirmed (Hemmingsen & Sørensen, 1979).

Drug replacement therapy

One approach that has been taken for the treatment of physical dependence, as expressed by a withdrawal syndrome, is the use of drugs that have similar mechanisms of action as the drug on which the patient is dependent, but either the drugs have no dependence liability or the withdrawal syndrome associated with them is less severe. The most common example of this type of treatment, called drug replacement therapy, is the use of methadone to treat patients dependent on heroin.

As discussed in Chapters 1 and 2, a number of short-chain aliphatic alcohols have similar actions on membranes. Since ethanol suppresses the withdrawal syndrome, there is a possibility that alcohols other than ethanol may have efficacy in treating an ethanol withdrawal syndrome. So far, there has been little research suggesting that this approach may have any therapeutic implications. One group of alcohols that has been studied is the aliphatic diols, which are alcohols containing two hydroxyl groups.

Aliphatic diols induce intoxication in animals identical to that obtained after ethanol administration (McCreery & Hunt, 1978). Since the diol 1,3-butandiol has been suggested as a source of calories to supplement the nutrition of humans and animals (Tobin, Mehlman, Kies, Fox, & Soeldner, 1975), based on its lack of toxicity (Dymsza, 1975), it has been tested for its efficacy to suppress the ethanol withdrawal syndrome. A 4-g/kg oral dose of 1,3-butandiol was found to suppress completely the withdrawal syndrome without inducing sedation (Majchrowicz et al., 1976). Other diols were also effective, with their potencies directly related to their lipid solubilities (Hunt & Majchrowicz, 1980). The use of 1,3-butandiol for the clinical management of ethanol withdrawal, however, will probably have little value, since it can induce physical dependence equivalent to that of ethanol (Frye, Chapin, Vogel, Mailman, Kilts, Mueller, & Breese, 1981). Also, its lack of potency would make it difficult to administer adequate amounts to a patient.

Another approach to drug replacement therapy is the use of drug classes in addition to alcohols that are cross-tolerant and cross-dependent to ethanol. In this case, when tolerance to and dependence on ethanol have developed, tolerance to and dependence on these drug classes also exist. This particular approach has been used extensively in the clinical management of ethanol withdrawal.

Barbiturates, paraldehyde, and chloral hydrate have been used in order to reduce the ethanol withdrawal syndrome. However, well-controlled studies are lacking to determine if they are more effective than other drugs (Sellers & Kalant, 1976). The efficacy of barbiturates might be expected, in part because of an action in common with ethanol on the GABA–benzodiazepine–ionophore receptor complex (Ticku, 1980a; Ticku & Davis, 1981). The largest disadvantage in using barbiturates is their high dependence liability. There is no evidence that any of these drugs is superior to benzodiazepines.

Commentary

Because ethanol is a drug with a simple molecular structure, it has a diverse array of actions that are nonspecific in nature. Although ethanol may act through interactions with membranes, these interactions result in many biological consequences characteristic of the properties of the cell. The mechanisms that underlie the expression of these biological consequences may be manifold and unrelated to the primary action of ethanol. Consequently, the development of experimental approaches for the treatment of ethanol-related disorders may not be predictable, based on the primary mechanism of action of ethanol.

Assuming that ethanol acts by disordering membranes, there is no straightforward way of reversing this effect, compared to a receptor-mediated response. The use of hyperbaric environments and induced hypothermia might help reduce the consequences of membrane disordering, but would not likely restore the membrane to its original state. Nonetheless, this approach for treating ethanol overdoses is an interesting one.

Since neuronal excitation and synaptic transmission in the brain are the bases of the expression of behavior, altering behavior through manipulation of these processes might be a possible therapeutic approach. The usefulness of this approach for treating ethanol-related problems has not been encouraging. Reversing the effects of a single dose of ethanol by altering the activity of receptors for neurotransmitters has not been consistent. Ethanol seems to have little direct effect on transmitter receptors in physiologically compatible concentrations. Consequently, stimulating or inhibiting these receptors would have to be based on the neuronal pathways responsible for expressing the biological effects of ethanol. Which pathways are involved is not well understood.

Treating an ethanol withdrawal syndrome is even more complex. Since this syndrome probably reflects the adaptive mechanisms that have been activated in response to chronic depression of the nervous system by ethanol and is expressed in phases, the problem in finding suitable ways to intervene in neuronal transmission is especially difficult. To date, the neural pathways involved in the expression of an ethanol withdrawal syndrome have not been identified. Successful treatment may involve using different drugs at different phases of withdrawal. For example, benzodiazepines may be valuable during the tremulous and convulsive phases of withdrawal, while β-adrenergic blockers may be useful during delirium tremens to suppress autonomic hyperactivity.

In conclusion, it is doubtful that much progress toward the treatment of ethanol-related disorders will be made before a better understanding of the underlying mechanisms of ethanol intoxication and dependence has been obtained. At this stage of knowledge, symptomatic treatment may be the best that can be accomplished.

9. Summary

Throughout this book, we have addressed the ways in which alcohols can interact with membranes. Various interdisciplinary approaches have been taken in many laboratories in order to determine the specific sites of action of alcohols and the functional entities that may be modified leading ultimately to an observable biological or behavioral change. Based on what has been presented, we now have a clearer picture of the mechanisms underlying the actions of alcohols. However, deficiencies exist.

In Chapter 1, a number of criteria were presented that should be satisfied if a possible mechanism of action for alcohols on the brain is to be viable. The effects of alcohols on a number of systems satisfy most of these criteria. The basis of all of these actions appears to relate to the interactions of alcohols with membrane lipids.

No evidence has appeared to suggest that alcohols act on their own specific receptor in the normal pharmacological sense. However, alcohols are not diffusely distributed throughout membranes. Although the exact localization of alcohols within membranes is not known, alcohols may occupy a particular region of the membrane. This may represent a receptor in a more abstract sense.

The bulk of the data supports the hypothesis that alcohols interact with membranes by first dissolving in them. Their presence in membranes expands their volume and disorders the lipid constituents. This disordering effect is greatest in the central core of the membrane, which is intrinsically more fluid. Alcohols may directly interact with proteins as well, although the evidence is not yet conclusive.

The disordering effect of ethanol, although consistent across laboratories, is quite small (generally less than 5%) at physiologically compatible concentrations. Pharmacologically, such a small effect is generally not thought to be significant. However, in this case, this small effect may be amplified into a larger one, involving a functional, physiological mechanism, such as ion flux. In fact, this possibility has been suggested for interactions of anesthetics and neurons.

So far, all the studies that have examined the disordering effect of alcohols on membranes have dealt with bulk lipids. Whether such an effect has functional significance is not clear. It appears intuitive to expect that disordering membranes should have some consequences on functional units embedded in membranes. A few studies have addressed this issue by dem-

156

onstrating that a number of agents that disorder membranes also alter ion flux and enzymatic activity, as in the case of sodium and calcium uptake and adenylate cyclase activity. Some of the functional entities of membranes require a lipid environment of a given composition and properties. Perhaps alcohols interact with these environments, and this interaction may or may not relate to their actions on bulk lipids.

One of the nagging problems with the hypothesis that disordering lipids can explain the intoxicating effects of ethanol is the inability of obtaining similar effects by changing body temperature. Elevating body temperature increases membrane fluidity and vice versa. Elevating body temperature can alter the depressant effects of ethanol, but does not in itself induce intoxication. It is possible that temperature effects on membrane fluidity are different than those induced by ethanol. For example, temperature changes may affect the total membrane, while alcohols may alter the properties of only part of the membrane. This may have different consequences on cellular function.

Another problem is the effect of ethanol on aged animals. Although these animals are more sensitive to the depressant effects of ethanol than young animals, membranes are disordered to a lesser extent by ethanol. Although this might be perceived as a major discrepancy to the membrane model of ethanol intoxication, the possibility that in aged animals other mechanisms underlying intoxication are considerably more sensitive to ethanol cannot yet be discounted.

Although alcohols can disorder membranes, it is not clear whether this effect directly initiates the chain of events that leads to alcohol intoxication. At present, there is no direct evidence linking a change in fluidity to a change in behavior. The consequences of disordering membranes may be extensive and varied, some of which may have little or no biological significance.

Ethanol has a multitude of effects on the functional properties of membranes. Electrical as well as biochemical properties have been examined. The basis of neural activity is the ability of ions to flow through membranes at appropriate times after the initiation of appropriate stimuli. Changes in this property of neurons should have profound effects on the ability of neurons to function properly.

Ethanol can alter the stimulus-induced increases in the movements of sodium and calcium into and potassium out of neurons *in vitro*. These effects have been demonstrated both with biochemical and electrophysiological techniques. In biochemical studies, the effects of ethanol are observable at concentrations that are compatible with life. Some of these effects might be related to an increase of the binding of calcium onto the interior surface of the neuronal plasma membrane.

Changes in membrane order could have profound effects on the ion movements that underlie electrical activity in neurons. An increase or a decrease in the availability of important molecular sites on ion channels could alter the flow of ions through membranes during excitation and recovery. The changes in stimulus-induced sodium and calcium influx and calcium-stimulated potassium efflux could be mediated by changes in membrane order. For example, disordering the membrane could increase or decrease the availability of important sites in functional components of the membrane, so that the effects of normal stimuli are altered.

Electrophysiological techniques have provided some additional support *in vitro* for ethanol-induced changes in ion flux, but studies *in vivo* have yielded more complex results. Both excitation and depression of cellular electrical activity have been observed in the hippocampus and cerebellum, depending on the design of the experiments. The relevance of these observations to the intoxicating properties of ethanol is inconclusive. On the other hand, the findings in several laboratories that orthodromically stimulated activity is more sensitive to disruption by ethanol than antidromically stimulated activity suggest a greater sensitivity of ethanol on synaptic transmission than on the neuronal cell bodies. The biochemical studies using synaptosomes support this point.

Functional entities such as enzymes and neurotransmitter receptors in membranes show some sensitivity to ethanol *in vitro*. However, the concentration of ethanol needed for an effect is high or the conditions involved are not clearly physiologically relevant. For example, inhibition of the Na-K-ATPase requires low potassium concentrations, and stimulation of adenylate cyclase requires the presence of GTP, whose biological relevance in the activity of the enzyme *in vivo* is not known. Transmitter receptors are generally not sensitive to ethanol at physiologically compatible concentrations, although there are a few promising exceptions including GABA, glutamate, and opiate receptors. The lack of a direct effect of ethanol on these entities is consistent with the observation suggesting that presynaptic terminals are more sensitive to ethanol than the dendrites and cell bodies of neurons.

The chronic effects of ethanol on membranes are difficult to interpret because of the inability in many cases to distinguish between the development of tolerance, physical dependence, a withdrawal syndrome, and brain damage. The presence of any one or more of these phenomena at the time measurements are made makes it difficult to determine the significance of any changes observed. In addition, most reported studies did not include a control group showing that a single dose of ethanol would not induce the same effect.

The alterations in membrane properties and function observed after chronic ethanol administration depend in part on how long exposure lasts. Some effects can occur in just a few days, while others require many months to develop. For example, the lipid-disordering effect of ethanol is reduced and an increased rigidity of membranes can be observed after just a few days of ethanol treatment. However, in order to obtain consistent effects on transmitter receptors, weeks to months of ethanol exposure are required. These effects may result from chronic alterations in presynaptic input.

The mechanisms underlying tolerance to the lipid-disordering properties of ethanol and the rigidifying effect on membranes after chronic ethanol treatment are unclear. It has been postulated that chronic exposure can lead to changes in the lipid composition of the membranes, especially in the cholesterol content and the ratio of saturated to unsaturated fatty acids. The evidence to date is not yet convincing that such changes account for the altered properties of the membrane, since reports from a number of laboratories indicated a variety of results, even though ethanol tolerance was evidence. In fact, some of the results reported are opposite from those expected.

Body temperature is a major variable that has not been controlled in chronic studies with ethanol. Considering that ethanol induces hypothermia, the presence of a reduced body temperature for a period of time might stimulate changes in the composition of membranes analogous to cold acclimation. Indeed, some of the effects on lipid composition found with animals are similar to those found in microorganisms incubated at lower temperatures.

Chronic ethanol treatment has been demonstrated to be associated with alterations in the properties of receptors for neurotransmitters. This effect is most pronounced as the duration of ethanol exposure increases. No studies have been reported that directly implicate these changes in the development of any of the consequences of chronic ethanol ingestion. However, one can speculate on some possibilities. For example, the reduction of the binding of GABA and benzodiazepines to their receptors would be consistent with their involvement in withdrawal-associated seizures. The efficacy of GABA agonists and benzodiazepines to block these seizures provides further support.

Research has clearly shown that brain damage can occur after a sufficient period of chronic ethanol treatment. The damage has been found in the hippocampus and cerebellum. These are logical areas in which to find damage, considering that deficits in learning and memory and motor function are associated with brain damage. Whether there is significant damage to other areas of the brain is unknown, since no systematic studies to address damage to the brain as a whole have been undertaken. The lack of studies is probably due to the labor-intensive nature of such studies.

Little progress toward improved treatment of ethanol-related disorders based on the research concerning ethanol–membrane interactions has been made. The best treatment for managing an ethanol withdrawal syndrome, the use of benzodiazepines, was implemented before information about the effect of ethanol on GABA and benzodiazepine receptors was reported.

In fairness, it takes time to incorporate basic research into clinically useful treatments. One promising treatment, though, is the use of hyperbaric environments and induced hypothermia for the treatment of ethanol overdoses. Although the procedures are not without difficulty or risk, they do offer improvements over existing treatments.

Alcohol research has become increasingly more exciting as the ways in which alcohols can exert actions on cells are unraveled. Many of the observed biological changes induced by alcohols may be important mechanisms by which alcohols disrupt cellular function. Others may not. An important area of future research will involve a more precise description of the interactions of alcohols with cells and linking these interactions with the biological consequences of alcohol ingestion.

References

Abdallah, A. H., & Roby, D. M. Antagonism of depressant activity of ethanol by DH-524; a comparative study with bemegride, doxapram and *d*-amphetamine (38640). *Proceedings of the Society for Experimental Biology and Medicine,* 1975, *148,* 819–822.

Abdul-Ghani, A.-S., Bruce, D., & Bradford, H. F. Effect of glutamate dimethyl ester and glutamate diethyl ester in delaying the onset of convulsions induced by pentylenetetrazole and strychnine. *Biochemical Pharmacology,* 1982, *31,* 3144–3146.

Abel, E. L., Jacobson, S., & Sherwin, B. T. *In utero* alcohol exposure; functional and structural brain damage. *Neurobehavioral Toxicology and Teratology,* 1983, *5,* 363–366.

Abel, E. L., Randall, C. L., & Riley, E. P. Alcohol consumption and prenatal development. In B. Tabakoff, P. B. Sutker, & C. L. Randall (Eds.), *Medical and social aspects of alcohol abuse.* New York: Plenum, 1983.

Abraham, W. C., & Hunter, B. E. An electrophysiological analysis of chronic ethanol neurotoxicity in the dentate gyrus: Distribution of entorhinal afferents. *Experimental Brain Research,* 1982, *47,* 61–68.

Abraham, W. C., Hunter, B. E., Zornetzer, S. E., & Walker, D. W. Augmentation of short-term plasticity of CA1 of rat hippocampus after chronic ethanol treatment. *Brain Research,* 1981, *221,* 271–287.

Abraham, W. C., Manis, P. B., Hunter, B. E., Zornetzer, S. F., & Walker, D. W. Electrophysiological analysis of synaptic distribution of rat hippocampus after chronic ethanol exposure. *Brain Research,* 1982, *237,* 91–105.

Aghajanian, G. K., Cedarbaum, J. M., & Wang, R. Y. Evidence for norepinephrine-mediated collateral inhibition of locus coeruleus neurons. *Brain Research,* 1977, *136,* 570–577.

Ahlquist, R. P. Study of adrenotropic receptors. *American Journal of Physiology,* 1948, *153,* 586–600.

Akera, T., Rech, R. H., Marquis, W. J., Tobin, T., & Brody, T. M. Lack of relationship between brain $(Na^+ + K^+)$-activated adenosine triphosphatase and the development of tolerance to ethanol in rats. *Journal of Pharmacology and Experimental Therapeutics,* 1973, *185,* 594–601.

Albuquerque, E. X., & Daly, J. W. Batrachotoxin, a selective probe for channels modulating sodium conductances in electrogenic membranes. In P. Cuatrecasas (Ed.), *Receptors and recognition.* London: Chapman & Hall, 1976.

Alger, B. E., & Nicoll, R. A. Epileptoform burst after hyperpolarization: Calcium-dependent potassium potential in hippocampal CA1 pyramidal cells. *Science,* 1980, *210,* 1122–1124.

Alkana, R. L., Finn, D. A., & Malcolm, R. D. Hyperbaric exposure precipitates withdrawal in ethanol dependent mice. *Alcoholism: Clinical and Experimental Research,* 1983, *7,* 104.

Alkana, R. L., & Malcolm, R. D. Antagonism of ethanol narcosis in mice by hyperbaric pressures of 4–8 atmospheres. *Alcoholism: Clinical and Experimental Research,* 1980, *4,* 350–353.

Alkana, R. L., & Malcolm, R. D. Low-level hyperbaric ethanol antagonism in mice: Dose and pressure response. *Pharmacology,* 1981, *22,* 199–208.

Alkana, R. L., & Malcolm, R. D. Hyperbaric ethanol in mice: Studies on oxygen, nitrogen, strain and sex. *Psychopharmacology*, 1982, *77*, 11-16. (a)

Alkana, R. L., & Malcolm, R. D. Hyperbaric ethanol in mice: Time course. *Substance and Alcohol Actions/Misuse*, 1982, *3*, 41-46. (b)

Alkana, R. L., & Noble, E. P. Amethystic agents: Reversal of acute ethanol intoxication in humans. In E. Majchrowicz & E. P. Noble (Eds.), *Biochemistry and pharmacology of ethanol.* (Vol. 2). New York: Plenum, 1979.

Alkana, R. L., Parker, E. S., Cohen, H. B., Birch, H., & Noble, E. P. Reversal of ethanol intoxication in humans: An assessment of the efficacy of propranolol. *Psychopharmacology*, 1976, *51*, 29-37.

Alkana, R. L., Parker, E. S., Cohen, H. B., Birch, H., & Noble, E. P. Reversal of ethanol intoxication in humans: An assessment of the efficacy of L-DOPA, aminophylline, and ephedrine. *Psychopharmacology*, 1977, *55*, 203-212.

Alkana, R. L., Parker, E. S., Malcolm, R. D., Cohen, H. B., Birch, H., & Noble, E. P. Interaction of apomorphine and amantadine with ethanol in men. *Alcoholism: Clinical and Experimental Research*, 1982, *6*, 403-411.

Alkana, R. L., & Syapin, P. J. Antagonism of ethanol narcosis in mice. In M. Galanter (Ed.), *Currents in alcoholism* (Vol. 5). New York: Grune & Stratton, 1979.

Alling, C., Liljequist, S., & Engel, J. The effect of chronic ethanol administration on lipids and fatty acids in subcellular fractions of rat brain. *Medical Biology*, 1982, *60*, 149-154.

Altshuler, H. L., Phillips, P. E., & Feinhandler, D. A. Alteration of ethanol self-administration by naltrexone. *Life Sciences*, 1980, *26*, 679-688.

Amaral, D. G., & Sinnamon, H. M. The locus coeruleus: Neurobiology of a central noradrenergic nucleus. *Progress in Neurobiology*, 1977, *9*, 147-196.

Amer, M. S. Cyclic AMP and gastric secretion. *American Journal of Digestive Diseases*, 1972, *17*, 945-953.

Andersen, P. Organization of hippocampal neurons and their interconnections. In R. L. Isaacson & K. H. Pribram (Eds.), *The hippocampus* (Vol. 1). New York: Plenum, 1975.

Andersen, P., Eccles, J. C., & Loyning, Y. Pathway of postsynaptic inhibition in the hippocampus. *Journal of Physiology*, 1964, *13*, 208-221.

Arbilla, S., Kamal, L., & Langer, S. Z. Presynaptic GABA autoreceptors on GABAergic nerve endings of the rat substantia nigra. *European Journal of Pharmacology*, 1979, *57*, 211-217.

Armbrecht, H. J., Wood, W. G., Wise, R. W., Walsh, J., Thomas, B. N., & Strong, R. Ethanol-induced disordering of membranes from different age groups of C57BL/6NNIA mice. *Journal of Pharmacology and Experimental Therapeutics*, 1983, *226*, 387-391.

Armstrong, C. M., & Binstock, L. The effects of several alcohols on the properties of the squid giant axon. *Journal of General Physiology*, 1964, *48*, 265-277.

Aston-Jones, G., Foote, S. L., & Bloom, F. E. Low doses of ethanol disrupt sensory responses of brain noradrenergic neurones. *Nature*, 1982, *296*, 857-860.

Bacopoulos, N. G., Bize, I., Levine, J., & Van Orden, L. S., III. Modification of ethanol intoxication by dopamine agonists and antagonists. *Psychopharmacology*, 1979, *60*, 195-201.

Badawy, A. A.-B., & Evans, M. The mechanism of the antagonism by naloxone of acute alcohol intoxication. *British Journal of Pharmacology*, 1981, *74*, 514-516.

Banerjee, S. P., Sharma, V. K., & Khanna, J. M. Alterations in beta-adrenergic receptor binding during ethanol withdrawal. *Nature (London)*, 1978, *276*, 407-408.

Banks, B. E. C., Brown, C., Burgess, G., Burnstock, G., Claret, M., Cocks, T. M., & Jenkinson, D. H. Apamin blocks certain neurotransmitter-induced increases in potassium permeability. *Nature*, 1979, *282*, 415-417.

Barbaccia, M. L., Reggiani, A., Spano, P. F., & Trabucchi, M. Ethanol effects on dopaminergic function: Modulation by the endogenous opioid system. *Pharmacology, Biochemistry, and Behavior*, 1980, *13, Supplement 1*, 303–306.

Barnes, D. E., & Walker, D. W. Prenatal ethanol exposure permanently reduces the number of pyramidal neurons in rat hippocampus. *Developmental Brain Research*, 1981, *1*, 333–340.

Barros, S. R., & Rodriguez, G. R. Naloxone as an antagonist in alcohol intoxication. *Anesthesiology*, 1981, *54*, 174.

Barry, H., III. Behavioral manifestations of ethanol intoxication and physical dependence. In E. Majchrowicz & E. P. Noble (Eds.), *Biochemistry and pharmacology of ethanol* (Vol. 2). New York: Plenum, 1979.

Bartus, R. T., Dean, R. L., III, Beer, B., & Lippa, A. S. The cholinergic hypothesis of geriatric memory dysfunction. *Science*, 1982, *217*, 408–417.

Basile, A., Hoffer, B., & Dunwiddie, T. Differential sensitivity of cerebellar Purkinje neurons to ethanol in selectively outbred lines of mice: Maintenance *in vitro* independent of synaptic transmission. *Brain Research*, 1983, *264*, 69–78.

Baudry, M., Oliver, M., Creager, R., Wieraszko, A., & Lynch, G. Increase in glutamate receptors following repetitive electrical stimulation in hippocampal slices. *Life Sciences*, 1980, *27*, 325–330.

Bauer-Moffett, C., & Altman, J. Ethanol-induced reductions in cerebellar growth of infant rats. *Experimental Neurology*, 1975, *48*, 378–382.

Bauer-Moffett, C., & Altman, J. The effect of ethanol chronically administered to preweanling rats on cerebellar development: A morphological study. *Brain Research*, 1977, *119*, 249–268.

Baumgold, J. ^{3}H-Saxitoxin binding to nerve membranes: Inhibition by phospholipase A_2 and by unsaturated fatty acids. *Journal of Neurochemistry*, 1980, *34*, 327–334.

Beaumont, A., & Hughes, J. Biology of opioid peptides. *Annual Reviews of Pharmacology and Toxicology*, 1979, *19*, 245–267.

Beazell, J. M., & Ivy, A. C. The influence of alcohol on the digestive tract. *Quarterly Journal of Studies on Alcohol*, 1940, *1*, 45–73.

Begleiter, H., & Platz, A. The effects of alcohol on the central nervous system in humans. In B. Kissin & H. Begleiter (Eds.), *The biology of alcoholism* (Vol. 2). New York: Plenum, 1972.

Bennett, A., & Fleshler, B. Prostaglandins and the gastrointestinal tract. *Gastroenterology*, 1970, *59*, 790–800.

Bennett, J. P., Jr. Methods in binding studies. In H. I. Yamamura, S. J. Enna, & M. J. Kuhar (Eds.), *Neurotransmitter receptor binding*. New York: Raven, 1978.

Bennett, J. P., Jr., & Snyder, S. H. Serotonin and lysergic acid diethylamide in rat brain membranes: Relationship to postsynaptic serotonin receptors. *Molecular Pharmacology*, 1976, *12*, 373–389.

Berger, T., French, E. D., Siggins, G. R., Shier, W. T., & Bloom, F. E. Ethanol and some tetrahydroisoquinolines alter the discharge of cortical and hippocampal neurons: Relationship to endogenous opioids. *Pharmacology, Biochemistry, and Behavior*, 1982, *17*, 813–821.

Bergmann, M. C., Klee, M. W., and Faber, D. S. Different sensitivities to ethanol of early transient voltage clamp currents of *Aplysia* neurons. *Pflügers Archives of Physiology*, 1974, *348*, 139–153.

Berkowitz, B. A., Finck, A. D., & Ngai, S. H. Nitrous oxide analgesia: Reversal by naloxone and development of tolerance. *Journal of Pharmacology and Experimental Therapeutics*, 1976, *203*, 539–547.

Berridge, M. J. The interaction of cyclic nucleotides and calcium in the control of cellular activity. In P. Greengard & G. A. Robison (Eds.), *Advances in cyclic nucleotide research* (Vol. 6). New York: Raven, 1975.

Berrie, C. P., Birdsall, N. J. N., Burgen, A. S. V., & Hulme, E. C. Guanine nucleotides modulate muscarinic receptor binding in the heart. *Biochemical and Biophysical Research Communications*, 1979, *87*, 1000-1005.

Berry, M. S., & Pentreath, V. W. The neurophysiology of alcohol. In M. Sandler (Ed.), *Psychopharmacology of alcohol*. New York: Raven, 1980.

Bignami, A., & Palladini, G. Experimentally produced cerebral status spongiosus and continuous pseudorhythmic electroencephalographic discharges with a membrane ATPase inhibitor. *Nature*, 1966, *209*, 413-414.

Bignami, A., Palladini, G., & Venturini, G. Effect of cardiazol on Na-K ATPase of the rat brain *in vivo*. *Brain Research*, 1966, *1*, 413-414.

Bills, C. E. A pharmacological comparison of six alcohols, singly and in admixture, on paramecium. *Journal of Pharmacology and Experimental Therapeutics*, 1924, *22*, 49-57.

Bing, R. J., Tillmanns, H. Fauvel, J. M., Seeler, K., & Mao, J. C. Effects of prolonged alcohol administration on calcium transport in heart muscle of the dog. *Circulation Research*, 1974, *35*, 33-38.

Björkqvist, S. E. Clonidine in alcohol withdrawal. *Acta Psychiatrica Scandinavica*, 1975, *52*, 256-263.

Black, R. F., Hoffman, P. L., & Tabakoff, B. Receptor-mediated dopaminergic function after ethanol withdrawal. *Alcoholism: Clinical and Experimental Research*, 1980, *4*, 294-297.

Blaustein, M. P. Effects of potassium, veratridine and scorpion venom on calcium accumulation and transmitter release by nerve terminals *in vitro*. *Journal of Physiology*, 1975, *247*, 617-655.

Blaustein, M. P., & Ector, A. C. Carrier-mediated sodium-dependent and calcium-dependent calcium efflux from pinched-off presynaptic nerve terminals (synaptosomes) *in vitro*. *Biochimica et Biophysica Acta*, 1976, *419*, 295-308.

Blaustein, M. P., & Oborn, C. J. The influence of sodium on calcium fluxes in pinched-off nerve terminals *in vitro*. *Journal of Physiology*, 1975, *247*, 657-686.

Blaustein, M. P., & Weismann, W. P. Effect of sodium ions on calcium movement in isolated synaptic terminals. *Proceedings of the National Academy of Sciences (USA)*, 1970, *66*, 664-671.

Blum, K., Briggs, A. H., Elston, S. F. A., Hirst, M., Hamilton, M. G., & Verebey, K. Common denominator theory for alcohol and opiate dependence. A review of similarities and differences. In H. Rigter & J. Crabbe (Eds.), *Alcohol tolerance and dependence*. Amsterdam: Elsevier, 1980.

Blum, K., Calhoun, W., Merritt, J., & Wallace, J. E. L-DOPA: Effect on ethanol narcosis and brain biogenic amines in mice. *Nature*, 1973, *242*, 407-409.

Blum, K., Eubanks, J. D., Wallace, J. E., & Schwertner, H. A. Suppression of ethanol withdrawal by dopamine. *Experientia*, 1976, *32*, 493-495.

Blum, K., & Wallace, J. E. Effects of catecholamine synthesis inhibition on ethanol-induced withdrawal symptoms in mice. *British Journal of Pharmacology*, 1974, *51*, 109-111.

Blum, K., Wallace, J. E., Calhoun, W., Tabor, R. G., & Eubanks, J. D. Ethanol narcosis in mice: Serotonergic involvement. *Experientia*, 1974, *30*, 1053-1054.

Blum, K., Wallace, J. E., Schwertner, H. A., & Eubanks, J. D. Enhancement of ethanol-induced withdrawal convulsions by blockade of 5-hydroxytryptamine receptors. *Journal of Pharmacy and Pharmacology*, 1976, *28*, 832-835.

Blum, K., Wallace, J. E., Schwertner, H. A., & Futterman, S. Naloxone-induced inhibition of ethanol dependence in mice. *Nature*, 1977, *256*, 49-51.

Blume, A. J. Interactions of ligands with the opiate receptors of brain membranes: Regulation by ions and nucleotides. *Proceedings of the National Academy of Sciences (USA)*, 1978, *75*, 1713-1717.

Boada, J., Feria, M., & Sanz, E. Inhibitory effect of naloxone on the ethanol-induced antinociception in mice. *Pharmacological Research Communications*, 1981, *13*, 673-678.

Bogdanski, D. F., Tissari, A., & Brodie, B. B. Role of sodium, potassium, ouabain, and reserpine in uptake, storage, and metabolism of biogenic amines in synaptosomes. *Life Sciences*, 1968, *7*, 419-428.

Boggan, W. O., Meyer, J. S., Middaugh, L. D., & Sparks, D. L. Ethanol, calcium, and naloxone in mice. *Alcoholism: Clinical and Experimental Research*, 1979, *3*, 158-161.

Bolton, J. R. Electron spin resonance theory. In H. M. Schwartz, J. R. Bolton, & D. C. Borg (Eds.), *Biological applications of electron spin resonance*. New York: Wiley (Interscience), 1972.

Booij, H. L., & Dijkshoorn, W. Studies on hemolysis II. The influence of alcohols on monomolecular films of stearic acid compared to that on hemolysis. *Acta Physiologica et Pharmacologica Neerlandica*, 1950, *1*, 631-637.

Borges, S., & Lewis, P. D. Effects of ethanol on postnatal cell acquisition in the rat cerebellum. *Brain Research*, 1983, *271*, 388-391.   (a)

Borges, S., & Lewis, P. D. The effect of ethanol on the cellular composition of the cerebellum. *Neuropathology and Applied Neurobiology*, 1983, *9*, 53-60.   (b)

Brand, L., & Gohlke, J. R. Fluorescence probes for structure. *Annual Review of Biochemistry*, 1972, *4*, 843-868.

Breese, G. R., Lundberg, D. B. A., Mailman, R. B., Frye, G. D., & Mueller, R. A. Effect of ethanol on cyclic nucleotides *in vivo*: Consequences of controlling motor and respiratory changes. *Drug and Alcohol Dependence*, 1979, *4*, 321-326.

Bretscher, M. S. Membrane structure: Some general principles. *Science*, 1973, *181*, 622-629.

Briley, M. S., & Langer, S. Z. Influence of GABA receptor agonists and antagonists on the binding of [^{3}H]-diazepam to the benzodiazepine receptor. *European Journal of Pharmacology*, 1978, *52*, 129-132.

Brink, F., & Posternak, J. M. Thermodynamic analysis of the relative effectiveness of narcotics. *Journal of Cellular and Comparative Physiology*, 1948, *32*, 211-233.

Brown, D. J., & Stone, W. E. Effects of convulsants on cortical ATPases. *Journal of Neurochemistry*, 1973, *20*, 1461-1467.

Burt, D. R., Creese, I., & Snyder, S. H. Antischizophrenic drugs: Chronic treatment elevates dopamine receptor binding in brain. *Science*, 1976, *196*, 326-328.

Bustos, G., & Roth, R. H. Effect of acute ethanol treatment on transmitter synthesis and metabolism in central dopaminergic neurons. *Journal of Pharmacy and Pharmacology*, 1976, *28*, 580-582.

Buttke, T. M., & Ingram, L. O. Ethanol-induced changes in lipid composition of *Escherichia coli*: Inhibition of saturated fatty acid synthesis *in vitro*. *Archives of Biochemistry and Biophysics,* 1980, *203*, 565-571.

Campochiaro, P., Schwarcz, R., & Coyle, J. T. GABA receptor binding in rat striatum: Localization and effects of denervation. *Brain Research*, 1977, *136*, 501-511.

Carey, V. C., & Ingram, L. O. Lipid composition of *Zymomonas mobilis*: Effects of ethanol and glucose. *Journal of Bacteriology*, 1983, *154*, 1291-1300.

Carlen, P. L., & Corrigall, W. A. Ethanol tolerance measured electrophysiologically in hippocampal slices and not in neuromuscular junctions from chronically ethanol-fed rats. *Neuroscience Letters*, 1980, *17*, 95-100.

Carlen, P. L., Gurevich, N., & Durand, D. Ethanol in low doses augments calcium-mediated mechanisms intracellularly in hippocampal neurons. *Science*, 1982, *215*, 306-309.

Carlsson, A., Engel, J., Strömbom, U., Svensson, T. H., & Waldeck, B. Suppression by dopamine-agonists of the ethanol-induced stimulation of locomotor activity and brain dopamine synthesis. *Naunyn-Schmiedeberg's Archives of Pharmacology*, 1974, *283*, 117-128.

Carlsson, A., Engel, J., & Svensson, T. H. Inhibition of ethanol-induced excitation in mice and rats by alpha-methyl-*p*-tyrosine. *Psychopharmacologia (Berlin)*, 1972, *26*, 307-312.

Catley, D. M., Jordan, C., Trith, C. D., Lehane, J. R., Rhodes, A. A., & Jones, J. G.

Alcohol-induced discoordination is not reversed by naloxone. *Psychopharmacology*, 1981, *75*, 65-68.

Catley, D. M., Lehane, J. R., & Jones, J. G. Failure of naloxone to reverse alcohol intoxication. *Lancet*, 1981, *1*, 1263.

Catterall, W. A. Neurotoxins that act on voltage-sensitive sodium channels in excitable membranes. *Annual Reviews of Pharmacology and Toxicology*, 1980, *20*, 15-43.

Chan, A. W. K., & Abel, E. L. Absence of long-lasting effects of brain receptors for neurotransmitters in rats prenatally exposed to alcohol. *Research Communications in Substances of Abuse*, 1982, *3*, 219-224.

Chang, H. H., & Michaelis, E. K. Effects of L-glutamic acid on synaptosomal and synaptic membrane Na^+ fluxes and (Na^+-K^+)-ATPase. *Journal of Biological Chemistry*, 1980, *255*, 2411-2417.

Chang, K.-J., Hazum, E., & Cuatrecasas, P. Multiple opiate receptors. *Trends in Neurosciences*, July 1980, 160-162.

Chignell, C. F. New application of electron spin resonance to problems in biochemistry and pharmacology. *Life Sciences*, 1973, *13*, 1299-1314.

Childers, S. R., & Snyder, S. H. Differential regulation by guanine nucleotides of opiate agonist and antagonist receptor interactions. *Journal of Neurochemistry*, 1980, *34*, 583-593.

Chin, J. H., & Goldstein, D. B. Effects of low concentrations of ethanol on the fluidity of spin-labeled erythrocyte and brain membranes. *Molecular Pharmacology*, 1977, *13*, 435-441. (a)

Chin, J. H., & Goldstein, D. B. Drug tolerance in biomembranes: A spin label study of the effects of ethanol. *Science*, 1977, *196*, 684-685. (b)

Chin, J. H., & Goldstein, D. B. Membrane-disordering action of ethanol: Variation with membrane cholesterol content and depth of the spin label probe. *Molecular Pharmacology*, 1981, *19*, 425-431.

Chin, J. H., Parsons, L. M., & Goldstein, D. B. Increased cholesterol content of erythrocyte and brain membranes in ethanol-tolerant mice. *Biochimica et Biophysica Acta*, 1978, *513*, 358-363.

Chin, J. H., Trudell, J. R., & Cohen, E. N. The compression-ordering and solubility-disordering effects of high pressure gases on phospholipid bilayers. *Life Sciences*, 1976, *18*, 489-498.

Chu, N.-S. Prevention of alcohol withdrawal seizures with phenytoin in rats. *Epilepsia*, 1981, *22*, 179-184.

Chweh, A. Y., & Leslie, S. W. Enhancement of $^{45}Ca^{++}$ binding to acidic lipids by barbiturates, diphenylhydantoin, and ethanol. *Journal of Neurochemistry*, 1981, *36*, 1865-1867.

Cohen, P. J., & Dripps, R. D. History and theories of general anesthetics. In L. S. Goodman & A. Gilman (Eds.), *The pharmacological basis of therapeutics*. New York: Macmillan, 1965.

Colangelo, W., & Jones, D. G. The fetal alcohol syndrome: A review and assessment of the syndrome and its neurological sequelae. *Progress in Neurobiology*, 1982, *19*, 271-314.

Cole, W. H., & Allison, J. B. Chemical stimulation by alcohols in the barnacle, the frog, and planaria. *Journal of General Physiology*, 1930, *14*, 71-86.

Colfer, H. F., & Essex, H. E. Distribution of total electrolyte potassium and sodium in cerebral cortex in relation to experimental convulsions. *American Journal of Physiology*, 1947, *150*, 27-36.

Collier, H. O. J., Hammond, M. D., & Schneider, C. Effects of drugs affecting endogenous amines or cyclic nucleotides. *British Journal of Pharmacology*, 1976, *58*, 9-16.

Collins, J. G., & Roppolo, J. R. Effects of pentobarbital and ethanol upon single-neuron activity in the primary somatosensory cortex of the rhesus monkey. *Journal of Pharmacology and Experimental Therapeutics*, 1980, *213*, 337-345.

Cook, W. J., & Robinson, J. D. Factors influencing calcium movements in rat brain slices. *American Journal of Physiology*, 1971, *221*, 218–225.

Cooper, B. R., Viik, K., Ferris, R. M., & White, H. L. Antagonism of the enhanced susceptibility to audiogenic seizures during alcohol withdrawal in the rat by GABA and "GABA-mimetic" agents. *Journal of Pharmacology and Experimental Therapeutics*, 1979, *209*, 396–403.

Cooper, J. R., Bloom, F. E., & Roth, R. H. *The biochemical basis of neuropharmacology* (4th ed.). New York: Oxford University Press, 1982.

Corne, S. J., Pickering, R. W., & Warner, B. T. A method for assessing the effects of drugs on the central actions of 5-hydroxytryptophan. *British Journal of Pharmacology*, 1963, *20*, 106–120.

Côté, L. Aging of the brain and dementia. In E. R. Kandel & J. H. Schwartz (Eds.), *Principles of neural science*. New York: Elsevier/North Holland, 1981.

Cowan, C. M., Cardeal, J. O., & Cavalheiro, E. A. Membrane Na^+K^+ ATPase activity: Changes using an experimental model of alcohol dependence and withdrawal. *Pharmacology, Biochemistry, and Behavior*, 1980, *12*, 333–335.

Cox, G. Neuropathological techniques. In J. D. Bancroft & A. Stevens (Eds.), *Theory and practice of histological techniques*. Edinburgh: Churchill Livingstone, 1982.

Creese, I., Sibley, D. R., Leff, S., & Hamblin, M. Dopamine receptors: Subtypes, localization, and regulation. *Federation Proceedings*, 1981, *40*, 147–152.

Creese, I., Usdin, T. B., & Snyder, S. H. Dopamine receptor binding regulated by guanine nucleotides. *Molecular Pharmacology*, 1979, *16*, 69–76.

Creveling, C. R., McNeal, E. T., Daly, J. W., & Brown, G. B. Batrachotoxin-induced depolarization and [^{3}H]batrachotoxin-A20 alpha-benzoate binding in a vesicular preparation from guinea pig cerebral cortex. *Molecular Pharmacology*, 1983, *23*, 350–358.

Crews, F. T., Majchrowicz, E., & Meeks, R. Changes in cortical synaptosomal plasma membrane fluidity and composition in ethanol-dependent rats. *Psychopharmacology*, 1983, *81*, 208–213.

Daniels, C. K., & Goldstein, D. B. Movement of free cholesterol from lipoproteins or lipid vesicles into erythrocytes: Acceleration by ethanol *in vitro*. *Molecular Pharmacology*, 1982, *21*, 694–700.

Darden, J. H., & Hunt, W. A. Reduction of striatal dopamine release during an ethanol withdrawal syndrome. *Journal of Neurochemistry*, 1977, *29*, 1143–1145.

Davidoff, R. A. Alcohol and presynaptic inhibition in an isolated spinal cord preparation. *Archives of Neurology*, 1973, *28*, 60–63.

Davis, K. L., & Yamamura, H. I. Cholinergic underactivity in human memory disorders. *Life Sciences*, 1978, *23*, 1729–1734.

Davis, W. C., & Ticku, M. J. Ethanol enhances [^{3}H]-diazepam binding at the benzodiazepine-GABA receptor–ionophore complex. *Molecular Pharmacology*, 1981, *20*, 287–294.

De Blasi, A., Cotecchia, S., & Mennini, T. Selective changes of receptor binding in brain regions of aged rats. *Life Sciences*, 1982, *31*, 335–340.

Dethier, V. G., & Chadwick, L. E. Rejection thresholds of the blowfly for a series of aliphatic alcohols. *Journal of General Physiology*, 1947, *30*, 247–253.

Deutsch, J. A., & Walton, N. Y. Diazepam maintenance of alcohol preference during alcohol withdrawal. *Science*, 1977, *198*, 307–309.

DeWeer, P. Aspects of the recovery processes in nerve. In C. C. Hunt (Ed.), *Physiology* (Vol. 3). Baltimore: University Park Press, 1975.

Dewey, S. L., & West, J. R. Evidence for altered lesion-induced sprouting in the dentate gyrus of adult rats exposed to ethanol in utero. *Alcohol*, 1984, *1*, 81–88.

Diamond, I., & Goldberg, A. L. Uptake and release of ^{45}calcium by brain microsomes, synaptosomes and synaptic vesicles. *Journal of Neurochemistry*, 1971, *18*, 1419–1431.

Diaz, J., & Samson, H. H. Impaired brain growth in neonatal rats exposed to ethanol. *Science*, 1980, *208*, 751–753.

Dickens, B. F., & Thompson, G. A., Jr. Rapid membrane response during low temperature acclimations: Correlation of early changes in the physical properties and lipid composition of *Tetrahymena* microsomal membranes. *Biochimica et Biophysica Acta*, 1981, *644*, 211–218.

Dinh, T. K. H., & Gailis, L. Effect of body temperature on acute ethanol toxicity. *Life Sciences*, 1979, *25*, 547–552.

Dinovo, E. C., Gruber, B., & Noble, E. P. Alterations of fast-reacting sufhydryl groups of rat brain microsomes by ethanol. *Biochemical and Biophysical Research Communications*, 1976, *68*, 975–981.

Dismukes, R. K., & Daly, J. W. Adaptive responses of brain cyclic AMP-generating systems to alterations in synaptic input. *Journal of Cyclic Nucleotide Research*, 1976, *2*, 321–336.

Dodson, R. A., & Johnson, W. E. Effects of general central nervous system depressants with and without calcium ionophore A23187 on rat cerebellar cyclic guanosine-3',5'-monophosphate. *Research Communications in Chemical Pathology and Pharmacology*, 1980, *29*, 265–280.

Dole, V. P., Fishman, J., Goldfrank, L., Khanna, J., & McGivern, R. F. Arousal of ethanol-intoxicated comatose patients with naloxone. *Alcoholism: Clinical and Experimental Research*, 1982, *6*, 275–279.

Dombek, K. M., & Ingram, L. O. Effects of ethanol on the *Escherichia coli* plasma membrane. *Journal of Bacteriology*, 1984, *157*, 233–239.

Dunbar, P. G., Harvey, D. J., McPherson, K., & Wing, D. R. The effect of chronic ethanol treatment on membrane lipids in the mouse. *Proceedings of the British Pharmacological Society*, 16–18, September 1981, 958P–959P.

Dreyfus, P. M. Diseases of the nervous system in chronic alcoholics. In B. Kissin & H. Begleiter (Eds.), *The biology of alcoholism* (Vol. 3). New York: Plenum, 1974.

Durand, D., & Carlen, P. L. Decreased neuronal inhibition in vitro after long-term administration of ethanol. *Science*, 1984, *224*, 1359–1361.

Durand, D., Corrigall, W. A., Kujtan, P., & Carlen, P. L. Effects of low concentrations of ethanol on CA1 hippocampal neurons *in vitro*. *Canadian Journal of Physiology and Pharmacology*, 1981, *59*, 979–984.

Dymsza, H. A. Nutritional application and implication of 1,3-butanediol. *Federation Proceedings*, 1975, *34*, 2167–2170.

Eccles, J. C. *The physiology of synapses*. New York: Springer-Verlag, 1977.

Eccles, J. C., Ito, M., & Szentágothai, J. *The cerebellum as a neuronal machine*. Berlin: Springer-Verlag, 1967.

Eccles, J. C., Nicoll, R. A., Oshima, T., & Rubia, F. J. The anionic permeability of the inhibitory postsynaptic membrane of hippocampal pyramidal cells. *Proceedings of the Royal Society of London, Series B — Biological Sciences*, 1977, *198*, 345–361.

Edidin, M. Rotational and translational diffusion in membranes. *Annual Review of Biophysics and Bioengineering*, 1974, *3*, 179–201.

Ehlert, F. J., Kokka, N., & Fairhurst, A. S. Altered [^{3}H]-quinuclidinyl benzilate binding in the striatum of rats following chronic cholinesterase inhibition with diisopropylfluorophosphate. *Molecular Pharmacology*, 1980, *17*, 24–30.

Ehlert, F. J., Roeske, W. R., Rosenberger, L. B., & Yamamura, H. I. The influence of guanyl-5'-yl imidodiphosphate and sodium on muscarinic receptor binding in the rat brain and longitudinal muscle of the rat ileum. *Life Sciences*, 1980, *26*, 245–252.

Ehlert, F. J., Roeske, W. R., & Yamamura, H. I. Muscarinic receptor: Regulation by guanine nucleotides, ions, and *N*-ethylmaleimide. *Federation Proceedings, 40*, 153–159.

Eidelberg, E., Bond, M. L., & Kelter, A. Effects of alcohol on cerebellar and vestibular neurones. *Archives Internationales de Pharmacodynamie et de Thérapie*, 1971, *192*, 213–219.

Eliasson, S. G., Kiessling, L. A., & Scarpellini, J. D. Ethanol-induced changes in cyclic guanosine-3',5'-phosphate metabolism in mouse vestibular region. *Neuropharmacology*, 1981, *20*, 397–403.

Engel, J., & Liljequist, S. The effect of long-term ethanol treatment on the sensitivity of the dopamine receptors in the nucleus accumbens. *Psychopharmacology*, 1976, *49*, 253–257.

Enna, S. J., & Snyder, S. H. Influences of ions, enzymes, and detergents on GABA receptor binding in synaptic membranes of rat brain. *Molecular Pharmacology*, 1977, *13*, 442–453.

Erickson, C. K., & Graham, D. J. The alteration of cortical and reticular acetylcholine release by ethanol *in vivo*. *Journal of Pharmacology and Experimental Therapeutics*, 1973, *185*, 583–593.

Erickson, C. K., Tyler, T. D., & Harris, R. A. Ethanol: Modification of acute intoxication by divalent cations. *Science*, 1978, *199*, 1219–1221.

Escueta, A. V., & Appel, S. H. Biochemical studies of synapses in vitro: II. Potassium transport. *Biochemistry*, 1969, *8*, 725–733.

Ewing, J. A., & McCarty, D. Are the endorphins involved in mediating the mood effect of ethanol? *Alcoholism: Clinical and Experimental Research*, 1983, *7*, 271–275.

Faber, D. S., & Klee, M. R. Ethanol suppresses collateral inhibition of the goldfish Mauthner cell. *Brain Research*, 1976, *104*, 347–353.

Ferguson, J. The use of chemical potentials as indices of toxicity. *Proceedings of the Royal Society of London, Series B—Biological Sciences*, 1939, *127*, 387–404.

Ferko, A. P., & Bobyock, E. A study on regional brain calcium concentrations following acute and prolonged administration of ethanol in rats. *Toxicology and Applied Pharmacology*, 1980, *55*, 179–187.

Festoff, B. W., & Appel, S. H. Effect of diphenylhydantoin on synaptosomal Na-K ATPase. *Jounal of Clinical Investigation*, 1968, *47*, 2752–2758.

Fleming, E. W., Tewari, S., & Noble, E. P. Effects of chronic ethanol ingestion on brain aminoacyl-tRNA synthetases and tRNA. *Journal of Neurochemistry*, 1975, *24*, 553–560.

Fontaine, O., Matsumoto, T., Goodman, D. B. P., & Rasmussen, H. Liponomic control of Ca^{2+} transport: Relationship to mechanism of action of 1,25-dihydroxy-vitamin D_3. *Proceedings of the National Academy of Sciences (USA)*, 1980, *78*, 1751–1754.

Fontaine, R. N., Harris, R. A., & Schroeder, F. Aminophospholipid asymmetry in murine synaptosomal plasma membrane. *Journal of Neurochemistry*, 1980, *34*, 269–277.

Foote, S. L., Bloom, F. E., & Aston-Jones, G. Nucleus locus ceruleus: New evidence of anatomical and physiological specificity. *Physiological Reviews*, 1983, *63*, 844–914.

Formby, B. The *in vivo* and *in vitro* effects of diphenylhydantoin on the Na-K ATPase in particulate membrane fractions from rat brain. *Journal of Pharmacy and Pharmacology*, 1970, *22*, 81–85.

Forney, E., & Klemm, W. R. Effect of ethanol on impulse activity in isolated cerebellum. *Research Communications in Chemical Pathology and Pharmacology*, 1976, *15*, 801–804.

Franks, N. P., & Lieb, W. R. Is membrane expansion relevant to anesthesia? *Nature*, 1981, *292*, 248–251.

Franks, N. P., & Lieb, W. R. Molecular mechanisms of general anaesthesia. *Nature*, 1982, *300*, 487–493.

Freed, W. J., & Michaelis, E. K. Glutamic acid and ethanol dependence. *Pharmacology, Biochemistry, and Behavior*, 1978, *5*, 509–514.

Freeman, J. A., & Nicholson, C. Experimental optimization of current source density technique for anuran cerebellum. *Journal of Neurophysiology*, 1975, *38*, 369–382.

French, S. W., & Palmer, D. S. Adrenergic supersensitivity during ethanol withdrawal. *Research Communications in Chemical Pathology and Pharmacology*, 1973, *6*, 651–662.

French, S. W., Palmer, D. S., & Narod, M. E. Effect of withdrawal from chronic ethanol ingestion on the cAMP response of cerebral cortical slices using the agonists histamine, serotonin, and other neurotransmitters. *Canadian Journal of Physiology and Pharmacology*, 1975, *53*, 248–255.

French, S. W., Palmer, D. S., & Narod, M. E. Noradrenergic subsensitivity of rat liver homogenates during chronic ethanol ingestion. *Research Communications in Chemical Pathology and Pharmacology*, 1976, *13*, 283–295.

French, S. W., Palmer, D. S., Narod, M. E., Reid, P. E., & Ramey, C. W. Noradrenergic sensitivity of the cerebral cortex after chronic ethanol ingestion and withdrawal. *Journal of Pharmacology and Experimental Therapeutics*, 1975, *194*, 319–326.

French, S. W., Reid, P. E., Palmer, D. S., Narod, M. E., & Ramey, C. W. Adrenergic subsensitivity of the rat brain during chronic ethanol ingestion. *Research Communications in Chemical Pathology and Pharmacology*, 1974, *9*, 575–578.

Freund, G. Chronic central nervous system toxicity of alcohol. *Annual Review of Pharmacology*, 1973, *13*, 217–227.   (a)

Freund, G. Hypothermia after acute ethanol and benzyl alcohol administration. *Life Sciences*, 1973, *13*, 345–349.   (b)

Freund, G. The prevention of ethanol withdrawal seizures in mice by lidocaine. *Neurology*, 1973, *23*, 91–94.   (c)

Freund, G. Prevention of ethanol withdrawal seizures in mice by local anesthetics and dextropropranolol. In M. M. Gross (Ed.), *Alcohol intoxication and withdrawal* (Vol. 3). New York: Plenum, 1977.

Freund, G. The effects of chronic alcohol and vitamin E consumption on aging pigments and learning performance in mice. *Life Sciences*, 1979, *24*, 145–152.

Freund, G. Benzodiazepine receptor loss in brains of mice after chronic ethanol consumption. *Life Sciences*, 1980, *27*, 987–992.   (a)

Fruend, G. Cholinergic receptor loss in brains of aging mice. *Life Sciences*, 1980, *26*, 371–375.   (b)

Freund, G. Interactions of aging and chronic ethanol consumption on the central nervous system. In W. G. Wood & M. F. Elias (Eds.), *Alcoholism and aging: Advances in research*. Boca Raton: CRC Press, 1982.

Fridovich, I. Oxygen radicals, hydrogen peroxide, and oxygen toxicity. In W. A. Pryer (Ed.), *Free radicals in biology* (Vol. 1). New York: Academic Press, 1976.

Friedman, M. B., Erickson, C. K., & Leslie, S. W. Effects of acute and chronic ethanol administration on whole mouse brain synaptosomal calcium influx. *Biochemical Pharmacology*, 1980, *29*, 1903–1908.

Frye, G. D., & Breese, G. R. GABAergic modulation of ethanol-induced motor impairment. *Journal of Pharmacology and Experimental Therapeutics*, 1982, *223*, 750–756.

Frye, G. D., Chapin, R. E., Vogel, R. A., Mailman, R. B., Kilts, C. D., Mueller, R. A., & Breese, G. R. Effects of acute and chronic 1,3-butanediol treatment on central nervous system function: A comparison with ethanol. *Journal of Pharmacology and Experimental Therapeutics*, 1981, *216*, 306–314.

Frye, G. D., Vogel, R. A., Mailman, R. B., Ondrusek, M. G., Wilson, J. H., Mueller, P. A., & Breese, G. R. A comparison of behavioral and neurochemical effects on ethanol and chlordiazepoxide. In R. G. Thurman (Ed.), *Alcohol and aldehyde metabolizing systems—IV*. New York: Plenum, 1980.

Funderburk, F. R., Allen, R. P., & Wagman, A. M. I. Residual effects of ethanol and chlordiazepoxide treatments for alcohol withdrawal. *Journal of Nervous and Mental Disease*, 1978, *166*, 195–203.

Fuxe, K., Hall, H., & Köhler, C. Evidence for an exclusive localization of [³H]-ADTN binding sites to postsynaptic nerve cells in the striatum of the rat. *European Journal of Pharmacology*, 1979, *58*, 515–517.

Garrett, K. M., & Ross, D. H. Effects of *in vivo* ethanol administration on Ca^{2+}/Mg^{2+} ATPase and ATP-dependent Ca^{2+} uptake activity in synaptosomal membranes. *Neurochemical Research*, 1983, *8*, 1013–1028.

Gatenbeck, S., & Ehrenberg, L. The influence of anesthetics on monomolecular films of cell lipids. *Arkhiv Kemi*, 1953, *5*, 333–340.

Gessner, P. K. Failure of diphenylhydantoin to prevent alcohol withdrawal convulsions in mice. *European Journal of Pharmacology*, 1974, *27*, 120–129.

Gessner, P. K. Drug therapy of the alcohol withdrawal syndrome. In E. Majchrowicz & E. P. Noble (Eds.), *Biochemistry and pharmacology of ethanol* (Vol. 2). New York: Plenum, 1979.

Ghez, C., & Fahn, S. The cerebellum. In E. R. Kandel & J. H. Schwartz (Eds.), *Principles of neural science*. New York: Elsevier/North Holland, 1981.

Gianutsos, G., & Lal, H. Alterations in the action of cholinergic and anticholinergic drugs after chronic haloperidol: Indirect evidence for cholinergic hyposensitivity. *Life Sciences*, 1976, *18*, 515–520.

Gilbert, P. E., & Martin, W. R. The effect of morphine- and nalorphine-like drugs in the non-dependent, morphine-dependent, and cyclazocine-dependent chronic spinal dog. *Journal of Pharmacology and Experimental Therapeutics*, 1976, *198*, 66–83.

Goldstein, A., & Judson, B. A. Alcohol dependence and opiate dependence: Lack of relationship in mice. *Science*, 1971, *172*, 290–292.

Goldstein, D. B. An animal model for testing effects of drugs on alcohol withdrawal reactions. *Journal of Pharmacology and Experimental Therapeutics*, 1972, *183*, 14–22.

Goldstein, D. B. Alcohol withdrawal reactions in mice: Effects of drugs that modify neurotransmission. *Journal of Pharmacology and Experimental Therapeutics*, 1973, *186*, 1–9.

Goldstein, D. B. Sodium bromide and sodium valproate: Effective suppressants of ethanol withdrawal reactions in mice. *Journal of Pharmacology and Experimental Therapeutics*, 1979, *208*, 223–227.

Goldstein, D. B., & Chin, J. H. Disordering effect of ethanol at different depths in the bilayer of mouse brain membranes. *Alcoholism: Clinical and Experimental Research*, 1981, *5*, 256–258.

Goldstein, D. B., Chin, J. H., & Lyon, R. C. Ethanol disordering of spin-labeled mouse brain membranes: Correlation with genetically determined ethanol sensitivity of mice. *Proceedings of the National Academy of Sciences (USA)*, 1982, *79*, 4231–4233.

Goldstein, D. B., Hungund, B. L., & Lyon, R. C. Increased surface glycoconjugates of synaptic membranes in mice during chronic ethanol treatment. *British Journal of Pharmacology*, 1983, *78*, 8–10.

Goldstein, D. B., & Israel, Y. Effects of ethanol on mouse brain (Na + K)-activated adenosine triphosphatase. *Life Sciences*, 1972, *11*, 957–963.

Gordon, L. M., Sauerheber, R. D., Esgate, J. A., Dipple, I., Marchmont, R. J., & Houslay, M. D. The increase in bilayer fluidity of rat liver plasma membranes achieved by the local anesthetic benzyl alcohol affects the activity of intrinsic membrane enzymes. *Journal of Biological Chemistry*, 1980, *255*, 4519–4527.

Gorman, R. E., & Bitensky, M. W. Selective activation by short chain alcohols of glucagon responsive adenyl cyclase in liver. *Endocrinology*, 1970, *87*, 1075–1081.

Goto, M., Banno, Y., Umeki, S., Kameyama, Y., & Nozawa, Y. Effects of chronic ethanol exposure on composition and metabolism of *Tetrahymena* membrane lipids. *Biochimica et Biophysica Acta*, 1983, *751*, 286–297.

Graham-Smith, D. G. Studies *in vivo* on the relationship between brain tryptophan, brain 5-HT synthesis and hyperactivity in rats treated with a monoamine oxidase inhibitor and L-tryptophan. *Journal of Neurochemistry*, 1971, *18*, 1053–1066.

Grant, K. A., & Samson, H. H. Development of physical dependence on *t*-butanol in rats: An examination using schedule-induced drinking. *Pharmacology, Biochemistry, and Behavior*, 1981, *14*, 633–637.

Greene, H. L., Herman, R. H., & Kraemer, S. Stimulation of jejunal adenyl cyclase by ethanol. *Journal of Laboratory and Clinical Medicine*, 1971, *78*, 336–342.

Greengard, P. *Cyclic nucleotides, phosphorylated proteins, and neuronal function.* New York: Raven, 1978.

Grevel, J., & Sadée, W. An opiate binding site in the rat brain is highly selective for 4,5-epoxymorphinans. *Science*, 1983, *221*, 1198–1201.

Grieve, S. J., & Littleton, J. M. Ambient temperature and the development of functional tolerance to ethanol by mice. *Journal of Pharmacy and Pharmacology*, 1979, *31*, 707–708.

Grieve, S. J., Littleton, J. M., Jones, P., & John, G. R. Functional tolerance to ethanol in mice: Relationship to lipid metabolism. *Journal of Pharmacy and Pharmacology*, 1979, *31*, 737–742.

Griffiths, P. J., Littleton, J. M., & Ortiz, A. Effect of *p*-chlorophenylalanine of brain monoamines and behavior during ethanol withdrawal in mice. *British Journal of Pharmacology*, 1974, *51*, 307–309.

Gripenberg, J., Heinonen, E., & Jansson, S.-E. Uptake of radiocalcium by nerve endings isolated from rat brain: Kinetic studies. *British Journal of Pharmacology*, 1980, *71*, 265–271.

Gross, M. M., Lewis, E., & Hastey, J. Acute alcohol withdrawal syndrome. In B. Kissin & H. Begleiter (Eds.), *The biology of alcoholism* (Vol. 3). New York: Plenum, 1974.

Gruber, B., Dinovo, E. C., Noble, E. P., & Tewari, S. Ethanol-induced changes in rat brain microsomal membranes. *Biochemical Pharmacology*, 1977, *26*, 2181–2185.

Gruol, D. L. Ethanol alters synaptic activity in cultured spinal cord neurons. *Brain Research*, 1982, *243*, 25–33.

Grupp, L. A. Biphasic action of ethanol on single units of the dorsal hippocampus and the relationship to the cortical EEG. *Psychopharmacology*, 1980, *70*, 95–103.

Grupp, L. A., & Perlanski, E. Ethanol-induced changes in the spontaneous activity of single units in the hippocampus of the awake rat: A dose–response study. *Neuropharmacology*, 1979, *18*, 63–70.

Guerrero-Figueroa, R., Merrill, M., & Rye, D. Electrographic and behavioral effects of diazepam during alcohol withdrawal stage in cats. *Journal of Pharmacology*, 1970, *9*, 143–150.

Guerri, C., Wallace, R., & Grisolia, S. The influence of prolonged ethanol intake on the levels and turnover of alcohol and aldehyde dehydrogenases and of brain (Na + K)-ATPase of rats. *European Journal of Biochemistry*, 1978, *86*, 581–587.

Guidotti, A., Toffano, G., & Costa, E. An endogenous protein modulates the affinity of GABA and benzodiazepine receptors in rat brain. *Nature*, 1978, *275*, 553–555.

Gustafsson, B., & Wigstrom, H. Evidence for two types of afterhyperpolarization in CA1 pyramidal cells in the hippocampus. *Brain Research*, 1981, *206*, 462–468.

Guttman, R. Stabilization of spider crab nerve membrane by alkaline earths, as manifested in resting potential measurement. *Journal of Physiology*, 1940, *23*, 346–364.

Hadházy, P., & Szerb, J. C. The effect of cholinergic drugs on [^{3}H]-acetylcholine release from slices, of rat hippocampus, striatum, and cortex. *Brain Research*, 1977, *123*, 311–322.

Halsey, M. J. Effects of high pressure on the central nervous system. *Physiological Reviews*, 1982, *62*, 1341–1377.

Halsey, M. J., & Wardley-Smith, B. Pressure reversal of narcosis produced by anesthetics, narcotics and tranquilizers. *Nature*, 1975, *257*, 811–813.

Hanski, E., Rimon, G., & Levitzki, A. Adenylate cyclase activation by the beta-adrenergic receptors as a diffusion-controlled process. *Biochemistry*, 1979, *18*, 846–853.

Harman, D. The free-radical theory of aging. In W. A. Pryor (Ed.), *Free radicals in biology* (Vol. 5). New York: Academic Press, 1982.

Harmony, R., Urba-Holmgren, R., Urbay, C. M., & Szava, S. Na-K ATPase activity in experimental epileptogenic foci. *Brain Research*, 1968, *11*, 672-680.

Harper, A. A., MacDonald, A. G., & Wann, K. T. The effect of temperature on the nerve-blocking action of benzyl alcohol on the squid giant axon. *Journal of Physiology*, 1983, 51-60.

Harris, R. A. Alteration of alcohol effects by calcium and other inorganic cations. *Pharmacology, Biochemistry, and Behavior*, 1979, *10*, 527-534.

Harris, R. A. Ethanol and pentobarbital inhibition of intrasynaptosomal sequestration of calcium. *Biochemical Pharmacology*, 1981, *30*, 3209-3215.

Harris, R. A. Differential effects of membrane perturbants on voltage-activated sodium and calcium channels and calcium-dependent potassium channels. *Biophysical Journal*, 1984, *45*, 132-134.

Harris, R. A., & Bruno, P. Effects of ethanol and other intoxicant-anesthetics on voltage-dependent sodium channels of brain synaptosomes. *Journal of Pharmacology and Experimental Therapeutics*, 1985, *232*, 401-406.

Harris, R. A., & Fenner, D. Ethanol and synaptosomal calcium binding. *Biochemical Pharmacology*, 1982, *31*, 1790-1792.

Harris, R. A., Fenner, D., Feller, D., Sieckman, G., Lloyd, S., Mitchell, M., Dexter, J. D., Tumbelson, M. E., & Bylund, D. B. Neurochemical effects of long-term ingestion of ethanol by Sinclair (S-1) swine. *Pharmacology, Biochemistry, and Behavior*, 1983, *18*, 363-367.

Harris, R. A., & Hood, W. F. Inhibition of synaptosomal calcium uptake by ethanol. *Journal of Pharmacology and Experimental Therapeutics*, 1980, *213*, 562-568.

Harris, R. A., Schmidt, J., Hitzemann, B. A., & Hitzemann, R. J. Phosphatidate as a molecular link between depolarization and neurotransmitter release in the brain. *Science*, 1981, *212*, 1290-1291.

Harris, R. A., Schroeder, F. Ethanol and the physical properties of brain membranes: Fluorescence studies. *Molecular Pharmacology*, 1981, *20*, 128-137.

Harris, R. A., & Schroeder, F. Effects of barbiturates and ethanol on the physical properties of brain membranes. *Journal of Pharmacology and Experimental Therapeutics*, 1982, *223*, 424-431.

Heilbronn, E., & Bartfai, T. Muscarinic acetylcholine receptor. *Progress in Neurobiology*, 1978, *11*, 171-188.

Hemmingsen, R., & Sørensen, S. C. Absence of an effect of naloxone on ethanol intoxication and withdrawal. *Brain Research*, 1979, *173*, 259-269.

Hemminki, K. Calcium binding to brain plasma membranes. *Biochimica et Biophysica Acta*, 1974, *363*, 202-210.

Hendler, R. W. Biological membrane ultrastructure. *Physiological Reviews*, 1971, *51*, 66-97.

Herrero, A. A., & Gomez, R. F. Development of ethanol tolerance in *Clostridium thermocellum*: Effect of growth temperature. *Applied and Environmental Microbiology*, 1980, *40*, 571-577.

Hillbom, M. E. The prevention of withdrawal seizures in rats by dipropylacetate. *Neuropharmacology*, 1975, *14*, 755-761.

Hiller, J. M., Angel, L. M., & Simon, E. J. Multiple opiate receptors: Alcohol selectively inhibits binding to delta receptors. *Science*, 1981, *214*, 468-469.

Hiller, J. M., Angel, L. M., & Simon, E. J. Characterization of the selective inhibition of the delta subclass of opioid binding sites by alcohols. *Molecular Pharmacology*, 1984, *25*, 249-255.

Himwich, H. E., & Callison, D. A. The effects on evoked potentials of various parts of the central nervous system of the cat. In B. Kissin & H. Begleiter (Eds.), *The biology of alcoholism* (Vol. 2). New York: Plenum, 1972.

Hirsch, J. D. Selective inhibition of [³H]-lysergic acid diethylamide binding to mouse brain membranes by ethanol. *Journal of Pharmacy and Pharmacology*, 1981, *33*, 475-477.

Hobbs, A. S., & Albers, R. W. The structure of proteins involved in active membrane transport. *Annual Reviews of Biophysics and Bioengineering*, 1980, *9*, 259-291.

Hodgkin, A. L., & Huxley, A. F. A quantitative description of membrane current and its application to conduction and excitation in nerve. *Journal of Physiology (London)*, 1952, *117*, 500-544.

Hoffman, B. B., & Lefkowitz, R. J. Radioligand binding studies of adrenergic receptors: New insights into molecular and physiological regulation. *Annual Reviews of Pharmacology and Toxicology*, 1980, *20*, 581-608.

Hoffman, P. L., & Tabakoff, B. Alterations in dopamine receptor sensitivity by chronic ethanol treatment. *Nature (London)*, 1977, *268*, 551-553.

Hoffman, P. L., & Tabakoff, B. Effects of ethanol on Arrhenius parameters and activity of mouse striatal adenylate cyclase. *Biochemical Pharmacology*, 1982, *31*, 3101-3106.

Hoffman, P. L., Urwyler, S., & Tabakoff, B. Alterations in opiate receptor function after chronic ethanol exposure. *Journal of Pharmacology and Experimental Therapeutics*, 1982, *222*, 182-189.

Hong, J. S., Majchrowicz, E., Hunt, W. A., & Gillin, J. C. Reduction in cerebral methionine-enkephalin content during the ethanol withdrawal syndrome. *Substance and Alcohol Actions/Misuse*, 1981, *2*, 233-240.

Hood, W. F., & Harris, R. A. Effect of pentobarbital, ethanol and morphine on subcellular localization of calcium and magnesium in brain. *Biochemical Pharmacology*, 1979, *28*, 3075-3080.

Hossack, J. A., & Rose, A. H. Fragility of plasma membranes in *Saccharomyces cerevisiae* enriched with different sterols. *Journal of Bacteriology*, 1976, *127*, 67-75.

Hotson, J. R., & Prince, D. A. A calcium-activated hyperpolarization follows repetitive firing in hippocampal neurons. *Journal of Neurophysiology*, 1980, *43*, 409-419.

Hruska, R. E., & Silbergeld, E. K. Inhibition of [³H]-spiroperidol binding by *in vitro* addition of ethanol. *Journal of Neurochemistry*, 1980, *35*, 750-752.

Hunt, W. A. The effects of aliphatic alcohols on the biophysical and biochemical correlates of membrane function. In E. Majchrowicz (Ed.), *Biochemical pharmacology of ethanol*. New York: Plenum, 1975.

Hunt, W. A. Effects of acute and chronic administration of ethanol on cyclic nucleotides and related systems. In E. Majchrowicz & E. P. Noble (Eds.), *Biochemistry and pharmacology of ethanol* (Vol. 2). New York: Plenum, 1979.

Hunt, W. A. The effect of ethanol on GABAergic transmission. *Neuroscience and Biobehavioral Reviews*, 1983, *7*, 87-95.

Hunt, W. A., & Dalton, T. K. Neurotransmitter–receptor binding in various brain regions in ethanol-dependent rats. *Pharmacology, Biochemistry, and Behavior*, 1981, *14*, 733-739.

Hunt, W. A., & Majchrowicz, E. Alterations in neurotransmitter function after acute and dopamine in alcohol-dependent rats. *Journal of Neurochemistry*, 1974, *23*, 549-552.

Hunt, W. A., & Majchrowicz, E. Alterations in neurotransmitter functions after acute and chronic treatment with ethanol. In E. Majchrowicz & E. P. Noble (Eds.), *Biochemistry and pharmacology of ethanol* (Vol. 2). New York: Plenum, 1979.

Hunt, W. A., & Majchrowicz, E. Suppression of the ethanol withdrawal syndrome by aliphatic diols. *Journal of Pharmacology and Experimental Therapeutics*, 1980, *213*, 9-12.

Hunt, W. A., & Majchrowicz, E. Studies of neurotransmitter interactions after acute and chronic ethanol administration. *Pharmacology, Biochemistry, and Behavior*, 1983, *18, Supplement 1*, 371-374, 1983.

Hunt, W. A., Majchrowicz, E., & Dalton, T. K. Alterations in high-affinity choline uptake in brain after acute and chronic ethanol treatment. *Journal of Pharmacology and Experimental Therapeutics*, 1979, *210*, 259-267.

Hunt, W. A., Majchrowicz, E., Dalton, T. K., Swartzwelder, H. S., & Wixon, H. Alterations in neurotransmitter activity after acute and chronic ethanol treatment: Studies of transmitter interactions. *Alcoholism: Clinical and Experimental Research*, 1979, *3*, 359-363.

Hunt, W. A., Redos, J. D., Dalton, T. K., & Catravas, G. N. Alterations in brain cyclic guanosine-3',5'-monophosphate levels after acute and chronic treatment with ethanol. *Journal of Pharmacology and Experimental Therapeutics*, 1977, *201*, 103-109.

Hwang, D. H., LeBlanc, P., & Chanmugan, P. *In vitro* and *in vivo* effects of ethanol on the formation of endoperoxide metabolites in rat platelets. *Lipids*, 1981, *16*, 583-588.

Hyvarinen, J., Laakso, M., Roine, R., Leinonen, L., & Sippel, H. Effect of ethanol on neuronal activity in the parietal association cortex of alert monkeys. *Brain*, 1978, *101*, 701-715.

Ikeda, Y., Sasa, M., & Takaori, S. Selective effect of ethanol on the vestibular nucleus neurons in the cat. *Japanese Journal of Pharmacology*, 1980, *30*, 665-673.

Ingram, L. O. Adaptation of membrane lipids to alcohols. *Journal of Bacteriology*, 1976, *125*, 670-678.

Ingram, L. O. Preferential inhibition of phosphatidyl ethanolamine synthesis in *E. coli* by alcohols. *Canadian Journal of Microbiology*, 1977, *23*, 779-789.

Ingram, L. O., Carey, V. C., & Dombek, K. M. On the relationship between alcohol narcosis and membrane fluidity. *Substance and Alcohol Actions/Misuse*, 1982, *2*, 213-224.

Ingram, L. O., Dickens, B. F., & Buttke, T. M. Reversible effects of ethanol on *E. coli*. In H. Begleiter (Ed.), *Biological effects of alcohol*. New York: Plenum, 1980.

Ingram, L. O., Ley, K. D., & Hoffman, E. M. Drug-induced changes in lipid composition of *E. coli* and of mammalian cells in culture: ethanol, pentobarbital, and chlorpromazine. *Life Sciences*, 1978, *22*, 489-494.

Israel, M. A., Kimura, H., & Kuriyama, K. Changes in activity and hormonal sensitivity of brain adenyl cyclase following chronic ethanol administration. *Experientia*, 1972, *28*, 1322-1323.

Israel, M. A., & Kuriyama, K. Effect of *in vivo* ethanol administration on adenosine triphosphatase activity of subcellular fractions of mouse brain and liver. *Life Sciences*, 1971, *10*, 591-599.

Israel, Y., Kalant, H., & Laufer, I. Effects of ethanol on Na, K, Mg-stimulated microsomal ATPase activity. *Biochemical Pharmacology*, 1965, *14*, 1803-1814.

Israel, Y., Kalant, H., & LeBlanc, A. E. Effects of lower alcohols on potassium transport and microsomal adenosine-triphosphatase activity of rat cerebral cortex. *Biochemical Journal*, 1966, *100*, 27-33.

Israel, Y., Kalant, H., LeBlanc, A. E., Bernstein, J. C., & Salazar, I. Changes in cation transport and (Na + K)-activated adenosine triphosphatase produced by chronic administration of ethanol. *Journal of Pharmacology and Experimental Therapeutics*, 1970, *174*, 330-336.

Israel, Y., & Salazar, I. Inhibition of brain microsomal adenosine triphosphatases by general depressants. *Archives of Biochemistry and Biophysics*, 1967, *122*, 310-317.

Jacobs, B. L. An animal behavior model for studying central serotonergic synapses. *Life Sciences*, 1976, *19*, 777-785.

Jakobs, K. H., Saur, W., & Schultz, G. Inhibition of platelet adenylate cyclase by epinephrine requires GTP. *FEBS Letters*, 1978, *85*, 167-170.

Jarlstedt, J. Experimental alcoholism in rats: Protein synthesis in subcellular fractions from cerebellum, cerebral cortex and liver after long term treatment. *Journal of Neurochemistry*, 1972, *19*, 603-608.

Jarlstedt, J., & Hamberger, A. Experimental alcoholism. Effect of acute ethanol intoxication on the *in vitro* incorporation of [³H]leucine into neuronal and glial proteins. *Journal of Neurochemistry*, 1972, *19*, 2299-2306.

Järnefelt, J. Inhibition of the brain microsomal adenosine triphosphatase by depolarizing agents. *Biochimica et Biophysica Acta*, 1961, *48*, 111-116.

Jeffcoate, W. J., Herbert, M., Cullen, M. H., Hastings, A. G., & Walder, C. P. Prevention of effects of alcohol intoxication by naloxone. *Lancet*, 1979, *2*, 1157-1159.

Jeffreys, B., Flanagan, R. J., & Volans, G. N. Reversal of ethanol-induced coma with naloxone. *Lancet*, 1980, *1*, 308-309.

John, G. R., Littleton, J. M., & Jones, P. A. Membrane lipids and ethanol tolerance in the mouse. The influence of dietary fatty acid composition. *Life Sciences*, 1980, *27*, 545-555.

Johnson, D. A., Friedman, H. J., Cooke, R., & Lee, N. M. Adaptation of brain bilayers to ethanol-induced fluidization: Species and strain generality. *Biochemical Pharmacology*, 1980, *29*, 1673-1676.

Johnson, D. A., Lee, N. M., Cooke, R., & Loh, H. H. Ethanol-induced fluidization of brain lipid bilayers: Required presence of cholesterol in membranes for the expression of tolerance. *Molecular Pharmacology*, 1979, *15*, 739-746.

Johnson, D. A., Lee, N. M., Cooke, R., & Loh, H. Adaptation to ethanol-induced fluidization of brain lipid bilayers: cross-tolerance and reversibility. *Molecular Pharmacology*, 1980, *17*, 52-55.

Jope, R. S., & Jenden, D. J. Effects of acute ethanol treatment on cholinergic function in rats. *Substance and Alcohol Actions/Misuse*, 1981, *2*, 15-23.

Jørgensen, H. A., & Hole, K. Does ethanol stimulate brain opiate receptors? Studies on receptor binding and naloxone inhibition of ethanol-induced effects. *European Journal of Pharmacology*, 1981, *75*, 223-229.

Kalant, H., Mons, W., & Mahon, M. A. Acute effects of ethanol on tissue electrolytes in the rat. *Canadian Journal of Physiology and Pharmacology*, 1966, *44*, 1-12.

Kalant, H., & Rangaraj, N. Interaction of catecholamines and ethanol on the kinetics of rat brain $(Na^+ + K^+)$-ATPase. *European Journal of Pharmacology*, 1981, *70*, 157-166.

Kalant, H., Woo, N., & Endrenyi, L. Effect of ethanol on the kinetics of rat brain $(Na^+ + K^+)$ ATPase and K^+-dependent phosphatase with different alkali ions. *Biochemical Pharmacology*, 1978, *27*, 1353-1358.

Kamaya, H., Kaneshina, S., & Ueda, I. Partition equilibrium of inhalation anesthetics and alcohols between water and membranes of phospholipids with varying acyl chain-lengths. *Biochimica et Biophysica Acta*, 1981, *646*, 135-142.

Kandel, E. R. Synaptic transmission I: Postsynaptic factors controlling ionic permeability. In E. R. Kandel & J. H. Schwartz (Eds.), *Principles of neural science*. New York: Elsevier/North Holland, 1981.

Kao, C. Y. Tetrodotoxin, saxitoxin, and their significance in the study of excitation phenomena. *Pharmacological Reviews*, 1966, *18*, 997-1049.

Karobath, M., Rogers, J., & Bloom, F. Benzodiazepine receptors remain unchanged after chronic ethanol administration. *Neuropharmacology*, 1980, *19*, 125-128.

Karobath, M., Sperk, G., & Schönbeck, G. Evidence for an endogenous factor interfering with [³H]-diazepam binding to rat brain membranes. *European Journal of Pharmacology*, 1978, *49*, 323-326.

Karoum, F., Wyatt, R. J., & Majchrowicz, E. Brain concentrations of biogenic amine metabolites in acutely treated and ethanol-dependent rats. *British Journal of Pharmacology*, 1976, *56*, 403-411.

Karppanen, H., & Puurunen, J. Ethanol, indomethacin and gastric acid secretion in the rat. *European Journal of Pharmacology*, 1976, *35*, 221-223.

Karppanen, H., Puurunen, J., Kairaluoma, M., & Larmi, T. Effects of ethyl alcohol on the cyclic AMP system of the human gastric mucosa. *Scandinavian Journal of Gastro-enterology*, 1976, *11*, 603–607.

Keane, B., & Leonard, B. E. Changes in "open field" behaviour and in some membrane-bound enzymes following the chronic administration of ethanol to the rat. *Neuropharmacology*, 1983, *22*, 555–557.

Kebabian, J. W., & Calne, D. B. Multiple receptors for dopamine. *Nature*, 1979, *227*, 93–96.

Keegan, R., Wilce, P. A., Ruczkal-Pietrzak, E., & Shanley, B. C. Effect of ethanol on cholesterol and phospholipid composition of HeLa cells. *Biochemical and Biophysical Research Communications*, 1983, *114*, 985–990.

Khanna, J. M., Kalant, H., Lê, A. D., & LeBlanc, A. E. Reversal of tolerance to ethanol — a possible consequence of ethanol brain damage. *Acta Physiologica Scandinavica*, 1980, *62, Supplement 286*, 129–134.

Khawaja, J. A., Lindholm, D. B., & Niittylä, J. Selective inhibition of protein synthetic activity of cerebral membrane-bound ribosomes as a consequence of ethanol ingestion. *Research Communications in Chemical Pathology and Pharmacology*, 1978, *19*, 185–188.

Kiianmaa, K., Hoffman, P. L., & Tabakoff, B. Antagonism of the behavioral effects of ethanol by naltrexone in BALB/C, C57BL/6, and DBA/2 mice. *Psychopharmacology*, 1983, *79*, 291–294.

Kimball, C. D., Huang, S. M., Torget, C. E., & Houck, J. C. Plasma ethanol, endorphin, and glucose experiment. *Lancet*, 1980, *2*, 418–419.

Kimberg, D. V. Cyclic nucleotides and their role in gastrointestinal secretion. *Gastroenterology*, 1974, *67*, 1023–1064.

Kimizuka, H., & Koketsu, K. Binding of calcium ion to lecithin film. *Nature*. 1962, *196*, 995–996.

Klausner, R. D., Kleinfeld, A. M., Hoover, R. L., & Karnovsky, M. J. Lipid domains in membranes. Evidence derived from structural perturbations induced by free fatty acids and lifetime heterogeneity analysis. *Journal of Biological Chemistry*, 1980, *255*, 1286–1295.

Klemm, W. R. Effects of ethanol on nerve impulse activity. In E. Majchrowicz & E. P. Noble (Eds.), *Biochemistry and pharmacology of ethanol* (Vol. 2). New York: Plenum, 1979.

Klemm, W. R., Dreyfus, L. R., Forney, E., & Mayfield, M. A. Differential effects of low doses of ethanol on the impulse activity in various regions of the limbic system. *Psychopharmacology*, 1976, *50*, 131–138.

Klemm, W. R., Mallari, C. G., Dreyfus, L. R., Fiske, J. C., Forney, E., & Mikeska, J. A. Ethanol-induced regional and dose–response differences in multiple-unit activity in rabbits. *Psychopharmacology*, 1976, *49*, 235–244.

Klemm, W. R., & Stevens, R. E. Alcohol effects on EEG and multiple-unit activity in various brain regions of rats. *Brain Research*, 1974, *70*, 361–368.

Klepner, C. A., Lippa, A. S., Benson, D. I., Sano, M. C., & Beer, B. Resolution of two biochemically and pharmacologically distinct benzodiazepine receptors. *Pharmacology, Biochemistry, and Behavior*, 1979, *11*, 457–462.

Knox, W., Perrin, R. G., & Sen, A. K. Effect of chronic administration of ethanol on (Na^+K^+)-ATPase activity in six areas of the cat brain. *Journal of Neurochemistry*, 1972, *19*, 2882–2884.

Koblin, D. D., & Deady, J. E. Sensitivity to alcohol in mice with an altered brain fatty acid composition. *Life Sciences*, 1981, *28*, 1889–1896.

Koblin, D. D., & Wang, H. H. Chronic exposure to inhaled anesthetics increases cholesterol content in *Acholeplasma laidlawii*. *Biochimica et Biophysica Acta*, 1981, *649*, 717–725.

Kochman, R. L., Hirsch, J. D., & Clay, G. A. Changes in ^{3}H-diazepam receptor binding after subacute ethanol administration. *Research Communications in Substance Abuse*, 1981, *2*, 135–144.

Koester, J. Resting membrane potential. In E. R. Kandel & J. H. Schwartz (Eds.), *Principles of neural science.* New York: Elsevier/North Holland, 1981. (a)

Koester, J. Passive electrical properties of the neuron. In E. R. Kandel & J. H. Schwartz (Eds.), *Principles of neural science.* New York: Elsevier/North Holland, 1981. (b)

Koester, J. Active conductances underlying the action potential. In E. R. Kandel & J. H. Schwartz (Eds.), *Principles of neural science.* New York: Elsevier/North Holland, 1981. (c)

Kolde, T., & Matsushita, H. An enhanced sensitivity of muscarinic cholinergic receptor associated with dopaminergic receptor subsensitivity after chronic antidepressant treatment. *Life Sciences,* 1981, *28,* 1139–1145.

Koppenhofer, E., & Schmidt, H. Die Wirkung von Skorpiongift auf die Ionenströme des Ranvierschen Schnürrings. I. Die Unvollständige Natrium Inaktivierung. *Pflügers Archives of Physiology,* 1968, *303,* 133–149.

Kornguth, S. E., Rutledge, J. J., Sunderland, E., Siegel, F., Carlson, I., Smollens, J., Juhl, U., & Young, B. Impeded cerebellar development and reduced serum thyroxine levels associated with fetal alcohol intoxication. *Brain Research,* 1979, *177,* 347–360.

Korsten, M. A., Gordon, E. R., Klingenstein, J., & Lieber, C. S. Effects of chronic ethanol feeding and acetaldehyde metabolism on calcium transport by rat liver mitochondria. *Biochemical and Biophysical Research Communications,* 1983, *117,* 169–175.

Kosterlitz, H. W., & Hughes, J. Some thoughts on the significance of enkephalin, the endogenous ligand. *Life Sciences,* 1975, *17,* 91–96.

Kosterlitz, H. W., & Waterfield, A. A. *In vitro* models in the study of structure–activity relationships of narcotic analgesics. *Annual Reviews of Pharmacology,* 1975, *15,* 29–47.

Krawitt, E. L. Ethanol inhibits intestinal calcium transport in rats. *Nature,* 1973, *243,* 88–89.

Krnjevic, K. Chemical nature of synaptic transmission in vertebrates. *Physiological Reviews,* 1974, *54,* 418–540.

Kubanis, P., Zornetzer, S. F., & Freund, G. Memory and postsynaptic cholinergic receptors in aging mice. *Pharmacology, Biochemistry, and Behavior,* 1982, *17,* 313–322.

Kuriyama, K. Ethanol-induced changes in activities of adenylate cyclase, guanylate cyclase and cyclic 3', 5'-monophosphate dependent protein kinase in rat brain and liver. *Drug and Alcohol Dependence,* 1977, *2,* 335–348.

Kuriyama, K., & Israel, M. A. Effect of ethanol administration on cyclic 3', 5'-adenosine monophosphate metabolism in brain. *Biochemical Pharmacology,* 1973, *22,* 2919–2922.

Kuriyama, K., Muramatsu, M., Aiso, M., & Ueno, E. Alteration in beta-receptor binding in brain, lung, and heart during morphine and alcohol dependence and withdrawal. *Neuropharmacology,* 1981, *20,* 659–666.

Kuriyama, K., Nakagawa, K., Muramatsu, M., & Kakita, K. Alterations of cerebral protein kinase following ethanol administration. *Biochemical Pharmacology,* 1976, *25,* 2541–2542.

Kuriyama, K., Sze, P. Y., & Rauscher, G. E. Effects of acute and chronic ethanol administration of ribosomal protein synthesis in mouse brain and liver. *Life Sciences,* 1971, *10,* 181–189.

LaBella, F. S., Pinsky, C., Havlicek, V., & Queen, G. Effects of anesthetics *in vitro* on brain receptors for opiates, spiroperidol, and ouabain. In E. L. Way (Ed.), *Endogenous and exogenous opiate agonists and antagonists.* New York: Pergamon, 1979.

Lai, H., Carino, M. A., & Horita, A. Effects of ethanol on central dopamine function. *Life Sciences,* 1980, *27,* 299–304.

Lake, N., Yarbrough, G. G., & Phillips, J. W. Effects of ethanol on cerebral cortical neurons: Interactions with some putative transmitters. *Journal of Pharmacy and Pharmacology,* 1973, *25,* 582–584.

Lands, A. M., Arnold, A., McAuliff, J. P., Luduena, F. P., & Brown, T. C. Differentiation of receptor systems activated by sympathomimetic amines. *Nature,* 1967, *214,* 597–598.

Langer, S. Z. Presynaptic receptors and their role in the regulation of transmitter release. *British Journal of Pharmacology*, 1977, *60*, 481–497.

Langer, S. Z. Presynaptic receptors and modulation of neurotransmission: Pharmacological implications and therapeutic relevance. *Trends in Neurosciences*, May 1980, 110–112.

LeBlanc, A. E., & Kalant, H. Ethanol-induced cross tolerance to several homologous alcohols in the rat. *Toxicology and Applied Pharmacology*, 1975, *32*, 123–128.

Ledig, M., M'Paria, J. R., Louis, J.-C., Fried, R., & Mandel, P. Effect of ethanol on superoxide dismutase activity in cultured neural cells. *Neurochemical Research*, 1980, *5*, 1155–1162.

Ledig, M., M'Paria, J.-R., & Mandel, P. Superoxide dismutase activity in rat brain during acute and chronic alcohol intoxication. *Neurochemical Research*, 1981, *6*, 385–390.

Lee, K., Dunwiddie, T., Dietrich, R., Lynch, G., & Hoffer, B. Chronic ethanol consumption and hippocampal neuron dendritic spines: A morphometric and physiological analysis. *Experimental Neurology*, 1981, *71*, 541–549.

Lee, N. M., Friedman, H. J., & Loh, H. H. Effect of acute and chronic ethanol treatment on the rat brain phospholipid turnover. *Biochemical Pharmacology*, 1980, *29*, 2815–2818.

Leeb-Lundburg, F. A., Snowman, A., & Olsen, R. W. Barbiturate receptor sites are coupled to benzodiazepine receptors. *Proceedings of the National Academy of Sciences (USA)*, 1980, *77*, 7468–7472.

Lefkowitz, R. J., Limbard, L. E., Mukherjee, C., & Caron, M. G. The beta-adrenergic receptor and adenylate cyclase. *Biochimica et Biophysica Acta*, 1976, *457*, 1–39.

Lenaz, G., Curatola, G., Mazzanti, L., Bertoli, E., & Pastuszko, A. Spin label studies on the effect of anesthetics in synaptic membranes. *Journal of Neurochemistry*, 1979, *32*, 1689–1695.

Leslie, S. W., Barr, E., Chandler, J., & Farrar, R. P. Inhibition of fast- and slow-phase depolarization-dependent synaptosomal calcium uptake by ethanol. *Journal of Pharmacology and Experimental Therapeutics*, 1983, *225*, 571–575.

Levental, M., & Tabakoff, B. Sodium–potassium-activated adenosine triphosphatase activity as a measure of neuronal membrane characteristics in ethanol-tolerant mice. *Journal of Phamacology and Experimental Therapeutics*, 1980, *212*, 315–319.

Lever, M. J., Miller, K. W., Patton, W., & Smith, D. M. Pressure reversal of anesthesia. *Nature*, 1971, *231*, 368–371.

Levine, A. S., Hess, S., & Morley, J. E. Alcohol and the opiate receptor. *Alcoholism: Clinical and Experimental Research*, 1983, *7*, 83–92.

Lewin, E., & Bleck, V. B. The effect of diphenylhydantoin administration on Na-K ATPase in cortex. *Neurology*, 1971, *21*, 647–651.

Leysen, J. E., Niemegeers, C. J. E., Tollenaere, J. P., & Laduron, P. M. Serotonergic component of neuroleptic receptors. *Nature (London)*, 1978, *272*, 168–171.

Lichtschtein, H., Kaback, R., & Blume, A. J. Use of a lipophilic cation for the determination of membrane potential in neuroblastoma–glioma hybrid cell suspensions. *Proceedings of the National Academy of Sciences (USA)*, 1979, *76*, 650–645.

Liljequist, S. Changes in the sensitivity of dopamine receptors in the nucleus accumbens and in the striatum induced by chronic ethanol administration. *Acta Pharmacologica et Toxicologica*, 1978, *43*, 19–28.

Liljequist, S., & Engel, J. The effect for chronic ethanol administration on central neurotransmitter mechanisms. *Medical Biology*, 1979, *57*, 199–210.

Liljequist, S., & Engel, J. Effects of GABAergic agonists and antagonists on various ethanol-induced behavioral changes. *Psychopharmacology*, 1982, *78* , 71–75.

Lindsay, R. The effect of prolonged ethanol treatment on the sodium-plus-potassium-ion-stimulated adenosine triphosphatase content of cultured human and mouse cells. *Clinical Science and Molecular Medicine*, 1974, *47*, 639–642.

Ling, C. M., & Abdel-Latif, A. A. Studies on sodium transport in rat brain nerve-ending particles. *Journal of Neurochemistry*, 1968, *15*, 721–729.

Linnoila, M., Stowell, L., Marangos, P. J., and Thurman, R. G. Effect of ethanol and ethanol withdrawal on [³H]-muscimol binding and behaviour in the rat: A pilot study. *Acta Pharmacologica et Toxicologica*, 1981, *49*, 407–411.

Lipicky, R. J., Gilbert, D. L., & Stillman, I. M. Diphenylhydantoin inhibition of sodium conductance in squid giant axon. *Proceedings of the National Academy of Sciences (USA)*, 1972, *69*, 1758–1760.

Lippa, A. S., Critchett, D. J., Sano, M. C., Klepner, C. A., Greenblatt, E. N., Coupet, J., & Beer, B. Benzodiazepine receptors: Cellular and behavioral characteristics. *Pharmacology, Biochemistry, and Behavior*, 1979, *10*, 831–843.

Littleton, J. M., & John, G. Synaptosomal membrane lipids of mice during continuous exposure to ethanol. *Journal of Pharmacy and Pharmacology*, 1977, *29*, 579–580.

Littleton, J. M., John, G. R., & Grieve, S. J. Alterations in phospholipid composition in ethanol tolerance and dependence. *Alcoholism: Clinical and Experimental Research.* 1979. *3*, 50–56.

Littleton, J. M., John, G. R., Jones, P. A., & Grieve, S. J. The rapid onset of functional tolerance to ethanol — role of different neurotransmitters and synaptosomal membrane lipids. *Acta Psychologica Scandinavica*, 1980, *62, Supplement 286*, 137–151.

Llinas, R., & Volkind, R. A. The olivo-cerebellar system: Functional properties as revealed by harmaline-induced tremor. *Experimental Brain Research*, 1973, *18*, 64–87.

Logan, B. J., Laverty, R., & Peake, B. M. ESR measurements on the effects of ethanol on the lipid and protein conformation in biological membranes. *Pharmacology, Biochemistry, and Behavior*, 1983, *18, Supplement 1*, 31–35.

Loh, H. H., & Law, P. Y. The role of membrane lipids in receptor mechanisms. *Annual Reviews of Pharmacology and Toxicology*, 1980, *20*, 201–234.

Lomax, P., Bajorek, J. G., Chesarek, W. A., and Chaffee, R. R. J. Ethanol-induced hypothermia in the rat. *Pharmacology*, 1980, *21*, 288–294.

Lorber, S. H., Vincente, V. P., Jr., & Chey, W. Y. Diseases of the gastrointestinal tract. In B. Kissin & H. Begleiter (Eds.), *The biology of alcoholism*. New York: Plenum, 1974.

Lucchi, L., Bosio, A., Spano, P. F., & Trabucchi, M. Action of ethanol and salsolinol on opiate receptor function. *Brain Research*, 1981, *232*, 506–510.

Lundberg, D. B. A., Breese, G. R., Mailman, R. B., Frye, G. D., & Mueller, R. A. Depression of some drug-induced *in vivo* changes of cerebellar guanosine 3′, 5′-monophosphate by control of motor and respiratory responses. *Molecular Pharmacology*, 1979, *15*, 246–256.

Lust, W. D., & Robinson, J. D. Calcium accumulation by isolated nerve ending particle from brain: II. Factors influencing calcium movements. *Journal of Neurobiology*, 1970, *1*, 317–328.

Luthin, G. R., & Tabakoff, B. Activation of adenylate cyclase by alcohols requires the nucleotide-binding protein. *Journal of Pharmacology and Experimental Therapeutics*, 1984, *228*, 579–587.

Lyon, R. C., & Goldstein, D. B. Changes in synaptic membrane order associated with chronic ethanol treatment in mice. *Molecular Pharmacology*, 1983, *23*, 86–91.

Lyon, R. C., McComb, J. A., Schreurs, J., & Goldstein, D. B. A relationship between alcohol intoxication and the disordering of brain membranes by a series of short-chain alcohols. *Journal of Pharmacology and Experimental Therapeutics*, 1981, *218*, 669–675.

Mackenzie, A. I. Naloxone in alcohol intoxication. *Lancet*, 1979, *1*, 733–734.

Maggi, A., Schmidt, M. J., Ghetti, B., & Enna, S. J. Effect of aging on neurotransmitter receptor binding in rat and human brain. *Life Sciences*, 1979, *24*, 367–374.

Magour, S., Kristof, V., Baumann, M., & Assmann, G. Effect of acute treatment with cadmium on ethanol anesthesia, body temperature, and synaptosomal Na⁺-K⁺-ATPase of rat brain. *Environmental Research*, 1981, *26*, 381–391.

Majchrowicz, E. Induction of physical dependence upon ethanol and the associated behavioral changes in rats. *Psychopharmacologia*, 1975, *43*, 245-254.

Majchrowicz, E., Hunt, W. A., & Piantadosi, C. Suppression by 1,3-butanediol of the ethanol withdrawal syndrome in rats. *Science*, 1976, *194*, 1181-1182.

Majumdar, S. K., Shaw, G. K., & Thomson, A. D. Plasma vitamin E status in chronic alcoholic patients. *Drug and Alcohol Dependence*, 1983, *12*, 269-272.

Makman, M. H., Ahn, H. S., Thal, L. J., Sharpless, N. S., Dvorkin, B., Horowitz, S. G., & Rosenfeld, M. Aging and monoamine receptors in brain. *Federation Proceedings*, 1979, *38*, 1922-1926.

Malcolm, R. D., & Alkana, R. L. Temperature dependence of ethanol depression in mice. *Journal of Pharmacology and Experimental Therapeutics*, 1981, *217*, 770-775.

Malcolm, R. D., & Alkana, R. L. Hyperbaric ethanol antagonism: Role of temperature, blood and brain concentrations. *Pharmacology, Biochemistry, and Behavior*, 1982, *16*, 341-346.

Malcolm, R. D., & Alkana, R. L. Temperature dependence of ethanol lethality in mice. *Journal of Pharmacy and Pharmacology*, 1983, *35*, 306-311.

Marklund, S. L., Oreland, L., Perdahl, E., & Winblad, B. Superoxide dismutase activity in brains from chronic alcoholics. *Drug and Alcohol Dependence*, 1983, *12*, 209-215.

Marquis, J. K., & Mautner, H. G. The binding of thiol reagents to axonal membranes: The effect of electrical stimulation. *Biochemical and Biophysical Research Communications*, 1974, *57*, 154-161.   (a)

Marquis, J. K., & Mautner, H. G. The effect of electrical stimulation on the action of sulfhydryl reagents in the giant axon of squid: Suggested mechanisms for the role of thiol and disulfide groups in electrically induced conformational changes. *Journal of Membrane Biology*, 1974, *15*, 249-260.   (b)

Marsh, D. Electron spin resonance: Spin labels. In E. Grell (Ed.), *Membrane spectroscopy*. Berlin: Springer-Verlag, 1981.

Martin, I. L., & Candy, J. M. Facilitation of benzodiazepine binding by sodium chloride and GABA. *Neuropharmacology*, 1978, *17*, 993-998.

Martz, A., Deitrich, R. A., & Harris, R. A. Behavioral evidence for the involvement of gamma-aminobutyric acid in the actions of ethanol. *European Journal of Pharmacology*, 1983, *89*, 53-62.

Mashiter, K., Mashiter, G. D., & Field, J. B. Effects of prostaglandin E, ethanol and TSH on the adenylate cyclase activity of beef thyroid plasma membranes and cyclic AMP content of dog thyroid slices. *Endocrinology*, 1974, *94*, 370-376.

Massarelli, R., Syapin, P. J., & Noble, E. P. Increased uptake of choline by neural cell cultures chronically exposed to ethanol. *Life Science*, 1976, *18*, 397-404.

Massotti, M., & Guidotti, A. Endogenous regulators of benzodiazepine recognition sites. *Life Sciences*, 1980, *27*, 847-854.

Mastrangelo, C. J., Kenig, J. J., Trudell, J. R., & Cohen, E. N. Nerve membrane lipid fluidity: Opposing effects of high pressure and ethanol. *Undersea Biomedical Research*, 1979, *6*, 47-53.

Matchett, J. A., & Erickson, C. K. Alteration of ethanol-induced changes in locomotor activity by adrenergic blockers in mice. *Psychopharmacology*, 1977, *52*, 201-206.

Mattila, M. J., Nuotto, E., & Seppala, T. Naloxone is not an effective antagonist of ethanol. *Lancet*, 1981, *1*, 775-776.

Mayer, J. M., Khanna, J. H., & Kalant, H. A role for calcium in the acute and chronic actions of ethanol *in vitro*. *European Journal of Pharmacology*, 1980, *68*, 223-227.

McClearn, G. E., & Kakihana, R. Selective breeding for ethanol sensitivity in mice. *Behavioral Genetics*, 1973, *3*, 409-410.

McComb, J. A., & Goldstein, D. B. Additive physical dependence: Evidence for a common mechanism in alcohol dependence. *Journal of Pharmacology and Experimental Therapeutics*, 1979, *210*, 87–90. (a)

McComb, J. A., & Goldstein, D. B. Quantitative comparison of physical dependence on tertiary butanol and ethanol in mice: Correlation with lipid solubility. *Journal of Pharmacology and Experimental Therapeutics*, 1979, *208*, 113–117. (b)

McConnell, H. M., & McFarland, B. G. The flexibility gradient in biological membranes. *Annals of the New York Academy of Sciences*, 1972, *195*, 207–217.

McCreery, M. J., & Hunt, W. A. Physico-chemical correlates of alcohol intoxication. *Neuropharmacology*, 1978, *17*, 451–461.

Mead, J. F. Free radical mechanisms of lipid damage and consequences for cellular membranes. In W. A. Pryor (Ed.), *Free radicals in biology* (Vol. 1). New York: Academic Press, 1976.

Meech, R. W. Calcium-dependent potassium activation in nervous tissue. *Annual Reviews of Biophysics and Bioengineering*, 1978, *7*, 1–18.

Membery, J. H., & Link, E. A. Hyperbaric exposure of mice to pressures of 60 to 90 atmospheres. *Science*, 1964, *144*, 1241–1242.

Memo, M., Spano, P. F., & Trabucchi, M. Brain benzodiazepine receptor changes during aging. *Journal of Pharmacy and Pharmacology*, 1981, *33*, 64.

Mena, M. A., Salinas, M., Martín del Río, R., & Herrera, E. Effects of maternal ethanol ingestion on cerebral neurotransmitters and cyclic-AMP in the rat offspring. *General Pharmacology*, 1982, *13*, 241–248.

Mendelson, J. H., Rossi, M., Bernstein, J. G., & Kuehnle, J. Propranolol and behavior of alcohol addicts after acute alcohol ingestion. *Clinical Pharmacology and Therapeutics*, 1974, *15*, 571–578.

Messiha, F. S. Antagonism of ethanol-evoked responses by amantadine: A possible clinical application. *Pharmacology, Biochemistry, and Behavior*, 1978, *8*, 573–577.

Meyer, H. Welche Eigenschaft der Anasthetica bedingt ihre narkitische Wirkung? *Naunyn-Schmiedebergs Archiv für Experimentelle Pathologie und Pharmakologie*, 1899, *42*, 109–118.

Meyer, H. Zur Theorie der Alkolnarkose: Der Einfuss wechselnder Temperatur auf Wirkungsstarke und Theilungscoefficient der Narcotica. *Naunyn-Schmiedebergs Archiv für Experimentelle Pathologie und Pharmakologie*, 1901, *46*, 338–346.

Meyer, H. H., & Gottlieb, R. *Experimental pharmacology as a basis for therapeutics* (2nd ed.), Philadelphia: Lippincott, 1926.

Meyer, K. H. Contributions to the theory of narcosis. *Transactions of the Faraday Society*, 1937, *33*, 1062–1068.

Miceli, J. N., & Ferrell, W. J. Effects of ethanol on membrane lipids. III. Quantitative changes in lipid and fatty acid composition of nonpolar and polar lipids of mouse total liver, mitochondria, and microsomes following ethanol feeding. *Lipids*, 1973, *8*, 722–727.

Michaelis, E. K., Chang, H. H., Roy, S., McFaul, J. A., & Zimbrick, J. D. Ethanol effects of synaptic glutamate receptor function and on membrane lipid organization. *Pharmacology, Biochemistry, and Behavior*, 1983, *18*, Supplement 1, 1–6.

Michaelis, E. K., Michaelis, M. L., Belieu, R. M., Grubbs, R. D., & Magruder, C. Effects of *in vitro* ethanol addition on brain synaptic membrane glutamate binding. *Brain Research Bulletin*, 1980, *5, Supplement 2*, 647–651.

Michaelis, E. K., Michaelis, M. L., & Boyarsky, L. L. High-affinity glutamic acid binding in brain synaptic membranes. *Biochimica et Biophysica Acta*, 1974, *367*, 338–348.

Michaelis, E. K., Mulvaney, M. J., & Freed, W. J. Effects of acute and chronic ethanol intake on synaptosomal glutamate binding activity. *Biochemical Pharmacology*, 1978, *27*, 1685–1691.

Michaelis, E. K., & Myers, S. L. Calcium binding to brain synaptosomes: Effects of chronic ethanol intake. *Biochemical Pharmacology*, 1979, *28*, 2081–2087.

Michaelis, E. K., Zimbrick, J. D., McFaul, J. A., Lampe, R. A., & Michaelis, M. L. Ethanol effects on synaptic glutamate receptors and on liposomal membrane structure. *Phar-*

macology, Biochemistry, and Behavior, 1980, *13*, Supplement *1*, 197–202.

Michaelis, M. L., & Michaelis, E. K. Alcohol and local anesthetic effects on Na^+-dependent Ca^{2+} fluxes in brain synaptic membrane vesicles. *Biochemical Pharmacology*, 1983, *32*, 963–969.

Michaelis, M. L., Michaelis, E. K., & Tehan, T. Alcohol effects on synaptic membrane calcium ion fluxes. *Pharmacology, Biochemistry, and Behavior*, 1983, *18*, Supplement *1*, 19–29.

Middaugh, L. D., Read, E., & Boggan, W. D. Effects of naloxone on ethanol induced alterations of locomotion in C57BL/6 mice. *Pharmacology, Biochemistry, and Behavior*, 1978, *9*, 157–160.

Mikeska, J. A., & Klemm, W. R. Action of ethanol on cerebellar single unit activity with and without pretreatment with *d*-penicillamine. *Research Communications in Psychology, Psychiatry, and Behavior*, 1979, *4*, 457–466.

Miller, K. W., & Yu, S.-C. The dependence of the lipid bilayer membrane: Buffer partition coefficient of pentobarbitone on pH and lipid composition. *British Journal of Pharmacology*, 1977, *61*, 57–63.

Minneman, K. P., & Molinoff, P. B. Classification and quantitation of beta-adrenergic receptor subtypes. *Biochemical Pharmacology*, 1980, *29*, 1317–1323.

Minocherhomjee, A. M., & Roufogalis, B. D. Mechanisms of coupling of the beta-adrenergic receptor to adenylate cyclase—an overview. *General Pharmacology*, 1982, *13*, 87–93.

Moore, J. W., Ulbricht, W., & Takata, M. Effect of ethanol on the sodium and potassium conductances of the squid axon membrane. *Journal of General Physiology*, 1964, *48*, 279–295.

Mrak, R. E. Calcium transport and fluorescence polarization of 1,6-diphenyl-1,3,5-hexatriene in sarcoplasmic reticulum from normal and ethanol-tolerant rats. *Experimental Neurology*, 1983, *80*, 573–581.

Mukherjee, C., Caron, M. G., & Lefkowitz, R. J. Catecholamine-induced subsensitivity of adenylate cyclase associated with loss of beta-adrenergic receptor binding sites. *Proceedings of the National Academy of Sciences (USA)*, 1975, *72*, 1945–1949.

Muller, P., Britton, R. S., & Seeman, P. The effects of long-term ethanol on brain receptors for dopamine, acetylcholine, serotonin and norepinephrine. *European Journal of Pharmacology*, 1980, *65*, 31–37.

Muller, P., & Seeman, P. Presynaptic subsensitivity as a possible basis for sensitization by long-term dopamine mimetics. *European Journal of Pharmacology*, 1979, *55*, 149–157.

Mullin, M. J., & Ferko, A. P. Alterations in dopaminergic function after subacute ethanol administration. *Journal of Pharmacology and Experimental Therapeutics*, 1983, *225*, 694–698.

Mullin, M. J., & Hunt, W. A. Ethanol inhibits veratridine-stimulated sodium uptake in synaptosomes. *Life Sciences*, 1984, *34*, 287–292.

Mullin, M. J., & Hunt, W. A. The actions of ethanol on voltage-sensitive sodium channels: Effects on neurotoxin-stimulated sodium uptake in synaptosomes. *Journal of Pharmacology and Experimental Therapeutics*, 1985, *232*, 413–419.

Mullins, L. J. Some physical mechanisms of narcosis. *Chemical Reviews*, 1954, *54*, 289–323.

Muñoz, C., & Guivernau, M. Antagonistic effects of propranolol upon ethanol-induced narcosis in mice. *Research Communications in Chemical Pathology and Pharmacology*, 1980, *29*, 57–65.

Murrin, L. C., Coyle, J. T., & Kuhar, M. J. Striatal opiate receptors: Pre- and postsynaptic localization. *Life Sciences*, 1980, *27*, 1175–1183.

Murrin, L. C., DeHaven, R. N., & Kuhar, M. J. On the relationship between [³H]-choline uptake activation and [³H]-acetylcholine release. *Journal of Neurochemistry*, 1977, *29*, 681–687.

Murrin, L. C., Gale, K., & Kuhar, M. J. Autoradiographic localization of neuroleptic and dopamine receptors in the caudate-putamen and substantia nigra. *European Journal of Pharmacology*, 1979, *60*, 229–235.

Mustala, O. O., & Azarnoff, D. L. Effect of oxygen tension on drug levels and pharmacological action in the intact animal. *Proceedings of the Society of Experimental Biology and Medicine*, 1969, *132*, 37–41.

Nachshen, D. A., & Blaustein, M. P. Some properties of potassium-stimulated calcium influx in presynaptic nerve endings. *Journal of General Physiology*, 1980, *76*, 709–728.

Nagy, J. I., Lee, T., Seeman, P., & Fibiger, H. C. Direct evidence for pre-synaptic and postsynaptic dopamine receptors in the brain. *Nature (London)*, 1978, *274*, 278–281.

Nandini-Kishore, S. G., Mattox, S. M., Martin, C. E., & Thompson, G. A. Membrane changes during growth of *Tetrahymena* in the presence of ethanol. *Biochimica et Biophysica Acta*, 1979, *551*, 315–327.

Narahashi, T. Chemicals as tools in the study of excitable membranes. *Physiological Reviews*, 1974, *54*, 813–889.

Narahashi, T., Moore, J. W., & Shapiro, B. I. Condylactis toxin: Interaction with nerve membrane ionic conductances. *Science*, 1969, *163*, 680–681.

Nathanson, J. A. Cyclic nucleotides and nervous system function. *Physiological Reviews*, 1977, *57*, 157–256.

Needham, L., & Houslay, M. D. The activity of dopamine-stimulated adenylate cyclase from rat brain striatum is modulated by temperature and the bilayer-fluidizing agent, benzyl alcohol. *Biochemical Journal*, 1982, *206*, 89–95.

Nestoros, J. N. Ethanol specifically potentiates GABA-mediated neurotransmission in feline cerebral cortex. *Science*, 1980, *209*, 708–710.   (a)

Nestoros, J. N. Ethanol selectively potentiates GABA-mediated inhibition of single feline cortical neurons. *Life Sciences*, 1980, *26*, 519–523.   (b)

Newlin, S. A., Mancillas-Trevino, J., & Bloom, F. E. Ethanol causes increases in excitation and inhibition in area CA3 of the dorsal hippocampus. *Brain Research*, 1981, *209*, 113–128.

Nicoll, R. A., & Alger, B. E. Synaptic excitation may activate a calcium dependent potassium conductance in hippocampus pyramidal cells. *Science*, 1981, *212*, 957–959.

Nikander, P., & Wallgren, H. Ethanol, electrical stimulation, and net movements of sodium and potassium in rat brain tissue *in vitro*. *Acta Physiologica Scandinavica*, 1970, *80*, 29A.

Noble, E. P., Gilles, R., Vigran, R., & Mandel, P. The modification of the ethanol withdrawal syndrome in rats by di-*n*-propylacetate. *Psychopharmacologia (Berlin)*, 1976, *46*, 127–131.

Noble, E. P., Syapin, P. J., Vigran, R., & Rosenberg, A. Neuraminidase-releasable surface sialic acid of cultured astroblasts exposed to ethanol. *Journal of Neurochemistry*, 1976, *27*, 217–221.

Nordberg, A., & Wahlström, G. Tolerance, physical dependence and changes in muscarinic receptor binding sites after chronic ethanol treatment in the rat. *Life Sciences*, 1982, *31*, 277–287.

Nuotto, E., Palva, E. S., & Lahdenranta, U. Naloxone fails to counteract heavy alcohol intoxication. *Lancet*, 1983, *2*, 167.

Oakes, S. G., & Pozos, R. S. Electrophysiologic effects of acute ethanol exposure. I. Alteration in the action potentials of dorsal root ganglia neurons in dissociated culture. *Developmental Brain Research*, 1982, *5*, 243–249.   (a)

Oakes, S. G., & Pozos, R. S. Electrophysiologic effects of acute exposure. II. Alterations in the calcium component of action potentials from sensory neurons in dissociated culture. *Developmental Brain Research*, 1982, *5*, 251–255.   (b)

Olney, J. W., Rhee, V., & Ho, O. L. Kainic acid: A powerful neurotoxic analogue of glutamate. *Brain Research*, 1974, *77*, 507–512.

Olsen, R. W. GABA–benzodiazepine–barbiturate receptor interactions. *Journal of Neurochemistry*, 1981, *37*, 1–13.

Olsen, R. W., Ticku, M. K., & Miller, T. Dihydropicrotoxinin binding to crayfish muscle sites probably related to GABA receptor ionophores. *Molecular Pharmacology*, 1978, *14*, 381-390.

Olsen, R. W., Ticku, M. K., Van Ness, P. C., & Greenlee, D. Effects of drugs on GABA receptors, uptake, release, and synthesis *in vitro*. *Brain Research*, 1978, *139*, 277-294.

Orenberg, E. K., Renson, J., & Barchas, J. D. The effects of alcohol on cyclic AMP in mouse brain. *Neurochemical Research*, 1976, *1*, 659-667.

Overstreet, D. H., & Yamamura, H. I. Receptor alterations and drug tolerance. *Life Sciences*, 1979, *25*, 1865-1878.

Overton, E. Über die osmotischen Eigenschaften der Zelle in ihrer Betdeutung für die Toxikologie und Pharmakologie. *Zeitschrift für physikalishe Chemie*, 1896, *22*, 189-209.

Overton, E. *Studien über die Narkose zugleich ein Beitrag zur allgemeinen Pharmakologie.* Jena: Verlag von Gustav Fischer, 1901.

Ozeki, M., Freeman, A. R., & Grundfest, H. The membrane components of crustacean neuromuscular systems. I. Immunity of different electrogenic components to tetrodotoxin and saxitoxin. *Journal of General Physiology*, 1966, *49*, 1319-1334.

Pang, K., Chang, T., & Miller, K. W. On the coupling between anesthetic induced membrane fluidization and cation permeability in lipid vesicles. *Molecular Pharmacology*, 1979, *15*, 729-738.

Pant, H. C., Virmani, M., & Majchrowicz, E. Changes in erythrocyte ghost protein phosphorylation associated with physical dependence upon ethanol. *Substance and Alcohol Actions/Misuse*, 1982, *3*, 343-351.

Parsons, L. A., Gallaher, E. J., & Goldstein, D. B. Rapidly developing functional tolerance to ethanol is accompanied by increased erythrocyte cholesterol in mice. *Journal of Pharmacology and Experimental Therapeutics*, 1982, *223*, 472-476.

Paterson, S. J., Butler, K. W., Huang, P., LaBelle, J., Smith, I. C. P., & Schneider, H. The effects of alcohols on lipid bilayers: Spin label study. *Biochimica et Biophysica Acta*, 1972, *266*, 597-602.

Peck, E. J., Jr. Receptors for amino acids. *Annual Reviews of Physiology*, 1980, *42*, 615-627.

Pelham, R. W., Marquis, J. K., Kugelmann, K., & Munsat, T. L. Prolonged ethanol consumption produces persistent alterations of cholinergic function in rat brain. *Alcoholism: Clinical and Experimental Research*, 1980, *4*, 282-287.

Pentney, R. J. Quantitative analysis of ethanol effects on Purkinje cell dentritic tree. *Brain Research*, 1982, *249*, 397-401.

Peroutka, S. J., Lebovitz, R. M., & Snyder, S. H. Serotonin receptors affected differentially by guanine nucleotides. *Molecular Pharmacology*, 1979, *16*, 700-708.

Peroutka, S. J., Lebovitz, R. M., & Snyder, S. H. Two distinct central serotonin receptors with different physiological functions. *Science*, 1981, *212*, 827-829.

Peroutka, S. J., & Snyder, S. H. Multiple serotonin receptors: differential binding of [^{3}H]-serotonin, [^{3}H]-lysergic acid diethylamide and [^{3}H]-spiroperidol. *Molecular Pharmacology*, 1979, *16*, 687-699.

Peroutka, S. J., & Snyder, S. H. Two distinct serotonin receptors: Regional variations in receptor binding in mammalian brain. *Brain Research*, 1981, *208*, 339-347.

Peroutka, S. J., U'Prichard, D. C., Greenberg, D. A., & Snyder, S. H. Neuroleptic drug interactions with norepinephrine alpha receptor binding sites in rat brain. *Neuropharmacology*, 1977, *16*, 549-556.

Pert, C. B. Type 1 and type 2 opiate receptor distribution in brain—what does it tell us? In J. B. Martin, S. Reichlin, & K. L. Blick (Eds.), *Neurosecretion and brain peptides*. New York: Raven, 1981.

Pesce, A. J., Rosén, C.-G., & Pasby, T. L. *Fluorescence spectroscopy: An introduction for biology and medicine*. New York: Dekker, 1971.

Pfeiffer, A., & Herz, A. Discrimination of three opiate receptor binding sites with the use of a computerized curve-fitting technique. *Molecular Pharmacology*, 1982, *21*, 266–271.

Pfeiffer, A., Seizinger, B. R., & Herz, A. Chronic ethanol imbibition with delta-, but not with mu-opiate receptors. *Neuropharmacology*, 1981, *20*, 1229-1232.

Phillips, M. C. The physical state of phospholipids and cholesterol in monolayers, bilayers and membranes. *Progress in Surface Membrane Science*, 1972, *5*, 139-221.

Phillips, M. C., & Finer, E. G. The stoichiometry and dynamics of lecithin–cholesterol clusters in bilayer membranes. *Biochimica et Biophysica Acta*, 1974, *356*, 199-206.

Phillips, S. C., & Cragg, B. G. Chronic consumption of alcohol by adult mice: Effect of hippocampal cells and synapses. *Experimental Neurology*, 1983, *80*, 218-226.

Pincus, J. H. Diphenylhydantoin and ion flux in lobster nerve. *Archives of Neurology*, 1972, *26*, 4-10.

Placheta, P., & Karobath, M. Regional distribution of Na^+-independent GABA and benzodiazepine binding sites in rat CNS. *Brain Research*, 1979, *178*, 580-583.

Pohorecky, L. A. Biphasic action of ethanol. *Biobehavioral Reviews*, 1977, *1*, 231-240.

Pohorecky, L. A. Animal analog of alcohol dependence. *Federation Proceedings*, 1981, *40*, 2056-2064.

Pohorecky, L. A., & Brick, J. Activity of neurons in the locus coeruleus of the rat: Inhibition by ethanol. *Brain Research*, 1977, *131*, 174-179.

Pohorecky, L. A., Jaffe, L. S., & Berkeley, H. A. Ethanol withdrawal in the rat: Involvement of noradrenergic neurons. *Life Sciences*, 1974, *15*, 427-457.

Pohorecky, L. A., & Rizek, A. E. Biochemical and behavioral effects of acute ethanol in rats at different environmental temperatures. *Psychopharmacology*, 1981, *72*, 205-209.

Polak, R. L., & Meeuws, M. M. The influence of atropine on the release and uptake of acetylcholine by the isolated cerebral cortex of the rat. *Biochemical Pharmacology*, 1966, *15*, 989-992.

Ponnappa, B. C., Waring, A. J., Hoek, J. B., Rottenberg, H., & Rubin, E. Chronic ethanol ingestion increases calcium uptake and resistance to molecular disordering by ethanol in liver microsomes. *Journal of Biological Chemistry*, 1982, *257*, 10141-10146.

Pradham, S. N. Central neurotransmitters and aging. *Life Sciences*, 1980, *26*, 1643-1656.

Prasad, C., & Edwards, R. M. Increased phospholipid methylation in the myocardium of alcoholic rats. *Biochemical and Biophysical Research Communications*, 1983, *111*, 710-716.

Pringle, M. J., Brown, K. B., & Miller, K. W. Can the lipid theories of anesthesia account for the cut-off in anesthetic potency in homologous series of alcohols? *Molecular Pharmacology*, 1981, *19*, 49-55.

Pryer, W. A. The role of free radical reactions in biological systems. In W. A. Pryer (Ed.), *Free radicals in biology* (Vol. 1). New York: Academic Press, 1980.

Przewlocki, R., Hollt, V., Duka, T. H., Kleber, G., Gramsch, C. H., Haarmann, I., & Herz, A. Long-term morphine treatment decreases endorphin levels in rat brain and pituitary. *Brain Research*, 1979, *174*, 357-361.

Puurunen, J. Studies on the mechanism of the inhibitory effect of ethanol on the gastric acid output in the rat. *Naunyn-Schmiedeberg's Archives of Pharmacology*, 1978, *303*, 87-93.

Puurunen, J., Hiltunen, K., & Karppanen, H. Ethanol-induced changes in gastric mucosal content of cyclic AMP and ATP in the rat. *European Journal of Pharmacology*, 1977, *42*, 85-89.

Puurunen, J., & Karppanen, H. Effects of ethanol on gastric acid secretion and gastric mucosal cyclic AMP in the rat. *Life Sciences*, 1975, *16*, 1513-1520.

Puurunen, J., Karppanen, H., Kairaluoma, M., & Larmi, T. Effects of ethanol on the cyclic AMP system of the dog gastric mucosa. *European Journal of Pharmacology*, 1976, *38*, 275-279.

Rabin, R. A., & Molinoff, P. B. Activation of adenylate cyclase in mouse striatal tissue. *Journal of Pharmacology and Experimental Therapeutics*, 1981, *216*, 129–134.

Rabin, R. A., & Molinoff, P. B. Multiple sites of action of ethanol on adenylate cyclase. *Journal of Pharmacology and Experimental Therapeutics*, 1983, *227*, 551–556.

Rabin, R. A., Wolfe, B. B., Dibner, M. D., Zahniser, N. R., Melchior, C., & Molinoff, P. B. Effects of ethanol administration and withdrawal on neurotransmitter receptor systems in C57 mice. *Journal of Pharmacology and Experimental Therapeutics*, 1980, *213*, 491–496.

Rang, H. P. Unspecific drug action. The effects of a homologous series of primary alcohols. *British Journal of Pharmacology*, 1960, *15*, 185–200.

Rangaraj, N., & Kalant, H. Effects of ethanol withdrawal, stress and amphetamine on rat brain ($Na^+ + K^+$)-ATPase. *Biochemical Pharmacology*, 1978, *27*, 1139–1144.

Rangaraj, N., & Kalant, H. Interaction of ethanol and catecholamines on rat brain ($Na^+ + K^+$)-ATPase. *Canadian Journal of Physiology and Pharmacology*, 1979, *57*, 1098–1106.

Rangaraj, N., & Kalant, H. Alpha adrenoreceptor mediated alteration of ethanol effects on ($Na^+ + K^+$)-ATPase of rat neuronal membranes. *Canadian Journal of Physiology and Pharmacology*, 1980, *58*, 1342–1346.

Rangaraj, N., & Kalant, H. Effect of chronic ethanol treatment on temperature dependence and on norepinephrine sensitization of rat brain ($Na^+ + K^+$)-adenosine triphosphatase. *Journal of Pharmacology and Experimental Therapeutics*, 1982, *224*, 536–539.

Rasmussen, H., & Goodman, D. B. P. Relationships between calcium and cyclic nucleotides in cell activation. *Physiological Reviews*, 1977, *57*, 421–509.

Rawat, A. K. Ribosomal protein synthesis in the fetal and neonatal rat brain as influenced by maternal ethanol consumption. *Research Communications in Chemical Pathology and Pharmacology*, 1975, *12*, 723–732.

Rawson, M. D., & Pincus, J. H. The effect of diphenylhydantoin on the Na-K ATPase in microsomal fractions of rat and guinea-pig and on whole homogenates of human brain. *Biochemical Pharmacology*, 1968, *17*, 573–579.

Redos, J. D., Catravas, G. N., & Hunt, W. A. Ethanol-induced depletion of cerebellar guanosine 3′, 5′-cyclic monophosphate. *Science*, 1976, *193*, 58–59.

Redos, J. D., Hunt, W. A., & Catravas, G. N. Lack of alteration in regional brain adenosine-3′, 5′-cyclic monophosphate levels after acute and chronic treatment with ethanol. *Life Sciences*, 1976, *18*, 989–992.

Reggiani, A., Barbaccia, M. L., Spano, P. F., & Trabucchi, M. Acute and chronic ethanol treatment on specific [^{3}H]-GABA binding in different rat brain areas. *Psychopharmacology*, 1980, *67*, 261–264.   (a)

Reggiani, A., Barbaccia, M. L., Spano, P. F., & Trabucchi, M. Role of dopaminergic-enkephalinergic interactions in the neurochemical effects of ethanol. *Substance and Alcohol Actions/Misuse*, 1980, *1*, 151–158.   (b)

Reisine, T., & Soubrie, P. Loss of rat cerebral cortical opiate receptors following chronic desimipramine treatment. *European Journal of Pharmacology*, 1982, *77*, 39–44.

Reisine, T. D., Yamamura, H. I., Bird, E. D., Spokes, E., & Enna, S. J. Pre- and postsynaptic neurochemical alterations in Alzheimer's disease. *Brain Research*, 1978, *159*, 477–481.

Riffee, W. H., & Gerald, M. C. The effect of chronic administration and withdrawal of (+)-amphetamine on seizure threshold and endogenous catecholamine concentrations and rates of biosynthesis in mice. *Psychopharmacology*, 1977, *51*, 175–179.

Riley, J. N., & Walker, D. W. Morphological alterations in hippocampus after long-term alcohol consumption in mice. *Science*, 1978, *201*, 646–648.

Ritchie, J. M., & Greengard, P. On the mode of action of local anesthetics. *Annual Review of Pharmacology*, 1966, *6*, 405–430.

Ritzmann, R. F., & Springer, A. Age-differences in brain sensitivity and tolerance to ethanol in mice. *Age*, 1980, *3*, 15–17.

Roach, M. K., Davis, D. L., Pennington, W., & Nordyke, E. Effect of ethanol on the uptake by rat brain synaptosomes of [^{3}H]DL-norepinephrine, [^{3}H]-hydroxytryptamine, [^{3}H]GABA and [^{3}H]glutamate. *Life Sciences*, 1973, *12*, 433–441.

Roach, M. K., Khan, M. M., Coffman, R., Pennington, W., & Davis, D. L. Brain (Na$^+$ + K$^+$)-activated adenosine triphosphatase activity and neurotransmitter uptake in alcohol-dependent rats. *Brain Research*, 1973, *63*, 323–329.

Roberts, P. J. Glutamate receptor in the rat central nervous system. *Nature*, 1974, *252*, 399–401.

Roberts, P. J. Glutamate binding to synaptic membranes—detection of post-synaptic receptor sites? *Journal of Physiology (London)*, 1975, *247*, 44–45.

Rogers, J., Siggins, G. R., Aston-Jones, G., Koda, L. Y., & Bloom, F. E. Electrophysiological effects of acute ethanol on olivo-cerebellar neurotransmission. *Abstracts, Society for Neuroscience*, 1982, *8*, 597.

Rogers, J., Siggins, G. R., Schulman, J. A., & Bloom, F. E. Physiological correlates of ethanol intoxication, tolerance, and dependence in rat cerebellar Purkinje cells. *Brain Research*, 1980, *196*, 183–198.

Rosett, H. L. Clinical pharmacology of the fetal alcohol syndrome. In E. Majchrowicz & E. P. Noble (Eds.), *Biochemistry and pharmacology of ethanol* (Vol. 2). New York: Plenum, 1979.

Ross, D. H. Selective action of alcohols on cerebral calcium levels. *Annals of the New York Academy of Sciences*, 1976, *273*, 280–294.

Ross, D. H., Medina, M. A., & Cardenas, H. L. Morphine and ethanol: Selective depletion of regional brain calcium. *Science*, 1974, *186*, 63–65.

Roth, S., Physical mechanisms of anesthesia, In R. George, R. Okun, & A. K. Cho (Eds.), *Annual review of pharmacology and toxicology*. Palo Alto: Annual Reviews, 1979.

Roth, S., & Seeman, P. All lipid-soluble anesthetics protect red cells. *Nature (London)*, 1971, *231*, 284–285.

Roth, S., & Seeman, P. Anesthetics expand erythrocyte membranes without causing loss of K$^+$. *Biochimica et Biophysica Acta*, 1972, *255*, 190–198.

Roth, S., & Spero, L. Effects of a series of alcohols on the binding of a fluorescent dye to erythrocyte membranes. *Canadian Journal of Physiology and Pharmacology*, 1976, *54*, 35–41.

Rothstein, A. Membrane phenomena. *Annual Reviews of Physiology*, 1968, *30*, 15–72.

Rothstein, E. Prevention of alcohol withdrawal seizures: The roles of diphenylhydantoin and chlordiazepoxide. *American Journal of Psychiatry*, 1973, *130*, 1381–1382.

Rotrosen, J., Mandio, D., Segarnick, D., Traficante, L. J., & Gershon, S. Ethanol and prostaglandins E$_1$: Biochemical and behavioral interactions. *Life Sciences*, 1980, *26*, 1867–1876.

Rottenberg, H., Robertson, D. E., & Rubin, E. The effect of ethanol on the temperature dependence of respiration and ATPase activities of rat liver mitochondria. *Laboratory Investigation*, 1980, *42*, 318–326.

Rottenberg, H., Waring, A., & Rubin, E. Tolerance and cross-tolerance in chronic alcoholism: Reduced membrane binding of ethanol and other drugs. *Science*, 1981, *213*, 583–585.

Rowe, E. S. Lipid chain length and temperature dependence of ethanol–phosphatidylcholine interactions. *Biochemistry*, 1983, *22*, 3229–3305.

Rubin, E. Alcohol and the heart: Theoretical considerations. *Federation Proceedings*, 1982, *41*, 2460–2464.

Rubin, E., & Rottenberg, H. Ethanol-induced injury and adaptation in biological membranes. *Federation Proceedings*, 1982, *41*, 2465–2471.

Rubin, R. P. The role of calcium in the release of neurotransmitter substances and hormones. *Pharmacological Reviews*, 1970, *22*, 389–428.

Salinas, M., & Fernández, T. Effects of chronic ingestion of alcohol in the pregnant rat on catecholamine-sensitive adenylate cyclase in the brain of mothers and their offspring. *Neuropharmacology*, 1983, *11*, 1283-1288.

Sampliner, R., & Iber, F. L. Diphenylhydantoin control of alcohol withdrawal seizures: Results of a controlled study. *Journal of the American Medical Association*, 1974, *230*, 1430-1432.

Schlapfer, W. T., Woodson, P. B. J., Smith, G. A., Tremblay, J. P., & Barondes, S. H. Marked prolongation of post-tetanic potentiation at a transition temperature and its adaptation. *Nature*, 1975, *258*, 623-625.

Schmidt, M. J., Schmidt, D. E., & Robinson, G. A. Cyclic adenosine monophosphate in brain areas: Microwave irradiation as a means of tissue fixation. *Science*, 1971, *173*, 1142-1143.

Schreier, S., Polnaszek, C. F., & Smith, I. C. P. Spin labels in membranes: Problems in practice. *Biochimica et Biophysica Acta*, 1978, *515*, 375-436.

Schulz, R., Wüster, M., Duka, T., & Herz, A. Acute and chronic ethanol treatment changes endorphin levels in brain and pituitary. *Psychopharmacology*, 1980, *68*, 221-227.

Schulz, R., Wüster, M., & Herz, A. Endogenous ligands for kappa-opiate receptors. *Peptides*, 1982, *3*, 973-976.

Schwarcz, R., Creese, I., Coyle, J. T., & Snyder, S. H. Dopamine receptors localized in cerebral cortical afferents to rat corpus striatum. *Nature (London)*, 1978, *271*, 766-768.

Schwartz, A., Lindenmayer, G. E., & Allen, J. C. The sodium–potassium adenosine triphosphatase: Pharmacological, physiological, and biochemical aspects. *Pharmacological Reviews*, 1975, *27*, 3-134.

Schwartz, J. C., Costentin, J., Martes, M. P., Protais, P., & Baudry, M. Modulation of receptor mechanisms in the CNS: Hyper- and hyposensitivity to catecholamines. *Neuropharmacology*, 1978, *17*, 665-685.

Schwartz, J. R., & Vogel, W. Diphenylhydantoin: Excitability reducing action in single myelinated nerve fibres. *European Journal of Pharmacology*, 1977, *44*, 241-249.

Scott, B. S., & Edwards, B. A. V. Effect of chronic ethanol exposure on the electric membrane properties of DRG neurons in cell culture. *Journal of Neurobiology*, 1981, *12*, 379-390.

Scott, B. S., Engelbert, V. E., & Fischer, K. C. Morphological and electrophysiological characteristics of dissociated chick embryonic spinal ganglion cells in culture. *Experimental Neurology*, 1969, *23*, 230-248.

Seeber, U., & Kuschinsky, K. Dopamine-sensitive adenylate cyclase in homogenates of rat striata during ethanol and barbiturate withdrawal. *Archives of Toxicology*, 1976, *35*, 247-253.

Seeman, P. Erythrocyte membrane stabilization by steroids and alcohols: A possible model for anesthesia. *Biochemical Pharmacology*, 1966, *15*, 1632-1637.

Seeman, P. The membrane actions of anesthetics and tranquilizers. *Pharmacological Reviews*, 1972, *24*, 583-655.

Seeman, P. The membrane expansion theory of anesthesia: Direct evidence using ethanol and a high-precision density meter. *Experientia*, 1974, *30*, 759-760.

Seeman, P. Brain dopamine receptors. *Pharmacological Reviews*, 1980, *32*, 229-313.

Seeman, P., Chau, M., Goldberg, M., Sauks, T., & Sax, L. The binding of Ca^{2+} to the cell membrane increased by volatile anesthetics (alcohols, acetone, ether) which induce sensitization of nerve or muscle. *Biochimica et Biophysica Acta*, 1971, *225*, 183-193.

Seeman, P., Kwant, W. O., Sauks, T., & Argent, W., Membrane expansion of intact erythrocytes by anesthetics. *Biochimica et Biophysica Acta*, 1969, *183*, 490-498.

Seeman, P., & Roth, S. General anesthetics expand cell membranes at surgical concentrations. *Biochimica et Biophysica Acta*, 1972, *225*, 171-177.

Seil, F. J., Leiman, A. L., Herman, M. M., & Fisk, R. A. Direct effects of ethanol on central nervous system cultures: An electrophysiological and morphological study. *Experimental Neurology*, 1977, *55*, 390–404.

Sellers, E., M., & Kalant, H. Alcohol intoxication and withdrawal. *New England Journal of Medicine*, 1976, *294*, 757–762.

Seppälä, M., Räihä, N. C. R., & Tamminen, V. Ethanol elimination in a mother and her premature twins. *Lancet*, 1971, *1*, 1188–1189.

Shah, K. R., & West, M. Prenatal exposure to ethanol alters [^{3}H]naloxone binding in rat striatum. *European Journal of Pharmacology*, 1983, *90*, 445–447.

Shanes, A. M. Electrochemical aspects of physiological and pharmacological action in excitable cells. Part I. The resting cell and its alteration by extrinsic factors. *Pharmacological Reviews*, 1958, *10*, 59–164.

Sharif, N. A., & Roberts, P. J. Effect of guanine nucleotides on binding of L-[^{3}H]-glutamate to cerebellar synaptic membranes. *European Journal of Pharmacology*, 1980, *61*, 213–214.

Sharma, V. K., & Banerjee, S. P. Effect of chronic ethanol treatment on specific [^{3}H]ouabain binding to ($Na^+ + K^+$)-ATPase in different areas of cat brain. *European Journal of Pharmacology*, 1979, *56*, 297–304.

Shen, A., Jacobyansky, A., Pathman, D., & Thurman, R. G. Changes in brain cyclic AMP levels during chronic ethanol treatment and withdrawal in the rat. *European Journal of Pharmacology*, 1983, *89*, 103–110.

Shepherd, G. M. *The synaptic organization of the brain: An introduction* (2nd ed.). New York: Oxford University Press, 1979.

Shinitzky, M., & Barenholz, Y. Fluidity parameters of lipid regions determined by fluorescence polarization. *Biochimica et Biophysica Acta*, 1978, *515*, 367–394.

Siggins, G. R., & Bloom, F. E. Alcohol-related electrophysiology. *Pharmacology, Biochemistry, and Behavior*, 1980, *13*, Supplement 1, 203–211.

Siggins, G. R., & French, E. Central neurons are depressed by iontophoretic and micropressure application of ethanol and tetrahydropapaveroline. *Drug and Alcohol Dependence*, 1979, *4*, 239–243.

Silver, L. H., & Treistman, S. N. Effects of alcohols upon pacemaker activity in neurons of *Aplysia californica*. *Cellular and Molecular Neurobiology*, 1982, *2*, 215–226.

Sinclair, J. G., & Lo, G. F. The effects of ethanol on cerebellar Purkinje cell discharge pattern and inhibition evoked by local surface stimulation. *Brain Research*, 1981, *204*, 465–471.

Sinclair, J. G., & Lo, G. F. Ethanol effects on rat cerebellar Purkinje cells. *General Pharmacology*, 1982, *13*, 449–451.

Sinclair, J. G., Lo, G. F., & Harris, D. P. Ethanol effects on the olivocerebellar system. *Canadian Journal of Physiology and Pharmacology*, 1982, *60*, 610–614.

Sinclair, J. G., Lo, G. F., & Harris, D. P. Ethanol inhibits inferior olive neurones. *Proceedings of the Western Pharmacological Society*, 1983, *26*, 155–156.

Sinclair, J. G., Lo, G. F., & Tien, A. F. The effects of ethanol on cerebellar Purkinje cells in naive and alcohol-dependent rats. *Canadian Journal of Physiology and Pharmacology*, 1980, *58*, 429–432.

Sinensky, M., Minneman, K. P., & Molinoff, P. B. Increased membrane acyl chain ordering activates adenylate cyclase. *Journal of Biological Chemistry*, 1979, *254*, 9135–9141.

Singer, S. J., & Nicholson, G. L. The fluid mosaic model of the structure of cell membranes. *Science*, 1972, *175*, 720–731.

Skolnick, P., Rice, K. C., Barker, J. L., & Paul, S. N. Interactions of barbiturates with benzodiazepine receptors in the central nervous system. *Brain Research*, 1982, *233*, 143–156.

Skolnick, P., Stalvey, L. P., Daly, J. W., Hoyler, E., & Davis, J. N. Binding of alpha- and beta-adrenergic ligands to cerebral cortical membranes: Effect of 6-hydroxydopamine treatment and relationship to the responsiveness of cyclic AMP-generating systems in two rat strains. *European Journal of Pharmacology*, 1978, *47*, 201–210.

Skou, J. C. Relation between the ability of various compounds to block nervous conduction and their penetration into a monomolecular layer of nerve-tissue lipoids. *Biochimica et Biophysica Acta*, 1958, *30*, 625-629.

Slotkin, T. A., Schanberg, S. M., & Kuhn, C. M. Synaptic development in brains of rats exposed perinatally to ethanol. *Experientia*, 1980, *36*, 1005-1007.

Sloviter, R. S., Drust, E. G., & Connor, J. D. Specificity of a rat behavioral model for serotonin receptor activation. *Journal of Pharmacology and Experimental Therapeutics*, 1978, *206*, 339-347.

Smith, A., Hayashida, K., & Kim, Y. Inhibition by propranolol of ethanol-induced narcosis. *Journal of Pharmacy and Pharmacology*, 1970, *22*, 644-645.

Smith, T. C. The effect of chronic ethanol feeding on the cAMP generating system of mouse brain. *Proceedings of the Western Pharmacological Society*, 1981, *24*, 37-39.

Smith, T. L., & Gerhart, M. J. Alterations in brain lipid composition of mice made physically dependent to ethanol. *Life Sciences*, 1982, 1419-1425.

Smith, T. L., Jacobyansky, A., Shen, A., Pathman, D., & Thurman, R. G. Adaptation of cyclic AMP generating system in rat cerebral cortical slices during chronic ethanol treatment and withdrawal. *Neuropharmacology*, 1981, *20*, 67-72.

Snyder, S. H., Bruns, R. F., Daly, J. W., & Innis, R. B. Multiple neurotransmitter receptors in the brain: Amines, adenosine, and cholecystokinin. *Federation Proceedings*, 1981, *40*, 142-146.

Snyder, S. H., & Innis, R. B. Peptide neurotransmitters. *Annual Reviews of Biochemistry*, 1979, *48*, 755-782.

Sorensen, S., Carter, D., Marwaha, J., Baker, R., & Freedman, R. Disinhibition of rat cerebellar Purkinje neurons from noradrenergic inhibition during rising blood ethanol. *Journal of Studies on Alcohol*, 1981, *42*, 908-917.

Sorensen, S., Dunwiddie, T., McClearn, G., Freedman, R., & Hoffer, B. Ethanol-induced depression in cerebellar and hippocampal neurons of mice selectively bred for difference in ethanol sensitivity: An electrophysiological study. *Pharmacology, Biochemistry, and Behavior*, 1981, *14*, 227-234.

Sorensen, S., Palmer, M., Dunwiddie, T., & Hoffer, B. Electrophysiological correlates of ethanol-induced sedation in differentially sensitive lines of mice. *Science*, 1980, *210*, 1143-1145.

Sørensen, S. C., & Mattisson, K. Naloxone as an antagonist in severe alcohol intoxication. *Lancet*, 1978, *2*, 688-689.

Spuhler, K., Hoffer, B., Weiner, N., & Palmer, M. Evidence for genetic correlation of hypnotic effects and cerebellar Purkinje neuron depression in response to ethanol in mice. *Pharmacology, Biochemistry, and Behavior*, 1982, *17*, 569-578.

Squires, R. F., Benson, D. I., Braestrup, C., Coupet, J., Klepner, C. A., Myers, V., & Beer, B. Some properties of brain specific benzodiazepine receptors: New evidence for multiple receptors. *Pharmacology, Biochemistry, and Behavior*, 1979, *10*, 825-830.

Stahl, W. L., & Swanson, P. D. Movements of calcium and other cations in isolated cerebral cortex. *Journal of Neurochemistry*, 1971, *18*, 415-427.

Starke, K. Regulation of noradrenaline release by presynaptic receptor systems. *Reviews of Physiology, Biochemistry, and Pharmacology*, 1977, *77*, 1-124.

Stock, K., & Schmidt, M. Effects of short-chain alcohols on adenylate cyclase in plasma membranes of adipocytes. *Naunyn-Schmiedeberg's Archives of Pharmacology*, 1978, *302*, 37-48.

Stokes, J. A., & Harris, R. A. Alcohols and synaptosomal calcium transport. *Molecular Pharmacology*, 1982, *22*, 99-104.

Stoltenburg-Didinger, G., & Spohr, H. L. Fetal alcohol syndrome and mental retardation: Spine distribution of pyramidal cells in prenatal alcohol-exposed rat cerebral cortex; a Golgi study. *Developmental Brain Research*, 1983, *11*, 119-123.

Straub, R. Die Wirkung von Veratridin auf das Membran Potential von markhaltigen Nervenfasern des Frosches. *Helvetica Physiologie und Pharmacologie*, 1954, *14*, 1–28.

Strong, R., Samorajski, T., & Gottesfeld, Z. Regional mapping of neostriatal neurotransmitter systems as a function of aging. *Journal of Neurochemistry*, 1982, *39*, 831–836.

Study, R. E., & Barker, J. L. Diazepam and (–)-pentobarbital: Fluctuation analysis reveals different mechanisms for potentiation of GABA responses in cultured central neurons. *Proceedings of the National Academy of Sciences (USA)*, 1981, *78*, 7180–7184.

Suga, M. Effect of long-term L-DOPA administration on the dopaminergic and cholinergic (muscarinic) receptors of striatum in 6-hydroxydopamine lesioned rats. *Life Sciences*, 1980, *27*, 877–882.

Sun, A. Y., & Samorajski, T. Effects of ethanol on the activity of adenosine triphosphatases and acetylcholinesterase in synaptosomes isolated from guinea-pig brain. *Journal of Neurochemistry*, 1970, *17*, 1365–1372.

Sun, A. Y., & Samorajski, T. The effects of age and alcohol on $(Na^+ + K^+)$-ATPase activity of whole mouse and human brain. *Journal of Neurochemistry*, 1975, *24*, 161–164.

Sun, G. Y., Creech, D. M., Corbin, D. R., & Sun, A. Y. The effect of chronic ethanol administration on arachidonyl transfer to 1-acyl-glycerophosphorylcholine in rat brain synaptosomal fraction. *Research Communications in Chemical Pathology and Pharmacology*, 1977, *18*, 753–756.

Sun, G. Y., & Sun, A. Y. Effect of chronic ethanol administration on phospholipid acyl groups of synaptic plasma membrane fraction isolated from guinea pig brain. *Research Communications in Chemical Pathology and Pharmacology*, 1979, *24*, 405–408.

Sun, G. Y., & Sun, A. Y. Chronic ethanol administration induced an increase in phosphatidylserine in guinea pig synaptic plasma membranes. *Biochemical and Biophysical Research Communications*, 1983, *113*, 262–268.

Supavilai, P., & Karobath, M. Ethanol and other CNS depressants decrease GABA synthesis in mouse cerebral cortex and cerebellum *in vivo*. *Life Science*, 1980, *27*, 1035–1040.

Swartz, M. H., Tepke, D. I., Katz, A. M., & Rubin, E. Effects of ethanol on calcium binding and calcium uptake by cardiac microsomes. *Biochemical Pharmacology*, 1974, *23*, 2369–2371.

Syapin, P. J., Stefanovic, V., Mandel, P., & Noble, E. P. The chronic and acute affects of ethanol on adenosine triphosphatase activity in cultured astroblast and neuroblastoma cells. *Journal of Neuroscience Research*, 1976, *2*, 147–155.

Syapin, P. J., Stefanovic, V., Mandel, P., & Noble, E. P. Stimulation of the plasma membrane enzyme, 5′-nucleotidase, by ethanol exposure to neural cells in culture. *Progress in Neuro-Psychopharmacology*, 1980, *4*, 19–30. (a)

Syapin, P. J., Stefanovic, V., Mandel, P., & Noble, E. P. Stimulation of rat C6 glioma ecto-5′-nucleotidase by chronic ethanol treatment. *Biochemical Pharmacology*, 1980, *29*, 2279–2284. (b)

Tabakoff, B., & Hoffman, P. L. Alterations in receptors controlling dopamine synthesis after chronic ethanol ingestion. *Journal of Neurochemistry*, 1978, *31*, 1223–1229.

Tabakoff, B., & Hoffman, P. L. Development of functional dependence on ethanol in dopaminergic systems. *Journal of Pharmacology and Experimental Therapeutics*, 1979, *208*, 216–222.

Tabakoff, B., & Hoffman, P. L. Alcohol interactions with brain opiate receptors. *Life Sciences*, 1983, *32*, 197–204.

Tabakoff, B., Hoffman, P. L., & Ritzman, R. F. Dopamine receptor function after chronic ingestion of ethanol. *Life Sciences*, 1978, *23*, 643–648.

Tabakoff, B., Munoz-Marcus, M., & Fields, J. Z. Chronic ethanol feeding produces an increase in muscarinic cholinergic receptors in mouse brain. *Life Sciences*, 1979, *25*, 2173–2180.

Tabakoff, B., Urwyler, S., & Hoffman, P. L. Ethanol alters kinetic characteristics and function of striatal morphine receptors. *Journal of Neurochemistry*, 1981, *37*, 518–521.

Tague, L. L., & Shanbour, L. L. Effects of ethanol on bicarbonate-stimulated ATPase, ATP, and cyclic AMP in canine gastric mucosa. *Proceedings of the Society for Experimental Biology and Medicine*, 1977, *154*, 37–40.

Tamkun, M. M., & Catterall, W. A. Ion flux studies of voltage-sensitive sodium channels in synaptic nerve-ending particles. *Molecular Pharmacology*, 1981, *19*, 78–86.

Tanford, C. *The hydrophobic effect: Formation of micelles and biological membranes.* New York: Wiley, 1973.

Tasaki, I., Carbone, E., Sisco, K., & Singer, I. Spectral analyses of extrinsic fluorescence of the nerve membrane labeled with aminonaphthalene derivatives. *Biochimica et Biophysica Acta*, 1973, *323*, 220–233.

Tasaki, I., Watanabe, A., & Hallett, M. Properties of squid axon membrane as revealed by a hydrophobic probe, 2-*p*-toluidinylnaphthalene-6-sulfonate. *Proceedings of the National Academy of Sciences (USA)*, 1971, *68*, 938–941.

Tavares, M. A., & Paula-Barbosa, M. M. Alcohol-induced granule cell loss in the cerebellar cortex of the adult rat. *Experimental Neurology*, 1982, *78*, 574–582.

Tavares, M. A., & Paula-Barbosa, M. M. Lipofuscin granules in Purkinje cells after long-term alcohol consumption in rats. *Alcoholism: Clinical and Experimental Research*, 1983, *7*, 302–306.

Tewari, S., Fleming, E. W., & Noble, E. P. Alterations in brain RNA metabolism following chronic ethanol ingestion. *Journal of Neurochemistry*, 1975, *24*, 561–569.

Tewari, S., Murray, S., & Noble, E. P. Studies of the effects of chronic ethanol ingestion on the properties of rat brain ribosomes. *Journal of Neuroscience Research*, 1978, *3*, 375–387.

Tewari, S., & Noble, E. P. Ethanol and brain protein synthesis. *Brain Research*, 1971, *26*, 469–474.

Tewari, S., & Noble, E. P. Effects of ethanol on cerebral protein and ribonucleic acid synthesis. In E. Majchrowicz & E. P. Noble (Eds.), *Biochemistry and pharmacology of ethanol* (Vol. 2). New York: Plenum, 1979.

Thadani, P. V., Kulig, B. M., Brown, F. C., & Beard, J. D. Acute and chronic ethanol-induced alterations in brain norepinephrine metabolites in the rat. *Biochemical Pharmacology*, 1976, *25*, 93–94.

Thadani, P. V., & Truitt, E. B., Jr. Effect of acute ethanol or acetaldehyde on the uptake, release, metabolism, and turnover rate of norepinephrine in the rat brain. *Biochemical Pharmacology*, 1977, *26*, 1147–1150.

Thomas, D. S., Hossack, J. A., & Rose, A. H. Plasma-membrane lipid composition and ethanol tolerance in *Saccharomyces cervesiae*. *Archives of Microbiology*, 1978, *117*, 239–245.

Thompson, W. L. Management of alcohol withdrawal syndromes. *Archives of Internal Medicine*, 1978, *138*, 278–283.

Thulborn, K. R., & Sawyer, W. H. Properties and locations of a set of fluorescent probes sensitive to the fluidity gradient of the lipid bilayer. *Biochimica et Biophysica Acta*, 1978, *511*, 125–140.

Thulborn, K. R., Tilley, L. M., Sawyer, W. H., and Treloar, E. The use of *n*-(9-anthroyloxy) fatty acids to determine fluidity and polarity gradients in phospholipid bilayers. *Biochimica et Biophysica Acta*, 1979, *558*, 166–178.

Thurman, R. G., & Pathman, D. E. Withdrawal symptoms from ethanol: Evidence against the involvement of acetaldehyde. In K. O. Lindros & C. J. P. Eriksson (Eds.), *The role of acetaldehyde in the actions of ethanol.* Helsinki: Finnish Foundation for Alcohol Studies, 1975.

Ticku, M. K. Interaction of depressant, convulsant, and anticonvulsant barbiturates with the [^{3}H]-diazepam binding site of the benzodiazepine–GABA-receptor–ionophore complex. *Biochemical Pharmacology*, 1980, *30*, 1573–1579. (a)

Ticku, M. K. The effects of acute and chronic ethanol administration and its withdrawal on GABA receptor binding in rat brain. *British Journal of Pharmacology*, 1980, *70*, 403-410.   (b)

Ticku, M. K., Ban, M., & Olsen, R. W. Binding of [^{3}H]-dihydropicrotoxinin, GABA synaptic antagonist, to rat brain membranes. *Molecular Pharmacology*, 1978, *14*, 391-402.

Ticku, M. K., & Burch, T. Alterations in GABA receptor sensitivity following acute and chronic ethanol treatments. *Journal of Neurochemistry*, 1980, *34*, 417-423.

Ticku, M. K., & Davis, W. C. Evidence that ethanol and pentobarbital enhances [^{3}H]-diazepam binding at the benzodiazepine-GABA receptor-ionophore complex indirectly. *European Journal of Pharmacology*, 1981, *71*, 521-522.

Tilley, F. W., & Schaffer, J. M. Relation between the chemical constitution and germicidal activity of the monohydric alcohols and phenols. *Journal of Bacteriology*, 1926, *12*, 303-309.

Tilley, F. W., & Schaffer, J. M. Chemical constitution and germicidal activity of amines, ketones, and aldehydes. *Journal of Bacteriology*, 1928, *16*, 279-285.

Tjeol, S., Bianchi, C. P., & Haugaard, N. The function of ATP in calcium uptake by rat brain mitochondria. *Biochimica et Biophysica Acta*, 1970, *216*, 270-273.

Tobin, R. B., Mehlman, M. A., Kies, C., Fox, H. M., & Soeldner, J. S. Nutritional and metabolic studies in humans with 1,3-butanediol. *Federation Proceedings*, 1975, *34*, 2171-2176.

Toffano, G., Guidotti, A., & Costa, E. Purification of an endogenous protein inhibitor of the high-affinity binding of GABA to synaptic membranes of rat brain. *Proceedings of the National Academy of Sciences (USA)*, 1978, *75*, 4024-4028.

Tran, V. T., Snyder, S. H., Major, F. L., & Hawley, R. J. GABA receptors are increased in brain of alcoholics. *Annals of Neurology*, 1981, *9*, 289-292.

Traube, J. Über die wirkung lipoidölicher Stoffe auf rote Blutkörperchen. *Biochemische Zeitschrift*, 1908, *10*, 371-379.

Traynor, A. E., Schlapfer, W. T., & Barondes, S. H. Stimulation is necessary for the development of tolerance to a neuronal effect of ethanol. *Journal of Neurobiology*, 1980, *11*, 633-637.

Traynor, M. E., Schlapfer, W. T. Woodson, P. B. J., & Barondes, S. H. Tolerance to a specific synaptic effect of ethanol in *Aplysia*. In E. Majchrowicz & E. P. Noble (Eds.), *Biochemistry and pharmacology of ethanol* (Vol. 2). New York: Plenum, 1979.

Traynor, M. E., Woodson, P. B. J., Schlapfer, W. T., & Barondes, S. H. Sustained tolerance to a specific effect of ethanol in post-tetanic potentiation in *Aplysia*. *Science*, 1976, *193*, 510-511.

Trudell, J. R. A unitary theory of anesthesia based on lateral phase separations in nerve membranes. *Anesthesiology*, 1977, *46*, 5-10.

Ulbricht, W. The effect of veratridine on excitable membranes of nerve and muscle. *Ergebnisse der Physiologie, Biologischen Chemie und Experimentellen Pharmakologie*, 1969, *61*, 18-71.

Unwin, J. W., & Taberner, P. V. Sex and Strain differences in GABA receptor binding after chronic ethanol drinking in mice. *Neuropharmacology*, 1980, *19*, 1257-1259.

Urwyler, S., & Tabakoff, B. Stimulation of dopamine synthesis and release by morphine and D-Ala^2, D-Leu^5-enkephalin in the mouse striatum *in vivo*. *Life Sciences*, 1981, *28*, 2277-2286.

Vanderkooi, J. M. Effect of ethanol on membranes: A fluorescent probe study. *Alcoholism: Clinical and Experimental Research*, 1979, *3*, 60-63.

Veloso, D., Passaneau, J. V., & Veech, R. L. The effects of intoxicating doses of ethanol upon intermediary metabolism. *Journal of Neurochemistry*, 1972, *19*, 2679-2686.

Vesely, D. L., Lehotay, D. C., & Levey, G. S. Effects of ethanol on myocardial guanylate and adenylate cyclase activity and on cyclic GMP and AMP levels. *Journal of Studies on Alcohol*, 1978, *39*, 842-847.

Vesely, D. L., & Levey, G. S. Ethanol-induced inhibition of guantylate cyclase in liver, pancreas, stomach, and intestine. *Research Communications in Chemical Pathology and Pharmacology*, 1977, *17*, 215-224.

Victor, M., & Adams, R. D. The effect of alcohol on the nervous system. In H. H. Merritt & C. C. Hare (Eds.), *Metabolic and toxic diseases of the nervous system*. Baltimore: Williams & Wilkins, 1953.

Victor, M., Adams, R. D., & Collins, H. G. *The Wernicke-Korsakoff syndrome*. Philadelphia: F. A. Davis, 1971.

Villegas, R. Barnola, F. V., & Camejo, G. Ionic channels and nerve membrane lipids: Cholesterol-tetrodotoxin interaction. *Journal of General Physiology*, 1970, *55*, 548-561.

Vincent, M., de Foresta, B., Gallay, J., & Alfsen, A. Fluorescence anisotropy decays of *n*-(9-anthroyloxy) fatty acids in dipalmitoyl phosphatidylcholine vesicles. Localization of the effects of cholesterol addition. *Biochemical and Biophysical Research Communications*, 1982, *107*, 914-921.

Vogel, R. A., Frye, G. D., Koepkem, K. M., Mailman, R. B., Mueller, R. A., & Breese, G. R. Differential effects of TRH, amphetamine, naloxone, and fenmetozole on ethanol actions: Attenuation of the effect of punishment and impairment of aerial righting reflex. *Alcoholism: Clinical and Experimental Research*, 1981, *5*, 386-392.

Volicer, L. GABA levels and receptor binding after acute and chronic ethanol administration. *Brain Research Bulletin*, 1980, *5, Supplement 2*, 809-813.

Volicer, L., & Biagioni, T. M. Effect of ethanol administration and withdrawal on benzodiazepine receptor binding in the rat brain. *Neuropharmacology*, 1982, *21*, 283-286. (a)

Volicer, L., & Biagioni, T. M. Effect of ethanol administration and withdrawal on GABA receptor binding in rat cerebral cortex. *Substance and Alcohol Actions/Misuse*, 1982, *3*, 31-39. (b)

Volicer, L., & Gold, B. I. Effect of ethanol on cyclic AMP levels in the rat brain. *Life Sciences*, 1973, *13*, 269-280.

Volicer, L., & Hurter, B. P. Effects of acute and chronic ethanol administration and withdrawal on adenosine 3':5'-monophosphate and guanosine 3':5'-monophosphate levels in the rat brain. *Journal of Pharmacology and Experimental Therapeutics*, 1977, *200*, 298-305.

von Hungen, K., & Baxter, C. F. Sensitivity of rat brain adenylate cyclase to activation by calcium and ethanol after chronic exposure to ethanol. *Biochemical and Biophysical Research Communications*, 1982, *106*, 1078-1082.

Waddington, J. L., & Cross, A. J. Denervation supersensitivity in the striatonigral GABA pathway. *Nature*, 1978, *276*, 618-620.

Waggoner, A. S., & Stryer, L. Fluorescent probes of biological membranes. *Proceedings of the National Academy of Sciences (USA)*, 1970, *67*, 579-589.

Wahlström, G. The effects of cyclic 3',5' adenosine monophosphate on the acute tolerance induced by ethanol in male rats. *Life Sciences*, 1975, *17*, 1655-1662.

Walker, D. W., Barnes, D. E., Riley, J. N., Hunter, B. E., & Zornetzer, S. F. Neurotoxicity of chronic alcohol consumption: An animal model. In M. Sandler (Ed.), *Psychopharmacology of alcohol*. New York: Raven, 1980.

Walker, D. W., Barnes, D. E., Zornetzer, S. F., Hunter, B. E., & Kubanis, P. Neuronal loss in hippocampus induced by prolonged ethanol consumption in rats. *Science*, 1980, *209*, 711-713.

Walker, D. W., Hunter, B. E., & Abraham, W. C. Neuroanatomical and functional deficits subsequent to chronic ethanol administration in animals. *Alcoholism: Clinical and Experimental Research*, 1981, *5*, 267-282.

Wallgren, H. Relative intoxicating effects on rats of ethyl, propyl and butyl alcohols. *Acta Pharmacologica et Toxicologica*, 1960, *16*, 217-222.

Wallgren, H., Kosunen, A. L., & Ahtee, L. Technique for producing an alcohol withdrawal syndrome in rats. *Israel Journal of Medical Sciences*, 1973, *9, Supplement*, 63-71.

Wallgren, H., Nikander, P., von Boguslawsky, P., & Linkola, J. Effects of ethanol, tert.

butanol, and clomethiazole on net movements of sodium and potassium in electrically stimulated cerebral tissue. *Acta Physiologica Scandinavica*, 1974, *91*, 83–93.

Waltman, R., & Iniquez, E. S. Placental transfer of ethanol and its elimination at term. *Obstetrics and Gynecology*, 1972, *40*, 180–185.

Wang, Y. J., Salvaterra, P., & Roberts, E. Characterization of [^{3}H]muscimol binding to mouse brain membranes. *Biochemical Pharmacology*, 1979, *28*, 1123–1128.

Waring, A. J., Rottenberg, H., Ohnishi, T., & Rubin, E. Membranes and phospholipids of liver mitochondria from chronic alcoholic rats are resistant to membrane disordering by alcohol. *Proceedings of the National Academy of Sciences (USA)*, 1981, *78*, 2582–2586.

Waring, A. J., Rottenberg, H., Ohnishi, T., & Rubin, E. The effect of chronic ethanol consumption on temperature-dependent physical properties of liver mitochondrial membranes. *Archives of Biochemistry and Biophysics*, 1982, *216*, 51–61.

Watson, J. D. *Molecular biology of the gene* (3rd ed.). Menlo Park, Cal.: W. A. Benjamin, 1976.

West, J. R., Dewey, S. L., & Cassel, M. D. Prenatal ethanol exposure alters the post-lesion reorganization (sprouting) of acetylcholinesterase staining in the dentate gyrus of adult rats. *Development Brain Research*, 1984, *12*, 83–95.

West, J. R., Hodges, C. A., & Black, A. C., Jr. Prenatal exposure to ethanol alters to organization of hippocampal mossy fibers in rats. *Science*, 1981, *211*, 957–959.

West, J. R., Lind, M. D., Demuth, R. M., Parker, E. S., Alkana, R. L., Cassell, M., & Black, A. C., Jr. Lesion-induced sprouting in the rat dentate gyrus is inhibited by repeated ethanol administration. *Science*, 1982, *218*, 808–810.

Westcott, J. Y., & Weiner, H. Effect of ethanol on synaptosomal (Na$^+$ + K$^+$)-ATPase in control and ethanol-dependent rats. *Archives of Biochemistry and Biophysics*, 1983, *223*, 51–57.

Whalley, L. J., Freeman, C. P., & Hunter, J. Role of endogenous opioids in alcoholic intoxication. *Lancet*, 1981, *2*, 89.

White, A., Handler, P., & Smith, E. L. *Principles of biochemistry* (4th ed.). New York: McGraw-Hill, 1968.

Williams, L. T., & Lefkowitz, R. J. Slowly reversible binding of catecholamine to a nucleotide-sensitive state of the beta-adrenergic receptor. *Journal of Biological Chemistry*, 1977, *252*, 7207–7209.

Williams, M., & Rodnight, R. Protein phosphorylation in nervous tissue: Possible involvement in nervous tissue function and relationship to cyclic nucleotide metabolism. *Progress in Neurobiology*, 1977, *8*, 183–250.

Willow, M., & Catterall, W. A. Inhibition of binding of [^{3}H]batrachotoxin A 20-alpha-benzoate to sodium channels by the anticonvulsant drugs diphenylhydantoin and carbamazepine. *Molecular Pharmacology*, 1982, *22*, 627–635.

Wilson, D. E. Prostaglandins and the gastrointestinal tracts. *Prostaglandins*, 1972, *1*, 281–293.

Wimbish, G. H., Martz, R., & Forney, R. B. Combined effects of ethanol and propranolol on sleep time in the mouse. *Life Sciences*, 1977, *20*, 65–72.

Wing, D. R., Harvey, D. J., Hughes, J., Dunbar, P. G., McPherson, K. A., & Paton, W. D. M. Effects of chronic ethanol administration on the composition of membrane lipids in the mouse. *Biochemical Pharmacology*, 1982, *31*, 3431–3439.

Wixon, H. N., & Hunt, W. A. Effect of acute and chronic treatment on gamma-aminobutyric acid levels and on aminoxyacetic acid-induced GABA accumulation. *Substances and Alcohol Actions/Misuse*, 1980, *1*, 481–491.

Woo, E., & Greenblat, D. J. Massive benzodiazepine requirements during acute alcohol withdrawal. *American Journal of Psychiatry*, 1979, *136*, 821–823.

Wood, J. D. The role of GABA in the mechanism of seizures. *Progress in Neurobiology*, 1975, *5*, 77–95.

Wood, P. L., Stotland, M., Richard, J. W., & Rackham, A. Actions of mu, sigma, delta, and agonist/antagonist opiates on striatal dopaminergic function. *Journal of Pharmacology and Experimental Therapeutics*, 1980, *215*, 697-703.

Wood, W. G., & Armbrecht, H. J. Behavioral effects of ethanol in animals: Age differences and age changes. *Alcoholism: Clinical and Experimental Research*, 1982, *6*, 3-12.   (a)

Wood, W. G., & Armbrecht, H. J. Age differences in ethanol-induced hypothermia and impairment in mice. *Neurobiology of Aging*, 1982, *3*, 243-246.   (b)

Wood, W. G., Armbrecht, H. J., & Wise, R. W. Ethanol intoxication and withdrawal among three age groups of C57BL/6NNIA mice. *Pharmacology, Biochemistry, and Behavior*, 1982, *17*, 1037-1041.

Woodbury, D. M. Effect of diphenylhydantoin on electrolytes and radiosodium turnover in brain and other tissues in normal, hyponatremic, and postictal rats. *Journal of Pharmacology and Experimental Therapeutics*, 1955, *115*, 74-95.

Woodson, P. B. J., Traynor, M. E., Schlapfer, W. T., & Barondes, S. H. Increased membrane fluidity implicated in acceleration of decay of post-tetanic potentiation by alcohols. *Nature*, 1976, *260*, 797-799.

Yamamoto, H., & Harris, R. A. Calcium-dependent ^{86}Rb efflux and ethanol intoxication: Studies of human red blood cells and rodent brain synaptosomes. *European Journal of Pharmacology*, 1983, *88*, 357-363.   (a)

Yamamoto, H., & Harris, R. A. Effects of ethanol and barbiturates on Ca^{2+}-ATPase activity of erythrocyte and brain membranes. *Biochemical Pharmacology*, 1983, *32*, 2787-2791.   (b)

Yamamoto, H., Sutoo, D., & Misawa, S. Effect of cadmium on ethanol induced sleeping time in mice. *Life Sciences*, 1981, *28*, 2917-2923.

Yamamura, H. I., & Snyder, S. H. Muscarinic cholinergic receptor binding in rat brain. *Proceedings of the National Academy of Sciences (USA)*, 1974, *71*, 1725-1729.

Yamanaka, Y. Effects of brain biogenic amines on ethanol withdrawal reactions and the development of ethanol dependence in mice. *Japanese Journal of Phamacology*, 1982, *32*, 499-508.

Yoshikawa, K., Adachi, K., Halprin, K. M., & Levine, V. Effects of short chain alcohols and hydrocarbon compounds on the adenylate cyclase of the skin. *British Journal of Dermatology*, 1976, *94*, 611-614.

Yoshimura, K. Activation of Na-K activated ATPase in rat brain by catecholamines. *Journal of Biochemistry*, 1973, *74*, 389-391.

Zavoico, G. B., & Kutchai, H. Effects of *n*-alkanols of the membrane fluidity of chick embryo heart microsomes. *Biochimica et Biophysica Acta*, 1980, *600*, 263-269.

Zieglänsberger, W., Fry, J. P., Moroder, L., Herz, A., & Wunsch, E. Enkephalin-induced inhibition of cortical neurones and the lack of this effect in morphine tolerant/dependent rats. *Brain Research*, 1976, *115*, 160-164.

Zysset, T., Sutherland, E., & Simon, F. R. Studies on the differences in NaK-ATPase and lipid properties of liver plasma membranes in long sleep and short sleep mice. *Alcoholism: Clinical and Experimental Research*, 1983, *7*, 85-92.

Author index

Page numbers in italics represent material in figures.

Abdallah, A. H., 151, 161*n*.
Abdel-Latif, A. A., 67, 179*n*.
Abdul-Ghani, A.-S., 120, 161*n*.
Abel, E. L., 137-139, 161*n*., 166*n*.
Abraham, W. C., 51, 131, 133, 134, 161*n*., 195*n*.
Adachi, K., 91, 197*n*.
Adams, R. D., 130, 145, 195*n*.
Aghajanian, G. K., 57, 161*n*.
Ahlquist, R. P., 107, 161*n*.
Ahn, H. S., 136, 181*n*.
Ahtee, L., 11, 195*n*.
Aiso, M., 109, 178*n*.
Akera, T., 82, 84, 161*n*.
Albers, R. W., 81, 174*n*.
Albuquerque, E. X., 67, 161*n*.
Alfsen, A., 38, 195*n*.
Alger, B. E., 60, 71, 161*n*., 184*n*.
Alkana, R. L., 12, 27, 132, 146, 147, 151, 161*n*., 162*n*., 181*n*., 196*n*.
Allen, J. C., 81, 189*n*.
Allen, R. P., 150, 170*n*.
Alling, C., 31, 162*n*.
Allison, J. B., 9, 166*n*.
Altman, J., 138, 163*n*.
Altshuler, H. L., 123, 162*n*.
Amaral, D. G., 56, 162*n*.
Amer, M. S., 95, 162*n*.
Andersen, P., 47, 50, 162*n*.
Angel, L. M., 122, 173*n*.
Appel, S. H., 67, 87, 169*n*.
Arbilla, S., 114, 118, 162*n*.
Argent, W., 15, 189*n*.
Armbrecht, H. J., 28, 136, 137, 162*n*., 197*n*.
Armstrong, C. M., 45, 67, 162*n*.
Arnold, A., 107, 178*n*.
Assmann, G., 83, 180*n*.
Aston-Jones, G., 55-57, 162*n*., 169*n*., 188*n*.
Azarnoff, D. L., 12, 184*n*.

Bacopoulos, N. G., 151, 162*n*.
Badawy, A. A.-B., 152, 162*n*.
Bajorek, J. G., 38, 180*n*.
Baker, R., 53, 191*n*.
Ban, M., 114, 194*n*.
Banerjee, S. P., 84, 108, 135, 162*n*., 190*n*.
Banks, B. E. C., 69, 162*n*.
Banno, Y., 33, 171*n*.
Barbaccia, M. L., 108, 162*n*., 187*n*.
Barchas, J. D., 93, 94, 185*n*.
Barenholz, Y., 22, 26, 190*n*.
Barker, J. L., 115, 190*n*., 191*n*.
Barnes, D. E., 132, 133, 138, 163*n*., 195*n*.
Barnola, F. V., 75, 195*n*.
Barondes, S. H., 45, 46, 189*n*., 194*n*., 197*n*.
Barr, E., 72, 179*n*.
Barros, S. R., 124, 152, 163*n*.
Barry, H., 145, 163*n*.
Bartfai, T., 112, 173*n*.
Bartus, R. T., 136, 163*n*.
Basile, A., 61, 163*n*.
Baudry, M., 107, 121, 163*n*., 189*n*.
Bauer-Moffett, C., 138, 163*n*.
Baumann, M., 83, 163*n*., 180*n*.
Baumgold, J., 75, 163*n*.
Baxter, C. F., 91, 195*n*.
Beard, J. D., 97, 193*n*.
Beaumont, A., 121, 163*n*.
Beazell, J. M., 95, 163*n*.
Beer, B., 114, 136, 150, 163*n*., 177*n*., 180*n*., 191*n*.
Begleiter, H., 41, 163*n*.
Belieu, R. M., 120, 182*n*.
Bennett, A., 96, 163*n*.
Bennett, J. P., 104, 110, 163*n*.
Benson, D. I., 114, 150, 177*n*., 191*n*.
Berger, T., 50, 53, 163*n*.
Bergmann, M. C., 45, 67, 163*n*.
Berkley, H. A., 97, 186*n*.

Berkowitz, B. A., 123, 163*n*.
Bernstein, J. C., 84, 175*n*.
Bernstein, J. G., 151, 182*n*.
Berridge, M. J., 88, 163*n*.
Berrie, C. P., 113, 163*n*., 164*n*.
Berry, M. S., 41, 164*n*.
Bertoli, E., 26, 179*n*.
Biagioni, T. M., 115–117, 195*n*.
Bianchi, C. P., 70, 194*n*.
Bignami, A. G., 86, 87, 164*n*.
Bills, C. E., 9, 164*n*.
Bing, R. J., 75, 164*n*.
Binstock, L., 45, 67, 162*n*.
Birch, H., 151, 162*n*.
Bird, E. D., 136, 187*n*.
Birdsall, N. J. N., 113, 164*n*.
Bitensky, M. W., 91, 171*n*.
Bize, I., 151, 162*n*.
Bjökqvist, S. E., 152, 164*n*.
Black, A. C., 132, 138, 196*n*.
Black, R. F., 109, 164*n*.
Blaustein, M. P., 70, 72, 76, 164*n*., 184*n*.
Bleck, V. B., 87, 179*n*.
Bloom, F. E., 49, 50, 53, 55, 56, 60, 99,
   117, 162*n*., 163*n*., 167*n*., 169*n*., 176*n*.,
   184*n*., 188*n*., 190*n*.
Blum, K., 111, 124, 152, 164*n*.
Blume, A. J., 71, 121, 164*n*., 179*n*.
Boada, J., 123, 152, 164*n*.
Bobyock, E., 70, 169*n*.
Bogdanski, D. F., 99, 165*n*.
Boggan, W. O., 70, 152, 165*n*., 183*n*.
Bolton, J. R., 22, 165*n*.
Bond, M. L., 52, 169*n*.
Booij, H. L., 14, 165*n*.
Borges, S., 138, 165*n*.
Bosio, A., 122, 180*n*.
Boyarsky, L. L., 119, 182*n*.
Bradford, H. F., 120, 161*n*.
Braestrup, C., 114, 191*n*.
Brand, L., 22, 23, 164*n*.
Breese, G. R., 93, 94, 117, 118, 150, 152,
   153, 165*n*., 170*n*., 180*n*., 195*n*.
Bretschner, M. S., 6, 165*n*.
Brick, J., 56, 57, 186*n*.
Briggs, A. H., 124, 164*n*.
Briley, M. S., 115, 165*n*.
Brink, F., 8, 165*n*.
Britton, R. S., 108, 183*n*.
Brodie, B. B., 99, 165*n*.
Brody, T. M., 82, 161*n*.
Brown, C., 69, 162*n*.
Brown, D. J., 87, 165*n*.

Brown, F. C., 97, 193*n*.
Brown, G. B., 148, 167*n*.
Brown, K. B., 9, 186*n*.
Brown, T. C., 107, 178*n*.
Bruce, D., 120, 161*n*.
Bruno, P., 68, 173*n*.
Bruns, R. F., 105, 191*n*.
Burch, T., 115, 194*n*.
Burgen, A. S. V., 113, 164*n*.
Burgess, G., 69, 162*n*.
Burnstock, G., 69, 162*n*.
Burt, D. R., 107, 165*n*.
Bustos, G., 123, 165*n*.
Butler, K. W., 24, 185*n*.
Buttke, T. M., 32, 33, 165*n*., 175*n*.
Bylund, D. B., 28, 173*n*.

Calhoun, W., 111, 151, 164*n*.
Callison, D. A., 41, 173*n*.
Calne, D. B., 105, 106, 177*n*.
Camejo, G., 76, 195*n*.
Campochiaro, P., 115, 165*n*.
Candy, J. M., 115, 181*n*.
Carbone, E., 36, 193*n*.
Cardeal, J. O., 84, 167*n*.
Cardenas, H. L., 70, 188*n*.
Carey, V. C., 27, 33, 165*n*., 175*n*.
Carino, M. A., 108, 178*n*.
Carlen, P. L., 59, 60, 69, 134, 165*n*.,
   168*n*.
Carlson, I., 138, 178*n*.
Carlsson, A., 151, 165*n*.
Caron, M. G., 96, 107, 179*n*., 183*n*.
Carter, D., 53, 191*n*.
Cassel, M. D., 132, 138, 196*n*.
Catley, D. M., 124, 152, 165*n*., 166*n*.
Catravas, G. N., 93, 94, 175*n*., 187*n*.
Catterall, W. A., 66, 68, 76, 148, 166*n*.,
   193*n*., 196*n*.
Cavalheiro, E. A., 84, 167*n*.
Cederbaum, J. M., 57, 161*n*.
Chadwick, L. E., 9, 167*n*.
Chaffee, R. R., 38, 180*n*.
Chan, A. W. K., 139, 166*n*.
Chandler, J., 72, 179*n*.
Chang, H. H., 67, 120, 166*n*., 182*n*.
Chang, K.-J., 121, 166*n*.
Chang, T., 36, 185*n*.
Chanmugan, P., 32, 175*n*.
Chapin, R. E., 153, 170*n*.
Chau, M., 73, 189*n*.
Chesarek, W. A., 38, 180*n*.
Chey, W. Y., 95, 180*n*.

Chignell, C. F., 22, 166n.
Childers, S. R., 121, 166n.
Chin, J. H., 8, *19*, 24, 26, 28, 30, 76, 147, 166n., 171n.
Chu, N.-S., 148, 166n.
Chweh, A. Y., 73, 166n.
Claret, M., 69, 162n.
Clay, G. A., 117, 177n.
Cocks, T. M., 69, 162n.
Coffman, R., 84, 188n.
Cohen, E. N., 8, 27, 181n.
Cohen, H. B., 151, 162n.
Cohen, P. J., 7, 166n.
Colangelo, W., 137, 166n.
Cole, W. H., 9, 166n.
Colfer, H. F., 86, 166n.
Collier, H. O. J., 95, 152, 166n.
Collins, H. G., 130, 195n.
Collins, J. G., 47, 166n.
Connor, J. D., 111, 191n.
Cooke, R., 28, 176n.
Cooke, W. J., 70, 167n.
Cooper, B. R., 118, 150, 167n.
Cooper, J. R., 99, 167n.
Corbin, D. R., 99, 192n.
Corne, S. J., 111, 167n.
Corrigall, W. A., 59, 165n., 168n.
Costa, E., 114, 115, 172n., 194n.
Costentin, J., 107, 189n.
Côté, L., 136, 140, 167n.
Cotecchia, S., 136, 167n.
Coupet, J., 114, 180n., 191n.
Cowan, C. M., 84, 167n.
Cox, G., 130, 167n.
Coyle, J. T., 106, 115, 121, 165n., 183n., 189n.
Cragg, B. G., 132, 186n.
Creager, R., 120, 163n.
Creech, D. M., 99, 192n.
Creese, I., 105–107, 165n., 167n., 189n.
Creveling, C. R., 148, 167n.
Crews, F. T., 30, 167n.
Cricchett, D. J., 114, 180n.
Cross, A. J., 115, 195n.
Cuatrecasas, P., 121, 166n.
Cullen, M. H., 124, 176n.
Curatola, G., 26, 179n.

Dalton, T. K., 91, 93, 100, 108, 110, 111, 113, 114, 116, 127, 174n., 175n.
Daly, J. W., 67, 97, 105, 107, 148, 161n., 167n., 168n., 190n., 191n.
Daniels, C. K., 31, 167n.

Darden, J. H., 110, 167n.
Davidoff, R. A., 57, 167n.
Davis, D. L., 84, 100, 188n.
Davis, J. N., 107, 190n.
Davis, K. L., 136, 167n.
Davis, W. C., 116, 117, 154, 167n., 194n.
De Blasi, A., 136, 167n.
de Foresta, B., 38, 195n.
Deady, J. E., 32, 177n.
Dean, R. L., 136, 163n.
DeHaven, R. N., 100, 183n.
Demuth, R. M., 132, 196n.
Dethier, V. G., 9, 167n.
Deutsch, J. A., 150, 167n.
DeWeer, P., 81, 86, 167n.
Dewey, S. L., 138, 167n., 196n.
Dexter, J. D., 28, 173n.
Diamond, I., 70, 167n.
Diaz, J., 139, 168n.
Dibner, M. D., 91, 187n.
Dickens, B. F., 32, 33, 168n., 175n.
Dietrich, R. A., 51, 118, 179n., 181n.
Dijkshoorn, W., 14, 165n.
Dinh, T. K. H., 27, 147, 168n.
Dinovo, E. C., 34, 167n., 172n.
Dipple, I., 97, 171n.
Dismukes, R. K., 97, 168n.
Dodson, R. A., 94, 168n.
Dole, V. P., 152, 168n.
Dombeck, K. M., 27, 34, 168n., 175n.
Dreyfus, L. R., 47, 177n.
Dreyfus, P. M., 130, 168n.
Dripps, R. D., 7, 166n.
Drust, D., 111, 191n.
Duka, T. H., 125, 186n., 189n.
Dunbar, P. G., 31, 32, 168n., 196n.
Dunwiddie, T., 50–52, 61, 163n., 179n., 191n.
Durand, D., 59, 60, 134, 165n.
Dvorkin, B., 136, 181n.
Dymsza, H. A., 153, 168n.

Eccles, J. C., 50, 51, 60, 162n., 168n.
Ector, A. C., 70, 164n.
Edidin, M., 7, 168n.
Edwards, B. A. V., 62, 189n.
Edwards, R. M., 98, 186n.
Ehlert, F. J., 112, 113, 168n.
Ehrenberg, L., 14, 171n.
Eidelberg, E., 52, 55, 169n.
Eliasson, S. G., 93, 94, 169n.
Elston, S. F. A., 124, 164n.
Endrenyi, L., 82, 176n.

Engel, J., 31, 109, 118, 150, 151, 162*n.*, 165*n.*, 169*n.*, 179*n.*
Englebert, V. E., 62, 189*n.*
Enna, S. J., 114, 136, 169*n.*, 180*n.*, 187*n.*
Erickson, C. K., 71, 74, 113, 151, 169*n.*, 170*n.*, 181*n.*
Escueta, A. V., 67, 169*n.*
Esgate, J. A., 97, 171*n.*
Essex, H. E., 86, 166*n.*
Eubanks, J. D., 111, 152, 164*n.*
Evans, M., 152, 162*n.*
Ewing, J. E., 152, 169*n.*

Faber, D. S., 45, 50, 163*n.*, 169*n.*
Fahn, S., 51, *52*, 171*n.*
Fairhurst, A. S., 113, 168*n.*
Farrar, R. P., 72, 179*n.*
Farrell, W. J., 32, 182*n.*
Fauvel, J. M., 75, 164*n.*
Feinhandler, D. A., 123, 162*n.*
Feller, D., 28, 173*n.*
Fenner, D., 28, 73, 173*n.*
Ferguson, J., 8, 9, 169*n.*
Feria, M., 123, 152, 164*n.*
Ferko, A. P., 70, 100, 169*n.*, 183*n.*
Fernández, T., 139, 189*n.*
Ferris, R. M., 118, 167*n.*
Festoff, B. W., 87, 169*n.*
Fibiger, H. C., 106, 184*n.*
Field, J. B., 91, 181*n.*
Fields, J. Z., 113, 192*n.*
Finck, A. D., 123, 163*n.*
Finer, E. G., 39, 186*n.*
Finn, D. A., 12, 161*n.*
Fischer, K. C., 62, 189*n.*
Fishman, J., 152, 168*n.*
Fisk, R. A., 61, 189*n.*
Fiske, J. C., 47, 177*n.*
Flanagan, R. J., 124, 176*n.*
Fleming, E. W., 142, 169*n.*, 193*n.*
Fleshler, B., 96, 163*n.*
Fontaine, O., 76, 169*n.*
Fontaine, R. N., 6, 169*n.*
Foote, S. L., 56, 162*n.*, 169*n.*
Formby, B., 87, 169*n.*
Forney, E., 47, 52, 169*n.*, 177*n.*
Forney, R. B., 151, 196*n.*
Fox, H. M., 153, 194*n.*
Franks, N. P., 12, 15, 169*n.*
Freed, W. J., 119, 120, 169*n.*, 182*n.*
Freedman, R., 50, 191*n.*
Freeman, A. R., 67, 185*n.*
Freeman, C. P., 124, 152, 196*n.*

Freeman, J. A., 134, 170*n.*
French, E. D., 50, 55, 58, 163*n.*, 190*n.*
French, S. W., 92, 170*n.*
Freund, G., 38, 116, 130, 135, 136, 140, 144, 148-150, 170*n.*, 178*n.*
Fridovich, I., 141, 170*n.*
Fried, R., 141, 179*n.*
Friedman, H. J., 28, 98, 176*n.*, 179*n.*
Friedman, M. B., 71, 170*n.*
Frith, C. D., 124, 165*n.*
Fry, J. P., 125, 197*n.*
Frye, G. D., 93, 94, 116, 118, 150, 152, 153, 165*n.*, 170*n.*, 180*n.*, 195*n.*
Funderburk, F. R., 150, 170*n.*
Futterman, S., 124, 152, 164*n.*
Fuxe, K., 106, 171*n.*

Gailis, L., 27, 147, 168*n.*
Gale, K., 106, 183*n.*
Gallaher, E. J., 30, 185*n.*
Galley, J., 38, 195*n.*
Garrett, K. M., 72, 73, 171*n.*
Gatenbeck, S., 14, 171*n.*
Gerald, M. C., 110, 187*n.*
Gerhardt, M. J., 30, 31, 191*n.*
Gershon, S., 90, 188*n.*
Gessner, P. K., 146, 148, 152, 171*n.*
Ghetti, B., 136, 180*n.*
Ghez, C., 51, *52*, 171*n.*
Gianutsos, G., 128, 171*n.*
Gilbert, D. L., 148, 180*n.*
Gilbert, P. E., 121, 171*n.*
Gillies, R., 118, 184*n.*
Gillin, J. C., 125, 174*n.*
Gohlke, J. R., 22, 23, 165*n.*
Gold, B. I., 93, 195*n.*
Goldberg, A. L., 70, 167*n.*
Goldberg, M., 73, 189*n.*
Goldfrank, L., 152, 168*n.*
Goldstein, A., 124, 171*n.*
Goldstein, D. B., 11, *19*, 24-26, 28, 30, 31, 35, 38, 74, 82, 84, 97, 112, 118, 127, 128, 147, 150, 152, 166*n.*, 167*n.*, 171*n.*, 180*n.*-182*n.*, 185*n.*
Gomez, R. F., 33, 173*n.*
Goodman, D. B. P., 67, 88, 169*n.*, 187*n.*
Gordon, E. R., 74, 178*n.*
Gordon, L. M., 97, 171*n.*
Gorman, R. E., 91, 171*n.*
Goto, M., 33, 171*n.*
Gottesfeld, Z., 136, 192*n.*
Gottlieb, R., 1, 8, 182*n.*
Graham, D. J., 113, 169*n.*

Graham-Smith, D. G., 111, 171*n*.
Gramsch, C. H., 125, 186*n*.
Grant, K. A., 11, 172*n*.
Greenberg, D. A., 106, 185*n*.
Greenblatt, D. J., 150, 196*n*.
Greenblatt, E. N., 114, 180*n*.
Greene, H. L., 91, 172*n*.
Greengard, P., 87, 88, *89*, 148, 172*n*., 187*n*.
Greenlee, D., 114, 185*n*.
Grevel, J., 121, 172*n*.
Grieve, S. J., 30, 31, 38, 172*n*., 180*n*.
Griffiths, P. J., 112, 172*n*.
Gripenberg, J., 71, 72, 172*n*.
Grisola, S., 84, 172*n*.
Gross, M. M., 145, 172*n*.
Grubbs, R. D., 120, 182*n*.
Gruber, B., 34, 168*n*., 172*n*.
Grundfest, H., 67, 185*n*.
Gruol, D. L., 62, 172*n*.
Grupp, L. A., 49, 172*n*.
Guerrero-Figuero, R., 150, 172*n*.
Guerri, C., 84, 172*n*.
Guidotti, A., 114, 115, 117, 172*n*., 181*n*., 194*n*.
Guivernau, M., 151, 183*n*.
Gurevich, N., 60, 165*n*.
Gustafsson, B., 60, 172*n*.
Guttman, R., 14, 172*n*.

Haarmann, I., 125, 186*n*.
Hadházy, P., 113, 172*n*.
Hall, H., 106, 171*n*.
Hallett, M., 36, 193*n*.
Halprin, K. M., 91, 197*n*.
Halsey, J. M., 8, 12, 146, 172*n*.
Hamberger, A., 141, 175*n*.
Hamblin, M., 105, 167*n*.
Hamilton, M. G., 124, 164*n*.
Hammond, M. D., 95, 166*n*.
Handler, P., 79, 196*n*.
Hanski, E., 97, 172*n*.
Harman, D., 140, 173*n*.
Harmony, R., 86, 173*n*.
Harper, A. A., 45, 173*n*.
Harris, D. P., 53, 55, 190*n*.
Harris, R. A., 6, 26, 27, 68–74, 76, 118, 127, 169*n*., 173*n*., 174*n*., 181*n*., 191*n*., 197*n*.
Harvey, D. J., 31, 32, 168*n*., 196*n*.
Hastings, A. G., 124, 176*n*.
Hasty, J., 145, 172*n*.
Haugaard, N., 70, 194*n*.

Havicek, V., 122, 178*n*.
Hawley, R. J., 116, 194*n*.
Hayashida, K., 151, 191*n*.
Hazum, E., 121, 166*n*.
Heilbronn, E., 112, 173*n*.
Heinonen, E., 72, 172*n*.
Hemmingsen, R., 124, 127, 153, 173*n*.
Hemminki, K., 70, 76, 173*n*.
Hendler, R. W., 4, 173*n*.
Herbert, M., 124, 176*n*.
Herman, M. M., 61, 189*n*.
Herman, R. H., 91, 172*n*.
Herrera, E., 139, 182*n*.
Herrero, A. A., 33, 173*n*.
Herz, A., 121, 123, 125, 185*n*., 186*n*., 189*n*., 197*n*.
Hess, S., 122, 152, 179*n*.
Hillbom, M. E., 118, 150
Hiller, J. M., 122, 173*n*.
Hiltunen, K., 95, 186*n*.
Himwich, H. E., 41, 173*n*.
Hirsch, J. D., 111, 117, 174*n*., 177*n*.
Hirst, M., 124, 164*n*.
Hitzemann, B. A., 71, 173*n*.
Hitzemann, R. J., 71, 173*n*.
Ho, O. L., 120, 184*n*.
Hobbs, A. S., 81, 174*n*.
Hodges, C. A., 138, 196*n*.
Hodgkin, A. L., *43*, 66, 174*n*.
Hoek, J. B., 29, 186*n*.
Hoffer, B., 50–53, 61, 163*n*., 179*n*., 191*n*.
Hoffman, B. B., 105–107, 174*n*.
Hoffman, E. M., 32, 175*n*.
Hoffman, P. L., 90, 91, 97, 108, 109, 122–124, 152, 164*n*., 174*n*., 177*n*., 192*n*.
Hole, K., 124, 152, 176*n*.
Hollt, V., 125, 186*n*.
Hong, J. H., 125, 174*n*.
Hood, W. F., 70–72, 173*n*., 174*n*.
Hoover, R. L., 26, 177*n*.
Horita, A., 108, 178*n*.
Horowitz, S. G., 136, 181*n*.
Hossak, J. A., 39, 174*n*., 193*n*.
Hotson, J. R., 60, 174*n*.
Houck, J. C., 124, 177*n*.
Houslay, M. D., 90, 97, 171*n*., 184*n*.
Hoyler, E., 107, 190*n*.
Hruska, R. E., 108, 174*n*.
Huang, P., 24, 185*n*.
Huang, S. M., 124, 177*n*.
Hughes, J., 31, 121, 125, 163*n*., 178*n*., 196*n*.

Hulme, E. C., 113, 164*n*.
Hungund, B. L., 35, 171*n*.
Hunt, W. A., vii, 4, 9, 10, 37, 68, 76, 85, 91, 93, 94, 97, 100, 108, 110, 111, 113, 114, 116, 118, 119, 123, 125, 127, 148, 150, 153, 167*n*., 174*n*., 175*n*., 181*n*.-183*n*., 187*n*., 196*n*.
Hunter, B. E., 51, 131-134, 161*n*., 195*n*.
Hunter, J., 124, 152, 196*n*.
Hurter, P. B., 94, 195*n*.
Huxley, A. F., *43*, 66, 174*n*.
Hwang, D. H., 32, 175*n*.
Hyvarinen, J., 47, 175*n*.

Iber, F. L., 148, 189*n*.
Ikeda, Y., 55, 175*n*.
Ingram, L. O., 27, 32-34, 165*n*., 168*n*., 174*n*.
Iniquez, E. S., 143, 196*n*.
Innes, R. B., 105, 121, 191*n*.
Israel, M. A., 84, 88, 91, 94, 97, 175*n*., 178*n*.
Israel, Y., 69, 82-84, 171*n*., 175*n*.
Ito, M., 51, 168*n*.
Ivy, A. C., 95, 163*n*.

Jacobs, B. L., 111, 175*n*.
Jacobson, S., 138, 161*n*.
Jacobyansky, A., 92, 94, 190*n*., 191*n*.
Jaffe, L. S., 97, 186*n*.
Jakobs, K. H., 107, 175*n*.
Jansson, S.-E. 72, 172*n*.
Jarlstedt, J., 141, 175*n*.
Järnefelt, J., 82, 176*n*.
Jeffcoate, W. J., 124, 152, 176*n*.
Jeffreys, B., 124, 152, 176*n*.
Jenden, D. J., 100, 176*n*.
Jenkinson, G. H., 69, 162*n*.
John, G. R., 30-32, 172*n*., 176*n*., 180*n*.
Johnson, D. A., 28, 30, 176*n*.
Johnson, W. E., 94, 168*n*.
Jones, D. G., 137, 166*n*.
Jones, J. G., 124, 152, 165*n*., 166*n*.
Jones, P. A., 30, 32, 172*n*., 176*n*., 180*n*.
Jope, R. S., 100, 176*n*.
Jordan, C., 124, 165*n*.
Jørgensen, H. A., 124, 152, 176*n*.
Judson, B. A., 124, 171*n*.
Juhl, U., 138, 178*n*.

Kaback, R., 71, 179*n*.
Kairaluoma, M., 95, 176*n*., 186*n*.
Kakihana, R., 24, 181*n*.

Kakita, K., 92, 178*n*.
Kalant, H., 9, 11, 68, 69, 75, 82-85, 144, 146, 149, 152, 154, 175*n*.-177*n*., 179*n*., 181*n*., 187*n*., 190*n*.
Kamal, L., 114, 162*n*.
Kamaya, H., 39, 176*n*.
Kameyama, Y., 33, 171*n*.
Kandel, E. R., 43, 176*n*.
Kaneshina, S., 39, 176*n*.
Kao, C. Y., 67, 176*n*.
Karnovsky, M., 26, 177*n*.
Karobath, M., 114, 117, 118, 176*n*., 186*n*., 192*n*.
Karoum, F., 110, 123, 176*n*.
Karppanen, H., 95, 96, 176*n*., 186*n*.
Katz, A. M., 75, 192*n*.
Keane, B., 85, 177*n*.
Kebabian, J. W., 105, 106, 177*n*.
Keegan, R., 32, 177*n*.
Kelter, A., 52, 169*n*.
Kenig, J. J., 27, 181*n*.
Khan, M. M., 84, 188*n*.
Khanna, J. H., 75, 108, 144, 152, 162*n*., 168*n*., 177*n*., 181*n*.
Khawaja, J. A., 141, 177*n*.
Kies, C., 153, 194*n*.
Kiessling, L. A., 93, 169*n*.
Kiianmaa, K., 124, 152, 177*n*.
Kilts, C. D., 153, 170*n*.
Kim, Y., 151, 191*n*.
Kimball, C. D., 124, 152, 177*n*.
Kimberg, D. V., 95, 177*n*.
Kimizuka, H., 70, 76, 177*n*.
Kimura, H., 91, 175*n*.
Klausner, R. D., 26, 177*n*.
Kleber, G., 125, 186*n*.
Klee, M. W., 45, 50, 163*n*., 169*n*.
Kleinfield, A. M., 26, 177*n*.
Klemm, W. R., 41, 47, 49, 52, 169*n*., 177*n*., 183*n*.
Klepner, C. A., 114, 150, 177*n*., 180*n*., 191*n*.
Klingenstein, J., 74, 178*n*.
Knox, W., 84, 177*n*.
Koblin, D. D., 32, 177*n*.
Kochman, R. L., 117, 177*n*.
Koda, L. Y., 55, 188*n*.
Koepke, K. M., 152, 195*n*.
Koester, J., 41, 42, 178*n*.
Köhler, C., 106, 171*n*.
Koketsu, K., 70, 177*n*.
Kokka, A. N., 113, 168*n*.
Kolde, T., 128, 178*n*.

Koppenhofer, E., 67, 178n.
Kornguth, S. E., 138, 178n.
Korsten, M. A., 74, 178n.
Kosterlitz, H. W., 121, 125, 178n.
Kosunen, A. L., 11, 195n.
Kraemer, S., 91, 172n.
Krawitt, E. L., 75, 178n.
Kristof, V., 83, 180n.
Krnjevic, K., 112, 178n.
Kubanis, P., 132, 136, 178n., 195n.
Kuehnlie, J., 151, 182n.
Kugelmann, K., 108, 185n.
Kuhar, M. J., 100, 106, 183n.
Kuhn, C. M., 139, 191n.
Kujtan, P., 59, 168n.
Kulig, B. M., 97, 193n.
Kuriyama, K., 84, 88, 91–94, 98, 109,
    141, 175n., 178n.
Kuschinsky, K., 91, 189n.
Kutchai, H., 27, 197n.
Kwant, W. O., 15, 189n.

LaBella, F. S., 122, 178n.
LaBelle, J., 24, 185n.
Laakso, M., 47, 175n.
Laduron, P. M., 106, 179n.
Lahdenranta, U., 124, 152, 184n.
Lai, H., 108, 109, 178n.
Lake, N., 57, 58, 178n.
Lal, H., 128, 171n.
Lampe, R. A., 120, 182n.
Lands, A. M., 107, 178n.
Langer, S. Z., 106, 114, 115, 162n.,
    165n., 179n.
Larmi, T., 95, 176n., 186n.
Laufer, I., 82, 175n.
Laverty, R., 26, 180n.
Law, P. Y., 127, 180n.
Lê, A. D., 144, 177n.
LeBlanc, A. E., 9, 11, 69, 84, 144, 175n.,
    177n., 179n.
LeBlanc, P., 32, 175n.
Lebovitz, R. M., 111, 185n.
Ledig, M., 141, 179n.
Lee, K., 51, 132, 179n.
Lee, N. M., 28, 98, 176n., 179n.
Lee, T., 106, 184n.
Leeb-Lundberg, F. A., 115, 117, 179n.
Leff, S., 105, 167n.
Lefkowitz, R. J., 96, 105–107, 174n.,
    178n., 183n., 196n.
Lehane, J. R., 124, 152, 165n., 166n.
Lehotay, D. C., 91, 194n.

Leiman, A. L., 61, 189n.
Leinonen, L., 47, 175n.
Lenaz, G., 26, 179n.
Leonard, B. E., 85, 177n.
Leslie, S. W., 71–73, 166n., 170n., 179n.
Levental, M., 82, 84, 179n.
Lever, J. M., 8, 179n.
Levey, G. S., 91, 93, 194n.
Levine, A. S., 133, 152, 179n.
Levine, J., 151, 162n.
Levine, V., 91, 197n.
Levitzki, A., 97, 172n.
Lewin, E., 87, 179n.
Lewis, E., 145, 172n.
Lewis, P. D., 138, 165n.
Ley, K. D., 32, 175n.
Leysen, J. E., 106, 179n.
Lichtschtein, H., 71, 179n.
Lieb, W. R., 12, 15, 169n.
Lieber, C. S., 74, 178n.
Liljequist, S., 31, 109, 118, 150, 162n.,
    169n., 179n.
Limbard, L. E., 96, 179n.
Lind, M. D., 132, 196n.
Lindenmayer, G. E., 81, 189n.
Lindholm, D. B., 141, 177n.
Lindsay, R., 84, 179n.
Ling, C. M., 67, 179n.
Link, E., 12, 182n.
Linkola, J., 67, 195n.
Linnoila, M., 116, 180n.
Lipicky, R. J., 148, 180n.
Lippa, A. S., 114, 136, 150, 163n., 177n.,
    180n.
Littleton, J. M., 30–32, 38, 112, 172n.,
    176n., 180n.
Llinas, R., 55, 180n.
Lloyd, S., 28, 173n.
Lo, G. F., 53–55, 190n.
Logan, B. J., 26, 180n.
Loh, H. H., 28, 98, 127, 176n., 179n., 180n.
Lomax, P., 38, 180n.
Lorber, S. H., 95, 180n.
Louis, J.-C., 141, 179n.
Lucchi, L., 122, 180n.
Luduena, F. P., 107, 178n.
Lundberg, D. B. A., 93, 94, 165n., 180n.
Lust, W. D., 70, 180n.
Luthin, G. R., 90, 180n.
Lynch, G., 51, 121, 163n., 179n.
Lyon, R. C., 24, 25, 28, 31, 35, 38, 97,
    128, 171n., 180n.

MacDonald, A. G., 45, 173*n*.
Mackensie, A. I., 124, 152, 180*n*.
Maggi, A., 136, 180*n*.
Magour, S., 83, 180*n*.
Magruder, C., 120, 182*n*.
Mahon, M. A., 68, 176*n*.
Mailman, R. B., 93, 94, 116, 152, 153,
  165*n*., 170*n*., 180*n*., 195*n*.
Majchrowicz, E., 11, 30, 76, 91, 97, 99,
  100, 110, 113, 114, 123, 125, 150, 153,
  167*n*., 174*n*.-176*n*., 181*n*., 185*n*.
Major, F. L., 116, 194*n*.
Majumdar, S. K., 140, 181*n*.
Makman, M. H., 136, 181*n*.
Malcolm, R. D., 12, 27, 147, 161*n*.,
  162*n*., 181*n*.
Mallari, C. G., 47, 177*n*.
Mancillas-Trevino, J., 49, 184*n*.
Mandel, P., 84, 99, 118, 141, 150, 179*n*.,
  192*n*.
Mandio, D., 90, 188*n*.
Manis, P. B., 134, 161*n*.
Mao, J. C., 75, 164*n*.
Marchmont, R. J., 97, 171*n*.
Marangos, P. J., 116, 180*n*.
Marklund, S. L., 141, 181*n*.
Marquis, J. K., 37, 108, 181*n*., 185*n*.
Marquis, W. J., 82, 161*n*.
Marsh, D., *18*, 22, 181*n*.
Martin, C. E., 33, 184*n*.
Martin, I. L., 115, 181*n*.
Martin, W. R., 121, 171*n*.
Martín del Río, R., 139, 182*n*.
Martes, M. P., 107, 189*n*.
Martz, A., 118, 150, 181*n*.
Martz, R., 151, 196*n*.
Marwaha, J., 53, 191*n*.
Mashiter, G. D., 91, 181*n*.
Mashiter, K., 91, 181*n*.
Massarelli, R., 100, 181*n*.
Massotti, M., 114, 181*n*.
Mastrangelo, C. J., 27, 146, 181*n*.
Matchett, J. A., 151, 181*n*.
Matsumoto, T., 76, 169*n*.
Matsushita, H., 128, 178*n*.
Mattila, M. J., 124, 152, 181*n*.
Mattisson, K., 124, 152, 191*n*.
Mattox, S. M., 32, 184*n*.
Maunter, H. G., 37, 181*n*.
Mayer, J. M., 75, 181*n*.
Mayfield, M. A., 47, 177*n*.
Mazzanti, L., 26, 179*n*.
McAuliff, J. P., 107, 178*n*.

McCarty, D., 152, 169*n*.
McClearn, G. E., 24, 50, 181*n*., 191*n*.
McComb, J. A., 11, 24, *25*, 180*n*.-182*n*.
McConnell, H. M., 19, 182*n*.
McCreery, M. J., 9, 10, 37, 153, 182*n*.
McFarland, B. G., 19, 182*n*.
McFaul, J. A., 120, 182*n*.
McGivern, R. F., 152, 168*n*.
McNeal, E. T., 148, 167*n*.
McPherson, K. A., 31, 32, 168*n*., 196*n*.
Mead, J. F., 140, 182*n*.
Medina, M. A., 70, 188*n*.
Meech, R. W., 60, 69, 182*n*.
Meeks, R., 30, 167*n*.
Meeuws, M. M., 113, 186*n*.
Mehlman, M. A., 153, 194*n*.
Melchior, C., 91, 187*n*.
Membrey, J. H., 12, 182*n*.
Memo, M., 136, 182*n*.
Mena, M. A., 139, 182*n*.
Mendelson, J. H., 151, 182*n*.
Mennini, T., 136, 167*n*.
Merrill, M., 150, 172*n*.
Merritt, J., 151, 164*n*.
Messiha, F. S., 151, 182*n*.
Meyer, H. H., 1, 8, 182*n*.
Meyer, J. S., 70, 165*n*.
Meyer, K. H., 8, 182*n*.
Miceli, J. N., 32, 182*n*.
Michaelis, E. K., 67, 72-74, 119, 120,
  166*n*., 169*n*., 182*n*., 183*n*.
Michaelis, M. L., 72, 119, 120, 182*n*., 183*n*.
Middaugh, L. D., 70, 152, 165*n*., 183*n*.
Mikeska, J. A., 47, 52, 177*n*., 183*n*.
Miller, K. W., 8, 9, 36, 39, 179*n*., 183*n*.,
  185*n*., 186*n*.
Miller, T., 114, 185*n*.
Minnenan, K. P., 97, 105-107, 183*n*.,
  190*n*.
Minocherhomjee, A. M., 87, 183*n*.
Misawa, S., 83, 197*n*.
Mitchell, M., 28, 173*n*.
Molinoff, P. B., 88, 90, 91, 97, 105-108,
  183*n*., 187*n*., 190*n*.
Mons, W., 68, 176*n*.
Moore, J. M., 45, 67
Moore, J. W., 67, 183*n*., 184*n*.
Morley, J. E., 122, 152, 179*n*.
Moroder, L., 125, 197*n*.
M'Paria, J. R., 141, 179*n*.
Mrak, R. E., 29, 75, 183*n*.
Mueller, R. A., 93, 94, 116, 152, 153,
  165*n*., 170*n*., 180*n*., 195*n*.

Mukherjee, C., 96, 107, 179n., 183n.
Muller, P., 108, 110, 111, 183n.
Mullin, M. J., 68, 100, 183n.
Mullins, L. J., 8, 183n.
Mulvaney, M. J., 119, 183n.
Muñoz, C., 151, 183n.
Munoz-Marcus, M., 113, 192n.
Munsat, T. L., 108, 185n.
Muramatsu, M., 92, 109, 178n.
Murray, S., 142, 193n.
Murrin, L. C., 100, 106, 121, 183n.
Mustala, O. O., 12, 184n.
Myers, S. L., 73, 74, 182n.
Myers, V., 114, 191n.

Nachshen, D. A., 72, 184n.
Nagy, J. I., 106, 184n.
Nakagama, K., 92, 178n.
Nandini-Kishore, S. G., 32, 184n.
Narahashi, T., 67, 184n.
Narod, M. E., 92, 170n.
Nartres, M. P., 107
Nathanson, J. A., 87, 88, 90, 184n.
Needham, L., 90, 184n.
Nestoros, J. N., 58, 60, 184n.
Newlin, S. A., 49, 184n.
Ngai, S. H., 123, 163n.
Nicholson, C., 134, 170n.
Nicholson, G. L., 5, 190n.
Nicoll, R. A., 60, 71, 161n., 168n., 184n.
Niemegeers, C. J. E., 106, 179n.
Niittylä, J., 141, 177n.
Nikander, P., 67, 184n., 195n.
Noble, E. P., 34, 84, 99, 100, 118, 141,
  142, 146, 150, 151, 162n., 168n., 169n.,
  172n., 181n., 184n., 192n., 193n.
Nordberg, A., 113, 135, 184n.
Nordyke, E., 100, 188n.
Nozawa, Y., 33, 171n.
Nuotto, E., 124, 152, 181n., 184n.

Oakes, S. G., 62, 184n.
Oborn, C. J., 70, 164n.
Ohnishi, T., 29, 196n.
Oliver, M., 120, 163n.
Olney, J. W., 120, 184n.
Olsen, R. W., 114, 115, 179n., 184n.,
  185n., 194n.
Ondrusek, M. G., 116, 170n.
Oreland, L., 141, 181n.
Orenberg, E. K., 93, 185n.
Ortiz, A., 112, 172n.
Oshima, T., 60, 168n.

Overstreet, D. H., 127, 185n.
Overton, E., 8, 185n.
Ozeki, M., 67, 185n.

Palladini, G., 86, 87, 164n.
Palmer, D. S., 92, 170n.
Palmer, M., 52, 53, 191n.
Palva, E. A., 124, 152, 184n.
Pang, K., 36, 185n.
Pant, H. C., 99, 185n.
Parker, E. S., 132, 151, 162n., 196n.
Parsons, L. M., 30, 166n., 185n.
Pasby, T. L., 22, 185n.
Passaneau, J. V., 101, 194n.
Pastuszko, A., 26, 179n.
Paterson, S. J., 24, 185n.
Pathman, D. E., 11, 92, 94, 190n., 191n.,
  193n.
Paton, W. D. M., 31, 196n.
Patton, W., 8, 179n.
Paul, S. N., 115, 190n.
Paula-Barbosa, M. M., 133, 140, 193n.
Peake, B. M., 26, 180n.
Peck, E. J., 119, 185n.
Pelham, R. W., 108, 113, 135, 185n.
Pennington, W., 84, 100, 188n.
Pentley, R. J., 133, 185n.
Pentreath, V. W., 41, 164n.
Perdahl, E., 141, 181n.
Perlanski, E., 49, 172n.
Peroutka, S. J., 106, 110, 111, 185n.
Perrin, R. G., 84, 177n.
Pert, C. B., 121, 185n.
Pesce, A. J., 22, 185n.
Pfeiffer, A. A., 121, 123, 185n., 186n.
Phillips, M. C., 39, 186n.
Phillips, P. E., 123, 162n.
Phillips, S. C., 132, 186n.
Phillis, J. W., 57, 178n.
Piantadosi, C., 11, 181n.
Pickering, R. W., 111, 167n.
Pincus, J. H., 87, 148, 186n., 187n.
Pinsky, C., 122, 178n.
Placheta, P., 114, 186n.
Platz, A., 41, 163n.
Pohorecky, L. A., 3, 27, 56, 57, 97, 110,
  118, 128, 147, 186n.
Polak, R. L., 113, 186n.
Polnaszek, C. F., 22, 189n.
Ponnappa, B. C., 29, 74, 186n.
Posternak, J. M., 8, 165n.
Pozos, R. S., 62, 184n.
Pradhan, S. N., 136, 186n.

Prasad, C., 98, 186n.
Prince, D. A., 60, 174n.
Pringle, M. J., 9, 186n.
Protais, P., 107, 189n.
Pryer, W. A., 36, 186n.
Przewlocki, R., 125, 186n.
Puurunen, J., 95, 96, 101, 176n., 186n.

Queen, G., 122, 178n.

Rabin, R. A., 88, 90, 91, 108, 113, 187n.
Rackham, A., 123, 197n.
Räinä, N. C. R., 143, 190n.
Ramey, C. W., 92, 170n.
Randall, C. L., 137, 161n.
Rang, H. P., 9, 187n.
Rangaraj, N., 83–85, 176n., 187n.
Rasmussen, H., 76, 88, 169n., 187n.
Rauscher, G. E., 141, 178n.
Rawat, A. K., 141, 187n.
Rawson, M. D., 87, 187n.
Read, E., 152, 182n.
Rech, R. H., 82, 161n.
Redos, J. D., 93, 94, 175n., 187n.
Reggiani, A., 108, 116, 123, 162n., 187n.
Reid, P. E., 92, 170n.
Reisine, T., 128, 136, 187n.
Renson, J., 93, 185n.
Rhee, V., 120, 184n.
Rhodes, A. A., 124, 165n.
Rice, K. C., 115, 190n.
Richard, J. W., 123, 197n.
Riffee, W. H., 110, 187n.
Riley, E. P., 137, 161n.
Riley, J. N., 130, 132, 187n., 195n.
Rimon, G., 97, 172n.
Ritchie, J. M., 148, 187n.
Ritzmann, R. F., 28, 109, 137, 188n., 191n.
Rizek, A. E., 27, 147, 186n.
Roach, M. K., 84, 100, 188n.
Roberts, E., 114, 196n.
Roberts, P. J., 119, 188n., 190n.
Robertson, D. E., 29, 188n.
Robinson, G. A., 93, 189n.
Robinson, J. D., 70, 167n., 180n.
Roby, D. M., 151, 161n.
Rodnight, R., 88, 196n.
Rodreguez, G. R., 124, 152, 163n.
Roeske, W. R., 112, 113, 168n.
Rogers, J., 53–55, 117, 176n., 188n.
Roine, R., 47, 175n.
Roppolo, J. R., 47, 166n.

Rose, A. H., 39, 174n.
Rosén, C.-G., 22, 185n.
Rosenberg, A., 34, 184n.
Rosenberger, L. B., 113, 168n.
Rosenfeld, M., 136, 181n.
Rosett, H. L., 137, 188n.
Ross, D. H., 70–73, 171n., 188n.
Rossi, M., 151, 182n.
Roth, R. H., 99, 123, 165n.
Roth, S., 7, 14, 15, 23, 188n., 189n.
Rothstein, A., 70, 188n.
Rothstein, E., 148, 188n.
Rotrosen, J., 90, 188n.
Rottenberg, H., 29, 186n., 188n., 196n.
Roufogalis, B. D., 87, 183n.
Rowe, E. S., 15, 188n.
Roy, S., 120, 182n.
Rubia, F. J., 60, 168n.
Rubin, E., 29, 75, 186n., 188n., 192n., 196n.
Rubin, R. P., 70, 188n.
Ruczkal-Pietrzak, E., 32, 177n.
Rutledge, J. J., 138, 178n.
Rye, D., 150, 172n.

Sadée, W., 121, 172n.
Salazar, I., 82, 84, 175n.
Salinas, M., 139, 182n., 189n.
Salvaterra, P., 114, 196n.
Samorajski, T., 82, 83, 136, 137, 192n.
Sampliner, R., 148, 189n.
Samson, H. H., 11, 139, 168n., 172n.
Sano, M. C., 114, 150, 177n., 180n.
Sanz, E., 123, 152, 164n.
Sasa, M., 55, 175n.
Sauerheber, R. D., 97, 171n.
Sauks, T., 15, 73, 189n.
Saur, W., 107, 175n.
Sawyer, W. H., 22, 193n.
Sax, L., 73, 189n.
Scarpellini, J. D., 93, 169n.
Schaffer, J. M., 9, 194n.
Schanberg, S. M., 139, 191n.
Schlapfer, W. T., 45, 46, 189n., 194n., 197n.
Schmidt, D. E., 93, 189n.
Schmidt, H., 67, 178n.
Schmidt, J., 71, 173n.
Schmidt, M., 91, 191n.
Schmidt, M. J., 93, 136, 180n., 189n.
Schneider, C., 95, 166n.
Schneider, H., 24, 185n.
Schönbeck, G., 114, 176n.

Schreier, S., 22, 189n.
Schreurs, J., 24, 25, 180n.
Schroeder, F., 6, 26, 27, 169n., 173n.
Schulman, J. A., 53, 188n.
Schultz, G., 107, 175n.
Schultz, R., 121, 125, 189n.
Schwarcz, R., 106, 115, 165n., 189n.
Schwartz, A., 81, 189n.
Schwartz, J. C., 107, 189n.
Schwartz, J. R., 148, 189n.
Schwertner, H. A., 111, 124, 152, 153, 164n.
Scott, B. S., 62, 189n.
Seeber, U., 91, 189n.
Seeler, K., 75, 164n.
Seeman, P., 7, 8, 14, 15, 73, 105, 106, 108, 110, 183n., 184n., 188n., 189n.
Segarnick, D., 90, 188n.
Seil, F. J., 61, 189n.
Seizinger, B. R., 123, 186n.
Sellers, E. M., 146, 149, 152, 154, 190n.
Sen, A. K., 84, 177n.
Seppälä, M., 143, 190n.
Seppala, T., 124, 152, 181n.
Shah, K. R., 139, 189n.
Shanbour, L. L., 95, 101, 193n.
Shanes, A. M., 14, 190n.
Shanley, B. C., 32, 177n.
Shapiro, B. I., 67, 184n.
Sharif, N. A., 119, 190n.
Sharma, V. K., 84, 108, 162n., 190n.
Sharpless, N. S., 136, 181n.
Shaw, G. K., 140, 181n.
Shen, A., 92, 94, 190n., 191n.
Shepherd, G. M., 43, 190n.
Sherwin, B. T., 138, 161n.
Shier, W. T., 50, 163n.
Shinitzky, M., 22, 26, 190n.
Sibley, D. R., 105, 167n.
Sieckman, G., 28, 173n.
Siegel, F., 138, 178n.
Siggins, G. R., 50, 53, 55, 58, 60, 163n., 188n., 190n.
Silbergeld, E. K., 108, 174n.
Silver, L. H., 45, 190n.
Simon, E. J., 122, 173n.
Simon, F. R., 38, 197n.
Sinclair, J. G., 53–55, 190
Sinensky, M., 97, 190n.
Singer, I., 36, 193n.
Singer, S. J., 5, 190n.
Sinnamon, H. M., 56, 162n.
Sippel, H., 47, 175n.

Sisco, K., 36, 193n.
Skolnick, P., 107, 115, 117, 190n.
Skou, J. C., 14, 191n.
Slotkin, T. A., 139, 191n.
Sloviter, R. A., 111, 191n.
Smith, A., 151, 191n.
Smith, D. M., 8, 179n.
Smith, E. L., 79, 196n.
Smith, G. A., 46, 189n.
Smith, I. C. P., 22, 24, 185n., 189n.
Smith, T. C., 92, 98, 191n.
Smith, T. L., 30, 31, 92, 94, 191n.
Smollens, J., 138, 178n.
Snowden, A., 115, 179n.
Snyder, S. H., 105–107, 110–112, 114, 116, 121, 163n., 165n.–167n., 169n., 185n., 189n., 191n., 194n., 197n.
Soeldner, J. S., 153, 194n.
Sorensen, S., 50, 52, 53, 191n.
Sørensen, S. C., 124, 127, 152, 153, 173n., 191n.
Soubrie, P., 128, 187n.
Spano, P. F., 108, 122, 136, 162n., 180n., 182n., 187n.
Sparks, D. L., 70, 165n.
Sperk, G., 114, 176n.
Spero, L., 23, 188n.
Spohr, H. L., 139, 191n.
Spokes, E., 136, 187n.
Springer, A., 28, 137, 188n.
Spuhler, K., 53, 191n.
Squires, R. F., 114, 150, 191n.
Stahl, W. L., 70, 191n.
Stalvey, L. P., 107, 190n.
Starke, K., 107, 191n.
Stefanovic, V., 84, 99, 192n.
Stevens, R. E., 47, 177n.
Stillman, I. M., 148, 180n.
Stock, K., 91, 191n.
Stokes, J. A., 71, 191n.
Stoltenberg-Didinger, G., 139, 191n.
Stone, W. E., 87, 165n.
Stotland, M., 123, 197n.
Stowell, L., 116, 180n.
Straub, R., 67, 191n.
Ströbom, U., 5, 165n.
Strong, R., 28, 136, 162n., 192n.
Stryer, L., 21, 195n.
Study, R. E., 115, 192n.
Suga, M., 128, 192n.
Sun, A. Y., 31, 82–84, 99, 137, 192n.
Sun, G. Y., 31, 84, 99, 192n.
Sunderland, E., 138, 178n., 197n.

Supavilai, P., 118, 192*n*.
Sutherland, E., 38, 197*n*.
Sutoo, D., 83, 197*n*.
Svensson, T. H., 151, 165*n*.
Swanson, P. D., 70, 191*n*.
Swartz, M. H., 75, 192*n*.
Swartzwelder, H. S., 91, 113, 175*n*.
Syapin, P. J., 12, 34, 84, 99, 100, 146, 162*n*., 181*n*., 184*n*., 192*n*.
Szava, S., 86, 173*n*.
Sze, P. Y., 141, 178*n*.
Szentágothai, J., 51, 168*n*.
Szerb, C. J., 113, 172*n*.

Tabakoff, B., 82, 84, 90, 91, 97, 108, 109, 113, 122–124, 152, 174*n*., 177*n*., 179*n*., 180*n*., 192*n*., 194*n*.
Taberner, P. V., 115, 194*n*.
Tabor, R. T., 111, 164*n*.
Tague, L. L., 95, 101, 193*n*.
Takaori, S., 55, 175*n*.
Takata, M., 45, 183*n*.
Tamkun, M. M., 68, 193*n*.
Tamminen, V., 143, 190*n*.
Tanford, C., 6, 7, 193*n*.
Tasaki, I., 36, 193*n*.
Taveras, M. A., 133, 140, 193*n*.
Tehan, T., 72, 183*n*.
Tepke, D. I., 75, 192*n*.
Tewari, S., 34, 141, 142, 169*n*., 172*n*., 193*n*.
Thadani, P. V., 97, 100, 110, 193*n*.
Thai, L. J., 136, 181*n*.
Thomas, B. N., 28, 162*n*.
Thomas, D. S., 39, 193*n*.
Thompson, A. D., 140, 181*n*.
Thompson, G. A., 33, 168*n*., 184*n*.
Thompson, W. L., 146, 193*n*.
Thulborn, K. R., 22, 193*n*.
Thurman, R. G., 11, 92, 94, 116, 180*n*., 190*n*., 191*n*., 193*n*.
Ticku, M. K., 114–117, 154, 167*n*., 185*n*., 193*n*., 194*n*.
Tien, A. F., 53, 190*n*.
Tilley, L. M., 22, 193*n*., 194*n*.
Tillmanns, H., 75, 164*n*.
Tilly, F. W., 9
Tissari, A., 99, 165*n*.
Tjeol, S., 70, 194*n*.
Tobin, R. B., 153, 194*n*.
Tobin, T., 82, 161*n*.
Toffano, G., 114, 115, 172*n*., 194*n*.
Tollenaere, J. P., 106, 179*n*.

Torget, C. E., 124, 177*n*.
Trabucchi, M., 108, 123, 136, 162*n*., 180*n*., 182*n*., 187*n*.
Traficante, L. J., 90, 188*n*.
Tran, V. T., 116, 194*n*.
Traube, J., 14, 194*n*.
Traynor, M. E., 45, 46, 194*n*., 197*n*.
Treistman, S. N., 45, 190*n*.
Treloar, E., 22, 193*n*.
Tremblay, J. P., 46, 189*n*.
Trith, C. D., 124, 165*n*.
Trudell, J. R., 8, 9, 27, 166*n*., 181*n*., 194*n*.
Truitt, E. B., 100, 193*n*.
Tumbelson, M. E., 28, 173*n*.
Tyler, T. D., 74, 169*n*.

U'Prichard, D. S., 106, 185*n*.
Ueda, I., 39, 176*n*.
Ueno, E., 109, 178*n*.
Ulbricht, W., 45, 67, 183*n*., 194*n*.
Umeki, S., 33, 171*n*.
Unwin, J. W., 115, 194*n*.
Urba-Holmgren, R., 86, 173*n*.
Urbay, C. M., 86, 173*n*.
Urwyler, S., 122, 123, 174*n*., 192*n*., 194*n*.
Usden, T. M., 107, 167*n*.

Vanderkooi, J. M., 26, 27, 194*n*.
Van Ness, P. C., 114, 185*n*.
Van Orden, L. S., 151, 162*n*.
Veech, R. L., 101, 194*n*.
Veloso, D., 101, 194*n*.
Venturini, G., 87, 164*n*.
Verebey, K., 124, 164*n*.
Vesely, D. L., 91, 93, 194*n*.
Victor, M., 130, 145, 195*n*.
Vigran, R., 34, 118, 150, 184*n*.
Viik, K., 118, 167*n*.
Villegas, R., 75, 195*n*.
Vincent, M., 38, 195*n*.
Vincente, V. P., 95, 180*n*.
Virmani, M., 99, 185*n*.
Vogel, R. A., 116, 152, 153, 170*n*., 195*n*.
Vogel, W., 148, 189*n*.
Volans, G. N., 124, 176*n*.
Volicer, L., 93, 115–117, 195*n*.
Volkind, R. A., 55, 180*n*.
von Boguslawsky, P., 67, 195*n*.
von Hungen, K., 91, 195*n*.

Waddington, J. L., 115, 195*n*.
Waggoner, A. S., 21, 195*n*.

Wagman, A. M., 150, 170n.
Wahlström, G., 94, 113, 135, 184n., 195n.
Waldek, B., 151, 165n.
Walder, C. P., 124, 176n.
Walker, D. W., 51, 131-134, 138, 161n.,
    163n., 187n., 195n.
Wallace, J. E., 111, 124, 151-153, 164n.
Wallace, R., 84, 172n.
Wallgren, H., 9, 11, 67, 69, 184n., 195n.
Walsh, J., 28, 162n.
Waltman, R., 143, 196n.
Walton, N. Y., 150, 167n.
Wang, H. H., 32, 177n.
Wang, R. Y., 57, 161n.
Wang, Y. J., 114, 196n.
Wann, K. T., 45, 173n.
Wardley-Smith, B., 12, 146, 172n.
Waring, A. J., 29, 32, 38, 186n., 188n.,
    196n.
Warner, B. T., 111, 167n.
Watanabe, A., 36, 193n.
Waterfield, A. A., 121, 178n.
Watson, J. D., 142, 196n.
Weiner, H., 84, 196n.
Weiner, N., 53, 191n.
Weismann, W. P., 70, 164n.
West, J. R., 132, 138, 167n., 190n., 196n.
West, M., 139, 190n.
Westcott, J. Y., 84, 196n.
Whalley, L. J., 124, 152, 196n.
White, A., 79, 195n.
White, H. L., 118, 167n.
Wieraszko, A., 120, 163n.
Wigstrom, H., 60, 172n.
Wilce, P. A., 32, 177n.
Williams, L. T., 107, 196n.
Williams, M., 88, 196n.
Willow, M., 148, 196n.

Wilson, D. E., 96, 196n.
Wilson, J. H., 116, 170n.
Wimbish, G. H., 151, 196n.
Winblad, B., 141, 181n.
Wing, D. R., 31, 32, 168n., 196n.
Wise, R. W., 28, 162n., 197n.
Wixon, H. N., 91, 113, 118, 119, 175n.,
    196n.
Wolfe, B. B., 91, 187n.
Woo, E., 150, 196n.
Woo, N., 82, 176n.
Wood, J. D., 118, 196n.
Wood, P. I., 123, 197n.
Wood, W. G., 28, 136, 137, 162n., 197n.
Woodbury, D. M., 86, 197n.
Woodson, P. B. J., 45, 46, 189n., 194n.,
    197n.
Wunsch, E., 125, 197n.
Wüster, M., 121, 125, 189n.
Wyatt, R. J., 110, 176n.

Yamamoto, H., 68, 73, 76, 83, 197n.
Yamamura, H. I., 112, 113, 127, 136,
    167n., 168n., 185n., 187n., 197n.
Yamanaka, Y., 152, 197n.
Yarbrough, G. G., 57, 178n.
Yoshikawa, K., 91, 197n.
Yoshimura, K., 83, 197n.
Young, B., 138, 178n.
Yu, S.-C., 39, 183n.

Zahniser, N. R., 91, 187n.
Zavoico, G. B., 27, 197n.
Zieglänsberger, W., 125, 197n.
Zimbrick, J. D., 120, 182n.
Zornetzer, S. E., 51, 132-134, 136, 161n.,
    178n., 195n.
Zysset, T., 38, 197n.

Subject index

Acetylcholine, 57, 113, 114, 128
  receptors, 112–114, 127, 135
Aging, 28, 83, 136, 137, 143, 144, 157
  behavioral changes after ethanol, 137
  receptor changes, 136
Alcohols
  effects of lipid solubility, 24, 35, 46, 68, 69, 73, 82, 116, 122
  intoxication, characteristics of, 145
  lipid interactions, 14, 15, 23–28, 156
  overdoses, treatment of, 146, 147, 154, 160
  protein interactions, 26, 156
Aluminum, 86
Alzheimer's disease, 136
γ-Aminobutyric acid (see GABA)
Anesthetics, 1
  theories of, 7–9
8-Anilino-1-naphthalene-sulfonic acid (ANS) (see Molecular probes)
Animal models, 3
Anticonvulsants, use in treating ethanol withdrawal, 148
Astroblasts, 34, 85

Barbiturates, 39, 115, 154
Batrachotoxin, 67, 68
Benzodiazepines
  use in treating withdrawal syndrome, 148–150, 155
  receptors, 114, 116, 117, 135, 136, 159
Brain slices, 58–61, 64, 65, 91, 97

Cadmium, 74, 83, 84
Calcium, 46, 60, 74, 91
  afterhyperpolarization, 43, 60, 69
  antagonists, 74
  ATPase, 73
  binding, 73–76
  channels, 43, 62, 75, 94
  conductance, 45, 60
  content, 70
  sodium exchange, 72, 73
  transport, 70, 72, 73

  uptake, 29, 70–72, 74, 75, 157, 158
Catecholamine uptake, 100
Cell cultures, 61, 62, 64, 85, 86, 100, 141
Cerebellum, 51–56, 61, 94, 115, 130, 159
  anatomy, 51, 52
  Purkinje cells, 51–56, 61, 130, 133, 138, 143
Cerebral cortex, 47, 57, 58, 61, 71, 72, 84, 86, 122, 135, 139
Cesium, 82
Cholesterol (see Lipids)
Choline uptake, 100
Climbing fibers, 51–56
Corpus striatum, 71, 88–91, 100, 108, 111, 113, 122, 135
Cut-off phenomenon, 9, 10
Cyclic nucleotides, 87–98
  adenylate cyclase, 78, 87–97, 101, 109, 136, 157
  cAMP, 87, 88, 90–98
  cGMP, 87, 93–95
  guanylate cyclase, 87, 88, 93, 94
  phosphodiesterases, 87, 88, 93

Diols, 11, 153
1, 6-Diphenyl-1, 3, 5-hexatriene (DPH) (see Molecular probes)
Dopamine, 58, 83–85, 87, 88, 90, 91, 109, 110, 123
  agonists, 109, 151, 152
  antagonists, 109, 151, 152
  receptors, 103, 105, 106, 108, 109, 136

Ecto-5′-nucleotidase, 99
Electron paramagnetic resonance (EPR) (see Molecular probes)
Electrophysiology
  conductance, 42
  EEG, 41
  EPSPs, 43–45, 59, 60, 62, 133
  iontophoresis, 44, 57, 58
  IPSPs, 43, 44, 60, 61, 62, 134
  methods, 44, 47, 58, 59, 158
  pacemaker activity, 45

posttetanic potentiation, 45, 46, 51
potentials
    action, 42–45, 49, 50, 52, 53, 56–58,
        62–64, 66, 67, 148
    field, 47, 49, 51, 59, 133, 134
    resting, 42, 45, 62, 64, 71
    properties of membranes, 41–44
    recurrent collateral inhibition, 49–51, 59
Enzyme kinetics, methods, 78–81
Erythrocytes, 14, 15, 23, 24, 28, 30–32,
        69, 73
Ethanol
    properties of, 1, 2
    sensitivity, 24, 32
    structure of, 1

Fatty acids, 5, 7, 37, 99
    composition, 15, 31–34, 38
Fetal alcohol syndrome, 64, 137–139, 143
Fibroblasts, 85
Fish, 27, 32
Fluidity, 7, 9, 15–23, 35–38, 76, 96, 97,
        127, 128, 156–159
Fluorescence (see Molecular probes)
Free radicals, 137

GABA, 57, 58, 62, 118, 119, 149, 150
    agonists, 118, 150, 159
    antagonists, 118, 150
    uptake, 100
    receptors, 114–116, 126–128, 136, 158,
        159
Galactose, 34, 35
Gangliosides, 120
Genetic mouse strains, 24, 50, 52, 53, 61
Glioblasts, 100
Glutamate, 62, 67, 71
    agonists, 120
    antagonists, 120
    receptors, 119–121, 126, 158
    uptake, 100
Glycine, 58, 62
Guanine nucleotides, 87, 90, 91, 96, 106,
        107, 158

Heart, 27, 29
HeLa cells, 32, 85
Hippocampus, 47–51, 58–61, 84, 85, 100,
        111, 113, 121, 131–133, 138, 159
    anatomy, 47–49
    dentate fascia, 49
    pyramidal cells, 48–51, 59–61, 130–134,
        138, 143

Hyperbaric environments, 8, 12, 13, 27,
        146, 147, 160
Hypothermia, treatment for alcohol over-
        doses, 147, 160

Ileum, 75
Inferior olivary nucleus, 51–56
Intestinal absorption, 75
Invertebrates, 45, 67

Korsakoff's psychosis, 130

Learning and memory deficits, 131
Lipids, 5, 40, 96, 127, 159
    cholesterol, 6, 30–32, 38, 39, 97, 159
    lipofuscin, 140
    liposomes, 14, 15, 23, 31, 36
    peroxidation, 139, 140
    phospholipids, 5–7, 31–34, 38, 73, 84,
        98, 99
Local anesthetics, use in treating ethanol
        withdrawal, 148, 149
Locus ceruleus, 54, 56, 57
Liver, 29, 31, 74

Manganese, 74
Mauthner cell, 50
Membranes
    expansion, 8, 12, 14, 15
    structure of, 4–7
Microorganisms, 32–34, 39
Mitochondrial membranes, 29, 31
Molecular probes
    ANS, 21–23, 35
    DPH, 21–23, 26–28, 35
    EPR, methods, 16–19, 36
    fluorescence
        depolarization, 20, 21, 26–29, 33–36
        methods, 20–22
    spin labels, 16–19, 24–26, 28, 29, 35,
        36, 40
Morphine, 123

Na-K-ATPase, 67, 78, 81–88, 99, 101,
        137, 158
Neuroblastoma cells, 85, 86, 100
Norepinephrine, 54, 57, 58, 83–86, 87, 92,
        97, 101, 110, 128, 136
    α-adrenergic, 83, 90, 92, 106–108, 151, 152
    β-adrenergic, 83, 90, 92, 106–108, 127,
        135, 136, 151, 152, 155
    receptors, 87, 97, 101, 103, 106–108,
        127, 135, 136

Nucleic acids, 142

Oligosaccharides, 6
Opiates
    antagonists, 123, 124, 152
    receptors, 121-128, 158
Ouabain, 86
    binding, 84

Partition coefficient, 2, 29, 39, 40
Phospholipids (see Lipids)
Physical dependence, 3, 11, 74, 91, 92,
        95, 98, 100-112, 118, 124-127, 135,
        145, 146, 159
Platelets, 31, 32
Potassium, 82, 83, 86
    channels, 43
    conductance, 45, 60, 66
    efflux, calcium-induced, 68, 69, 76, 157
    transport, 67
Prostaglandins, 90, 96
Proteins, 5, 9, 34, 37, 40
    conformation, 34
    kinases, 88, 92, 98
    phosphorylation, 88, 99
    synthesis, 141, 142

Receptor binding methods, 103-105
Rubidium, 82
    efflux, 36, 69

Sarcoplasmic reticulum, 75
Serotonin, 57, 58, 87, 112
    agonists, 112
    antagonists, 111, 112

receptors, 110-112
Sialic acid, neuraminidase-releasable, 34
Skeletal muscle, 29
Sodium, 86, 121, 122
    channels, 42, 43, 66, 67, 76
    conductance, 45, 66, 67, 148
    transport, 67, 69
    uptake, 67, 68, 75, 157, 158
Startle reflex, 50
Stomach, 95, 96, 101
Sulfhydryl groups, 34, 37
Superoxide dismutase, 140, 141
Synaptosomes, 15, 68-74, 119
    plasma membranes, 24, 28-31,
        73, 119, 137

Temperature
    body, changes in, 12, 38, 147, 157, 159
    transition, 15, 22, 29, 46, 73, 82, 83,
        90, 120
Tetrodotoxin, 67, 68, 76
Thermodynamic activity, 8-10
Tolerance, 3, 11, 29, 30-32, 46, 53, 54,
        59, 72-75, 84-85, 94, 114, 135,
        144, 159

Veratridine, 67, 68, 71, 76
Vestibular nucleus, 56
Vitamin E, 140

Wernicke's encephalopathy, 130
Withdrawal syndrome
    characteristics of, 145, 146
    treatment of, 148-155, 159